SOURCEBOOK OF PHONOLOGICAL AWARENESS ACTIVITIES

VOLUME 4

CURRICULUM RELEVANT LITERATURE

SOURCEBOOK OF PHONOLOGICAL AWARENESS ACTIVITIES

VOLUME 4

CURRICULUM RELEVANT LITERATURE

Candace L. Goldsworthy, Ph.D.

Professor, Department of Speech-Language Pathology and Audiology
California State University—Sacramento, California
Partner in Speech Language Learning Associates—Sacramento, California
Co-Director, Sacramento Scottish Rite Childhood Language Disorders Center

Robert A. Pieretti, Ph.D.

Assistant Professor
Department of Speech-Language Pathology and Audiology
California State University—Sacramento, California
Language, Speech, and Hearing Specialist—Sacramento City
Unified School District

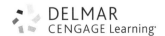

DELMAR
CENGAGE Learning·

Australia • Brazil • Japan • Korea • Mexico • Singapore • Spain • United Kingdom • United States

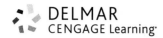
DELMAR
CENGAGE Learning·

Sourcebook of Phonological Awareness Activities, Volume 4
Curriculum Relevant Literature
Candace L. Goldsworthy, Ph.D.
Robert A. Pieretti, Ph.D.

Vice President, Editorial: Dave Garza

Director of Learning Solutions: Matthew Kane

Acquisitions Editor: Tom Stover

Managing Editor: Marah Bellegarde

Product Manager: Laura J. Wood

Editorial Assistant: Anthony Souza

Vice President, Marketing: Jennifer Ann Baker

Marketing Director: Wendy E. Mapstone

Associate Marketing Manager: Jonathan Sheehan

Production Director: Wendy A. Troeger

Production Manager: Andrew Crouth

Design Direction, Production Management, and Composition: PreMediaGlobal

For product information and technology assistance, contact us at
Cengage Learning Customer & Sales Support, 1-800-354-9706

For permission to use material from this text or product,
submit all requests online at **www.cengage.com/permissions.**
Further permissions questions can be e-mailed to
permissionrequest@cengage.com

Library of Congress Control Number: 2012937005

ISBN-13: 978-1-111-13870-7

ISBN-10: 1-111-13870-2

Delmar
5 Maxwell Drive
Clifton Park, NY 12065-2919
USA

Cengage Learning is a leading provider of customized learning solutions with office locations around the globe, including Singapore, the United Kingdom, Australia, Mexico, Brazil, and Japan. Locate your local office at:
international.cengage.com/region

Cengage Learning products are represented in Canada by Nelson Education, Ltd.

To learn more about Delmar, visit **www.cengage.com/delmar**

Purchase any of our products at your local college store or at our preferred online store **www.cengagebrain.com**

Notice to the Reader

Printed in the United States of America
1 2 3 4 5 6 7 16 15 14 13 12

Contents

The series of books entitled *Sourcebooks of Phonological Awareness Activities* have been widely accepted as rich resources for speech-language pathologists who choose to include phonological awareness training in oral/written language programs. The four Sourcebooks contain materials using words from a number of children's books which were selected because they are on a number of core reading lists for children in preschool through fifth grades. The *Sourcebooks of Phonological Awareness Activities* are being used around the country not only by speech-language specialists but by parents, regular and special education educators, and by some districts that have adopted the books district-wide for use in literacy programs.

Sourcebook of Phonological Awareness Activities: Curriculum Relevant Literature Volume 4 is new to the series of *Sourcebooks of Phonological Awareness Activities* volumes. It carries on the tradition of the other three volumes. Books covered are *Benny's Pennies*; *Bunny Cake*; *Chicken Soup with Rice*; *Chrysanthemum*; *From Head to Toe*; *Home for a Bunny*; *Liang and the Magic Paintbrush*; *Mice Squeak, We Speak*; *Miss Bindergarten Gets Ready for Kindergarten*; *The Garden*; *Tortillas and Lullabies*; and *The Three Little Pigs*.

Organization of Sourcebooks

Chapter 1 provides an introduction to phonological awareness, including key definitions. Chapter 2 offers teaching strategies for implementing the materials with clients.
The remaining chapters each profile phonological training activities that can be used with the various children's books mentioned above. An appendix offers forms for tracking student performance.

Features

Outstanding features of the Sourcebooks include:

- Offering speech-language specialists, special educators, and parents step-by-step guidance for helping children advance from oral language to print
- Mapping activities to children's books that appear on reading lists in preschools and schools throughout the country
- Providing instruction for using the materials, correcting errors, and tracking student progress

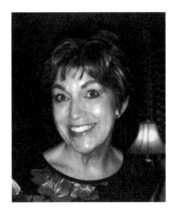

Candace L. Goldsworthy, Ph.D., is a professor of speech-language pathology at California State University–Sacramento. She received her doctorate in speech-language pathology from Case Western Reserve University in Ohio. Dr. Goldsworthy is co-director of the Sacramento Scottish Rite Childhood Language Disorders Center and is a partner in the private practice of Speech-Language-Learning Associates. She served as vice-chair of the Department of Speech-Language Pathology and Audiology at CSUS for 10 years. She is a frequent presenter on topics related to child language disorders and literacy. Her publications through Cengage include: *Developmental Reading Disabilities: A Language-Based Treatment Approach*; *Sourcebook of Phonological Awareness Activities: Children's Classic Literature*; *Sourcebook of Phonological Awareness Activities: Children's Core Literature*; and the co-authored *Sourcebook of Phonological Awareness Activities: Children's Core Literature Grades 3–5* with Robert Pieretti. *Linking the Strands of Language and Literacy: A Resource Manual*, with contributions by Katie Lambert, M.S., was published through Plural Publishing in 2010. Dr. Goldsworthy was named a fellow of the California Speech-Language-Hearing Association. She won the Outstanding Teaching Award for the College of Health and Human Services at California State University–Sacramento in spring 2001. She was honored as an Outstanding Alumna at California State University–Los Angeles in 2003 and received the first Distinguished Achievement award by the California Speech-Language Hearing Association at its annual conference in Long Beach in March 2009.

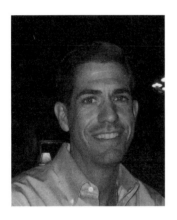

Robert Pieretti, Ph.D., is an assistant professor of speech-language pathology at California State University–Sacramento. He received his doctorate in the School of Education at the University of California–Davis with emphases in language, literacy, and culture and second language acquisition. Dr. Pieretti has been employed for the last 12 years as a language, speech, and hearing specialist in the Sacramento City Unified School District, formerly serving as the head language, speech, and hearing specialist for the district. Dr. Pieretti's scholarly interests include language disorders, language-based reading disorders, response to intervention (RTI) models, and English language learners (ELL). He co-authored *Sourcebook of Phonological Awareness Activities: Children's Core Literature Grades 3–5* with Candace Goldsworthy, Ph.D., in 2004 and has presented and co-presented numerous talks related to child language and literacy. He has served in various positions on the California Speech-Language-Hearing Association's (CSHA) Board of Directors, and he received the organization's District 2 Outstanding Service Award in 2009.

CHAPTER 1

Introduction

The *Sourcebooks of Phonological Awareness Activities* have been widely accepted as rich resources for practitioners who choose to include phonological awareness training in their oral/written language programs. *Sourcebook of Phonological Awareness Activities: Children's Classic Literature* (Goldsworthy, 1998, 2012) included training materials to be used with *Goldilocks and the Three Bears; Jack and the Beanstalk; Little Red Riding Hood; Rumpelstiltskin; Sleeping Beauty; Snow White and the Seven Dwarfs; The Gingerbread Boy;* and *Three Billy Goats Gruff. Sourcebook of Phonological Awareness Activities: Children's Core Literature* (Goldsworthy, 2001, 2012) included training materials to be used with *Blueberries for Sal; Corduroy; Happy Birthday, Moon; Harry and the Terrible Whatzit; Harry the Dirty Dog; Stone Soup; The Hungry Thing; The Little Red Hen; The Three Little Pigs; The Snowy Day;* and *The Very Hungry Caterpillar. Sourcebook of Phonological Awareness Activities: Children's Literature: Grades 3–5* (Goldsworthy & Pieretti, 2004, 2013) included training materials to be used with *Harry Potter and the Sorcerer's Stone; Tom Sawyer; Charlotte's Web; Little House on the Prairie;* A*melia Bedelia; Charlie and the Chocolate Factory; Sarah, Plain and Tall; The Indian in the Cupboard;* and *Henry Huggins.* The books included in the first two *Sourcebooks* were selected because they are on a number of core reading lists for children in preschool through third grade. The books included in the third *Sourcebook* were selected because they are on a number of core reading lists for children in third through fifth grades. The books selected for *Sourcebook IV* are frequently included in major kindergarten and first-grade curriculum adoptions used across the United States. Furthermore, a variety of various children's authors are expected to be more useful to parents and educators than the work of just one author. These *Sourcebooks* are being used around the country by parents, regular and special educators, and speech-language specialists, and in some school districts, they have been adopted school-wide for use in literacy programs. This has led to the revision of the first three *Sourcebooks* and the addition of this fourth volume.

Based on positive feedback from readers of the earlier books, the following sections have been updated and included in Chapter 1 in the *Sourcebooks*:

- Phonological awareness definitions
- Links between phonological awareness and reading
- Phonological awareness skill development
- New activities added under "Phonological Awareness at the Phoneme Level"

Phonological Awareness Defined

Phonological awareness refers to the ability to mentally manipulate the speech stream into smaller and smaller parts. Cabell et al. (2009) explained that phonological awareness is "an umbrella term that refers to children's metalinguistic understandings about the sound structure of language . . . [and] appears to develop in a general sequence: rhyme, alliteration, words, syllables, onset-rime, and phoneme" (p. 5). Phonological awareness is "most commonly defined as one's sensitivity to, or explicit awareness of, the phonological structure of words in one's language (Torgesen & Mathes, 2000, p. 2). According to Justice (2007), phonological awareness, print knowledge, and emergent writing are three high-priority targets and the best predictors of decoding ability. The National Early Literacy Panel (2004) identified the following key emergent literacy skills as the best predictors of later reading and spelling achievement:

- Oral language, including vocabulary and inferential language
- Phonological awareness
- Print awareness
- Alphabet knowledge
- Emergent writing

Because of their background in normal and disordered child language development, speech-language specialists are in a pivotal role to assess and treat phonological awareness problems and support literacy through moving from early phonological awareness into early print. Suggestions for working on the above areas are detailed in Goldsworthy's (2010, 2012) book *Linking the Strands of Language and Literacy: A Resource Manual.*

Links between Phonological Awareness and Reading

In their text on applied phonology, Hodson and Edwards (1997) defined these terms:

Phonological processing: using phonological information to process oral and written language

Phonological representation: stored knowledge about what a word sounds like (sufficient to recognize it when heard) and how to discriminate it from similar-sounding words

Phonological processing difficulties: problems with phonological input (auditory processing), lexical representation, and/or phonological output speech

Phonological deviations: broad simplifications (e.g., stopping, cluster reduction) that adversely affect intelligibility (p. 230)

During the development of speech, a child progresses through a series of stages. Articulatory gestures become integrated into automatic phonetic routines as the child practices producing speech (Stackhouse, 1997). Consequently, the phonologic code becomes a more efficient means for encoding and retrieving structures in verbal working memory. As phonemes begin to emerge as definite forms, the child becomes aware of them as structures in and of themselves. Becoming aware of these structures is critical for the language learner to develop strong, efficient phonological representations. A child comes to appreciate that phonemes can be "played with" as if they were mental toys. Words can be broken into parts; syllables and sounds within syllables can be added, deleted, and/or moved around in words. Becoming aware of phonemes-as-structures provides a solid foundation onto which a language learner can build. That is, the learner can add another layer of language—namely, a visual representation. A strongly stored phonological system allows a novice reader to have a much easier time mapping a visual, graphemic system onto it. Stated differently, the phonological code forms the foundation onto which the graphemic system will be laid. Phonological processing should naturally lead the way to phonological awareness, with the child's exposure to print facilitating this developing phonological awareness. As readers become more capable of accessing mental representations of words in phonological form, they will find it easier to decode print to sound: that is to read. According to the primary literacy standards (1999) of the National Center on Education and the Economy, "children who readily develop phonemic awareness in kindergarten probably will learn to read easily" (p. 52).

Phonological Awareness Skill Development

Signs of emerging phonological awareness appear during the preschool years in most normally developing children. According to Snow et al. (1998), even two- and three-year-olds occasionally correct speech errors and "play" with speech sounds—"e.g., pancakes, cancakes, canpakes" (p. 51). Perfetti (1991), Goldsworthy (2003), Stackhouse (1997), Snow et al. (1998), and Moats et al. (1998) have presented developmental perspectives for the emergence of phonological awareness skills in children. The following list provides current information about the developmental progression of phonological awareness.

At three years of age, children are usually able to:
- Recognize that two words rhyme (emerging).
- Recognize alliteration (words beginning with the same first sound), such as, "Mommy, Michele, they're the same."
- Recite known rhymes, such as, Jack and Jill.
- Produce rhyme by pattern, such as giving the word "cat" as a rhyming word for "hat."

At four years of age, children are usually able to:
- Segment syllables, such as know there are two parts to the word "cowboy."
- Count the number of syllables in words; 50% of four-year-olds can do this.

At five years of age, children are usually able to:
- Count syllables in words; 90% of five-year-olds can do this.
- Count phonemes within words; less than 50% of five-year-olds can do this.

At six years of age, children are usually able to:
- Match initial consonants in words, such as recognize that "shoe" and "sheep" begin with the same first sound.
- Blend two-to-three phonemes, such as recognize that the sounds /d/ /o/ /g/ form the word "dog."

- Count phonemes within words; 70% of six-year-olds can do this.
- Divide words by onset (first consonant or blend) and rime (rest of the word), such as dividing the word "stop" into /st/ /op/.

At seven years of age, children are usually able to:
- Blend phonemes to form words.
- Segment three-to-four phonemes within words.
- Spell phonetically.
- Delete phonemes from words, such as omit the /t/ sound in the word "cat."

The primary literacy standards (1999) of the National Center on Education and the Economy suggest that these specific phonemic awareness goals be met by the end of kindergarten:
- Produce rhyming words.
- Recognize pairs of rhyming words.
- Isolate initial consonants in single-syllable words, such as /t/ being the first sound in "top."
- Identify the onset (speech sounds before a vowel) and rime (vowel and what follows) in a one-syllable word, such as /k/ is the onset and (-at) is the rime in the word "cat."
- Begin to fully segment sounds in a one-syllable word, such as /k/ /a/ /t/.
- Blend onsets (/k/) and rimes (-at) to form words (cat).
- Begin to blend separate spoken phonemes (sounds) into one-syllable words, such as /k/ /a/ /t/ forming "cat" (p. 54).

The same primary literacy standards (1999) suggest that these specific phonemic awareness goals be met by the end of first grade:
- Segment the sounds in a word by saying each sound aloud, such as /k/ /a/ /t/.
- Blend separated spoken phonemes (sounds) into meaningful words (p. 96).
- The standards specifically state that "by the end of the year, first-grade students' phonemic awareness should be consolidated fully. They should be able to demonstrate, without difficulty, all the skills and knowledge expected at the end of kindergarten" (p. 96).

Phonological awareness has become recognized as a key literacy element that should be mastered early if students are to successfully decode words when reading. Many states include phonological awareness among their state standards for literacy development, and included in *Developmental Reading Disabilities: A Language Based Treatment Approach* (Goldsworthy, 2003) are samples of various states' reading/language arts standards and benchmarks for early grades. You should visit your state's department of education's online publications for up-to-date standards. Here are samples of California's phonemic awareness goals for kindergarten and first grade.

The California State Department of Education Language Arts content standards suggest specific phonemic awareness goals for kindergarten:

1.7. Track (move sequentially from sound to sound) and represent the number, sameness/difference, and order of two and three isolated phonemes (e.g., /f, s, th/, /j, d, j/).

1.8. Track (move sequentially from sound to sound) and represent changes in simple syllables and words with two and three sounds as one sound is added, substituted, omitted, shifted, or repeated (vowel-consonant, consonant-vowel, or consonant-vowel-consonant).

1.9. Blend vowel-consonant sounds orally to make words or syllables.

1.10. Identify and produce rhyming words in response to an oral prompt.

1.11. Distinguish orally stated one-syllable words and separate into beginning or ending sounds.

1.12. Track auditorily each word in a sentence and each syllable in a word.

1.13. Count the number of sounds in syllables and syllables in words.

The California State Department of Education Language Arts content standards suggest specific phonemic awareness goals for first grade:

1.4. Distinguish initial, medial, and final sounds in single-syllable words.

1.5. Distinguish long and short vowel sounds in orally stated single-syllable words (bit/bite).

1.6. Create and state a series of rhyming words, including consonant blends.

1.7. Add, delete, or change target sounds in order to change words (e.g., change cow to how; pan to an).

1.8. Blend two-to-four phonemes into a recognizable word (e.g., /c/a/t/ = cat; /f/l/a/t/ = flat).

1.9. Segment single-syllable words into their components (e.g., /c/a/t/ = cat; /s/p/l/a/t/ = splat; /r/i/ch/ = rich) (p. 86).

New Activities Added into All Four Sourcebooks under Phonological Awareness Activities at the Phoneme Level: from Phonological Awareness into Print

According to the American Speech-Language-Hearing Association's 2001 guidelines for speech pathologists' role in the support of literacy:

> "[R]egardless of their ages, children who struggle to learn word decoding and encoding require intervention focused on explicit awareness of phonemes in words, the association of phonemes with alphabetic symbols, and the ability to segment and blend phonemes in words and manipulate them in other ways" (p. 18).

Phonological awareness is necessary for children to successfully transition into reading, but it is not enough. Torgesen and Mathes (2000) supported research findings underscoring that the "effectiveness of oral language training in phonological awareness is significantly improved if, at some point in the training, children are helped to apply their newly acquired phonological awareness directly to very simple reading and spelling tasks" (p. 10). To facilitate the essential association of phonemes with graphemes (alphabetic symbols), six activities have been included under the phonological awareness at the phoneme level section in each of the four *Sourcebooks*. To provide the reader with an overview of these, the five activities and one example of each is provided here to allow the reader/user of these resources to be aware of their inclusion.

1. Substituting the initial sound/letter in words.

Stimulus items:

1.1 goat/boat

> **Task a.** "Say 'goat.' Instead of /g/, say /b/. What's your new word?" (boat). "Write/copy 'goat' and 'boat.'"
>
> **Task b.** "Circle the **letters** that make the words different." ([g], [b])
>
> **Task c.** "What **sounds** do these letters make?" (/g/, /b/)

2. Substituting the final sound/letter in words.

Stimulus items:

2.1 trap/tram

> **Task a.** "Say 'trap.' Instead of /p/, say /m/. What's your new word?" (tram). "Write/copy 'trap' and 'tram.'"
>
> **Task b.** "Circle the **letters** that make the words different." ([p], [m])
>
> **Task c.** "What **sounds** do these letters make?" (/p/, /m/)

3. Substituting the middle sound/letter in words.

Stimulus items:

3.1 trip/trap

> **Task a.** "Say 'trip.' Instead of /short I/, say /short A/. What's your new word?" (trap). "Write/copy 'trip' and 'trap.'"
>
> **Task b.** "Circle the **letters** that make the words different." ([i], [a])
>
> **Task c.** "What **sounds** do these letters make?" (should say/short I/, /short A/)

4. Supplying the initial sound/letter in words.

Stimulus items:

4.1 troll/roll

> **Task a.** "Say 'troll,' 'roll.' What sound did you hear in 'troll' that is missing in 'roll'?" (/t/). "Now we'll change the letter. Write/copy 'troll' and 'roll.'"
>
> **Task b.** "Circle the beginning **letter** that makes the words different." ([t])
>
> **Task c.** "What **sound** does this letter make?" (/t/)

5. Supplying the final sound/letter in words.

Stimulus items:

5.1 horns/horn

> **Task a.** "Say 'horns,' 'horn.' What sound did you hear in 'horns' that is missing in 'horn'?" (/z/). "Now we'll change the **letter.** Write/copy 'horns' and 'horn.'"
>
> **Task b.** "Circle the ending/last **letter** that makes the words different." ([s])
>
> **Task c.** "What **sound** does this letter make?" (/z/)

6. Switching the first sound and letter in words (ADVANCED).

Stimulus items:

6.1 billy goat

> **Task a.** "Say 'billy' and 'goat.' What sound do you hear at the beginning of 'billy'?" (/b/). "What sound do you hear at the beginning of 'goat'?" (/g/) "Switch the first sounds in those words." (gilly boat) "Now we'll change the **letters**. Write/copy 'billy goat' and 'gilly boat.'"
>
> **Task b.** "Circle the beginning **letters** that change the words." ([b] [g])
>
> **Task c.** "What **sounds** do those letters make?" (/b/ /g/)

The remainder of this book has been organized for maximum usefulness. Chapter 2 provides suggested teaching instructions and correction procedures to use with each of the training activities under word, syllable, and phoneme levels. The remaining chapters offer phonological awareness activities for the children's books included in each of the volumes. An appendix for suggested recordkeeping is included at the end of each *Sourcebook*.

CHAPTER 2

How the Materials Are Arranged and Suggestions for Using Them

From the activities suggested in *Developmental Reading Disabilities: A Language Based Treatment Approach* (Goldsworthy, 2003), 36 were selected for use in the first three *Sourcebooks*. Five activities are at the **word** level, 6 at the **syllable** level, and 25 at the **phoneme** level. In the revisions of the first three *Sourcebooks* and included in the fourth *Sourcebook* are six activities under the **phoneme** level to move from phonological **awareness into print**. Thus, each *Sourcebook* now contains 42 activities that use the vocabulary specific to each of the children's books selected.

Because there is a developmental progression of phonological awareness activities, users are encouraged to begin with the word level if the student needs to begin there and progress to the syllable and finally to the phoneme level. Activities included in each of the three levels have been arranged according to difficulty. For instance, some of the activities included at the **phoneme** level include lower level activities (such as rhyming in patterns) to higher, more difficult activities, including providing initial and final sounds in words, segmenting sounds, replacing sounds within words, phoneme switching (switching the first two phonemes in words, such as "feed me" becoming "meed fee"), and, finally, using pig Latin. It is suggested that a user begin with the first activity level under each category and move through the activities in the suggested sequence. However, as with other developmental sequences, children will vary in their acquisition of phonological awareness and consequently demonstrate skills for more difficult activities and have problems with what are considered more basic activities. Phonological awareness activities included in each of the four *Sourcebooks* are listed in the following section. Individual speech sounds, not alphabet letters, are placed between / /. Because phonetic notation is not used in this book, most vowel sounds are described as long or short—for example, /long A/ and /short U/. The user should pronounce the actual vowel sound and not describe, such as not saying "long A" or "short U."

Phonological Awareness Activities at the Word Level

1. Counting words.

What to say to the student: "We're going to count words."

> **EXAMPLE** "How many words do you hear in this sentence (or phrase)? 'her bear.' " (2)

2. Identifying the missing word from a list.

What to say to the student: "Listen to the words I say. I'll say them again. You tell me which word I leave out."

> **EXAMPLE** "Listen to the words I say: 'tin,' 'crow,' 'pail.' I'll say them again. You tell me which one I leave out: 'tin,' 'pail.'" (crow)

3. Identifying the missing word in a phrase or sentence.

What to say to the student: "Listen to the sentence I read. Tell me which word is missing the second time I read the sentence."

> **EXAMPLE** "Listen to the sentence I read: 'He was a big fat caterpillar.' Tell me which word is missing the second time I read the sentence: 'He was a big fat _____.'" (caterpillar)

4. Supplying missing word as an adult reads.

What to say to the student: "I want you to help me read the story. You fill in the words I leave out."

> **EXAMPLE** "I want you to help me read the story. You fill in the words I leave out: 'Blueberries for _____.'" (Sal)

5. Rearranging words.

What to say to the student: "I'll say some words out of order. You put them in the right order so they make sense."

> **EXAMPLE** "I'll say some words out of order. You put them in the right order so they make sense: 'size right.' Put those words in the right order." (right size)

Phonological Awareness Activities at the Syllable Level

1. Syllable counting.

What to say to the student: "We're going to count syllables (or parts) of words."

> **EXAMPLE** "How many syllables do you hear in '_____'?" (stimulus word) (e.g., "How many syllables do you hear in 'bear'?") (1)

2. Initial syllable deleting.

What to say to the student: "We're going to leave out syllables (or parts of words)."

> **EXAMPLE** "Say '_____.'" (stimulus word) "Say it again without '_____.'" (stimulus syllable) (e.g., "Say 'mouthful' without mouth.'") (ful)

3. Final syllable deleting.

What to say to the student: "We're going to leave out syllables (or parts of words)."

> **EXAMPLE** "Say '_____.'" (stimulus word) "Say it again without '_____.'" (stimulus syllable) (e.g., "Say 'around' without 'round.'") (a)

4. Initial syllable adding.

What to say to the student: "Now let's add syllables (or parts) to words."

> EXAMPLE   " Add '_____' " (stimulus syllable) "to the beginning of '_____.' " (stimulus syllable) (e.g., "Add 'mouth' to the beginning of 'ful.' ") (mouthful)

5. Final syllable adding.

What to say to the student: "Now let's add syllables (or parts) to words."

> EXAMPLE   "Add '_____' " (stimulus syllable) "to the end of '_____.' " (stimulus syllable) (e.g., "Add 'ing' to the end of 'can.' ") (canning)

6. Syllable substituting.

What to say to the student: "Let's make up some new words."

> EXAMPLE   "Say '_____.' " (stimulus word) "Instead of '_____' " (stimulus syllable) "say '_____.' " (stimulus syllable) (e.g., "Say 'inside.' Instead of 'side' say 'stead.' The new word is 'instead.' ")

Phonological Awareness Activities at the Phoneme Level

1. Counting sounds.

What to say to the student: "We're going to count sounds in words."

> EXAMPLE   "How many sounds do you hear in this word? 'can.' " (3)

2. Sound categorization or identifying rhyme oddity.

What to say to the student: "Guess which word I say does not rhyme with the other three words."

> EXAMPLE   "Tell me which word does not rhyme with the other three. '_____, _____, _____, _____.' " (stimulus words) (e.g., "'munch, bunch, crunch, gulp.' Which word doesn't rhyme?") (gulp)

3. Matching rhyme.

What to say to the student: "We're going to think of rhyming words."

> EXAMPLE   "Which word rhymes with '_____'?" (stimulus word) (e.g., "Which word rhymes with 'crow'? 'cold, Sal, grow, pail.' ") (grow)

4. Producing rhyme.

What to say to the student: "Now we'll say rhyming words."

> EXAMPLE   "Tell me a word that rhymes with '_____.' " (stimulus word) (e.g., "Tell me a word that rhymes with 'pick.' You can make up a word if you want.") (tick)

5. Sound matching (initial).

What to say to the student: "Now we'll listen for the first sound in words."

> **EXAMPLE** "Listen to this sound: / /." (stimulus sound) "Guess which word I say begins with that sound. '_____, _____, _____, _____.' " (stimulus words) (e.g., "Listen to this sound /b/. Guess which word I say begins with that sound: 'canning, munch, taste, bear.' ") (bear)

6. Sound matching (final).

What to say to the student: "Now we'll listen for the last sound in words."

> **EXAMPLE** "Listen to this sound: / /." (stimulus sound) "Guess which word I say ends with that sound. '_____, _____, _____, _____.' " (stimulus words) (e.g., "Listen to this sound /n/. Guess which word I say ends with that sound: 'berry, tin, with, pail.' ") (tin)

7. Identifying initial sound in words.

What to say to the student: "I'll say a word two times. Tell me what sound is missing. '_____, _____.' " (stimulus words)

> **EXAMPLE** "What sound do you hear in '_____' " (stimulus word) "that is missing in '_____'?" (stimulus word) (e.g., "What sound do you hear in 'time' that is missing in 'I'm'?") (/t/)

8. Identifying the final sound in words.

What to say to the student: "I'll say a word two times. Tell me what sound is missing. '_____,' '_____.' " (stimulus words)

> **EXAMPLE** "What sound do you hear in '_____' " (stimulus word) "that is missing in '_____'?" (stimulus word) (e.g., "What sound do you hear in 'time' that is missing in 'tie'?") (/m/)

9. Segmenting the initial sound in words.

What to say to the student: "Listen to the word I say and tell me the first sound you hear."

> **EXAMPLE** "What's the first sound in '_____'?" (stimulus word) (e.g., "What's the first sound in 'berry'?") (/b/)

10. Segmenting the final sound in words.

What to say to the student: "Listen to the word I say and tell me the last sound you hear."

> **EXAMPLE** "What's the last sound in the word '_____'?" (stimulus word) (e.g., "What's the last sound in the word 'took'?") (/k/)

11. Generating words from the story beginning with a particular sound.

What to say to the student: "Let's think of words from the story that start with certain sounds."

> **EXAMPLE** "Tell me a word from the story that starts with / /." (stimulus sound) (e.g., the sound /p/) (partridge)

12. Blending sounds in monosyllabic words divided into onset-rime beginning with two consonant cluster + rime.

What to say to the student: "Now we'll put sounds together to make words."

> **EXAMPLE** "Put these sounds together to make a word: / / + / /." (stimulus sounds) "What's the word?" (e.g., "gr + ow: What's the word?") (grow)

13. Blending sounds in monosyllabic words divided into onset/rime beginning with a single consonant + rime.

What to say to the student: "Let's put sounds together to make words."

> **EXAMPLE** "Put these sounds together to make a word: / / + / /." (stimulus sounds) "What's the word?" (e.g., "/d/ + /long A/: What's the word?") (day)

14. Blending sounds to form a monosyllabic word beginning with a continuant sound.

What to say to the student: "We'll put sounds together to make words."

> **EXAMPLE** "Put these sounds together to make a word: / / + / / + / /." (stimulus sounds) (e.g., /m/ + /long A/ + /k/) (make)

15. Blending sounds to form a monosyllabic word beginning with a noncontinuant sound.

What to say to the student: "We'll put sounds together to make words."

> **EXAMPLE** "Put these sounds together to make a word: / / + / / + / /." (stimulus sounds) (e.g., /p/ + /long A/ + /l/) (pail)

16. Substituting the initial sound in words.

What to say to the student: "We're going to change the beginning/first sound in words."

> **EXAMPLE** "Say '_____.' " (stimulus word) "Instead of / /" (stimulus sound), "say / /." (stimulus sound) (e.g., "Say 'bear.' Instead of /b/, say /ch/. What's your new word?") (chair)

17. Substituting the final sound in words.

What to say to the student: "We're going to change the ending/last sound in words."

> **EXAMPLE** "Say '_____.' " (stimulus word) "Instead of / /" (stimulus sound), "say / /." (stimulus sound) (e.g., "Say 'ate.' Instead of /t/, say /m/. What's your new word?") (aim)

18. Segmenting the middle sound in monosyllabic words.

What to say to the student: "Tell me the middle sound in the word I say."

> **EXAMPLE** "What's the middle sound in the word '_____'?" (stimulus word) (e.g., "What's the middle sound in the word 'feet'?") (/long E/)

19. Substituting the middle sound in words.

What to say to the student: "We're going to change the middle sound in words."

> **EXAMPLE**   "Say '_____.' " (stimulus word) "Instead of / /" (stimulus sound), "say / /."
> (stimulus sound) (e.g., "Say 'Sal.' Instead of /short A/, say /long E/. What's
> your new word?") (seal)

20. Identifying all sounds in monosyllabic words.

What to say to the student: "Now tell me all the sounds you hear in the word I say."

> **EXAMPLE**   "What sounds do you hear in the word '_____'?" (stimulus word)
> (e.g., "What sounds do you hear in the word 'Sal'?") (/s/ /short A/ /l/)

21. Deleting sounds within words.

What to say to the student: "We're going to leave out sounds in words."

> **EXAMPLE**   "Say '_____' " (stimulus word) "without / /." (stimulus sound)
> (e.g., "Say 'grains' without /r/.") (gains)

22. Substituting a consonant in words having a two-sound cluster.

What to say to the student: "We're going to substitute sounds in words."

> **EXAMPLE**   "Say '_____.' " (stimulus word) "Instead of / /" (stimulus sound), "say / /."
> (stimulus sound) (e.g., "Say 'climb.' Instead of /l/, say /r/.") (crime)

23. Phoneme reversing.

What to say to the student: "We're going to say words backward."

> **EXAMPLE**   "Say the word '_____' " (stimulus word) "backward." (e.g., "If you say
> 'gulp' backward, the word is 'plug.' ")

24. Phoneme switching.

What to say to the student: "We're going to switch the first sounds in two words."

> **EXAMPLE**   "Switch the first sounds in '_____' and '_____.' " (stimulus words)
> (e.g., "Switch the first sounds in 'sat down.' ") (dat sown)

25. Pig latin.

What to say to the student: "We're going to talk in a secret language using words from the story. In
pig latin, you take off the first sound of a word, put it at the end of the word, and add a /long A/
sound."

> **EXAMPLE**   "Say 'moon' in pig Latin." (oonmay)

From Phonological Awareness into Print

1. Substituting the initial sound/letter in words.
Stimulus items:

1.1 day/pay

> **Task a.** "Say 'day.' Instead of /d/, say /p/. What's your new word?" (pay) "Write/copy 'day' and 'pay.' "
>
> **Task b.** "Circle the **letters** that make the words different." ([d], [p])
>
> **Task c.** "What **sounds** do these letters make?" (/d/, /p/)

2. Substituting the final sound/letter in words.
Stimulus items:

2.1 kiss/kit

> **Task a.** "Say 'kiss.' Instead of /s/, say /t/. What's your new word?" (kit) "Write/copy 'kiss' and 'kit.' "
>
> **Task b.** "Circle the **letters** that make the words different." ([s], [s], [t])
>
> **Task c.** "What **sounds** do these letters make?" (/s/, /t/)

3. Substituting the middle sound/letter in words.
Stimulus items:

3.1 time/tame

> **Task a.** "Say 'time.' Instead of /long I/, say /long A/. What's your new word?" (tame) "Write/copy 'time' and 'tame.' "
>
> **Task b.** "Circle the **letters** that make the words different." ([i], [a])
>
> **Task c.** "What **sounds** do these letters make?" (/long I/, /long A/)

4. Supplying the initial sound/letter in words.
Stimulus items:

4.1 feast/east

> **Task a.** "Say 'feast,' 'east.' What sound did you hear in 'feast' that is missing in 'east'?" (/f/) "Now we'll change the **letter**. Write/copy 'feast' and 'east.' "
>
> **Task b.** "Circle the beginning **letter** that makes the words different." ([f])
>
> **Task c.** "What **sound** does this letter make?" (/f/)

5. Supplying the final sound/letter in words.
Stimulus items:

5.1 years/year

> **Task a.** "Say 'years,' 'year.' What sound did you hear in 'years' that is missing in 'year'?" (/z/) "Now we'll change the **letter**. Write/copy 'years' and 'year.' "
>
> **Task b.** "Circle the ending/last **letter** that makes the words different." ([s])
>
> **Task c.** "What **sound** does this letter make?" (/z/)

6. Switching the first sound and letter in words. (ADVANCED)

Stimulus items:

6.1 kissed her

> **Task a.** "Say 'kissed,' 'her.' What sound do you hear at the beginning of 'kissed'?" (/k/) "What sound do you hear at the beginning of 'her'?" (/h/) "Switch the first sounds in those words." (hissed ker) "Now we'll change the **letters.** Write/copy 'kissed her' and 'hissed ker.' "
>
> **Task b.** "Circle the beginning **letters** that change the words. ([k], [h])
>
> **Task c.** "What sounds do those **letters** make?" (/k/, /h/)

As mentioned in Chapter 1, the intent of the materials in this book is to promote phonological awareness activities by incorporating the richness of children's literature. To that end, numerous children's books were selected for use in the various *Sourcebooks*. Vocabulary was selected from the books and used as stimulus items for the phonological awareness activities at the word, syllable, and sound levels. Each of the 42 activities is repeated for all books in the *Sourcebooks* but individualized with the vocabulary specific to the children's books included in each *Sourcebook*. The purpose is twofold: to integrate phonological awareness activities into children's literature and to acquaint students with the vocabulary of these classic tales. Because the selected activities represent many critical word-, syllable-, and phoneme-level phonological awareness abilities, the redundancy of their inclusion for each story is believed to be important. As students become familiar with what is being requested—for example, "Now let's leave one syllable out of words"—their phonological awareness abilities will be strengthened as they simultaneously enjoy the stories and learn new vocabulary and semantic-syntactic constructions. One version of each children's book was used for vocabulary sources. Users of this book are encouraged to use the vocabulary from these versions or integrate vocabulary from other story versions into activities included in this book.

What Is Included in Each Activity

Four items are included in each activity:

1. **What to say to the student and an example.** For example, Activity 1: Counting Words under Phonological Awareness Activities at the Word Level for *Harry the Dirty Dog*:

What to say to the student: "We're going to count words."

> **EXAMPLE**   "How many words do you hear in this sentence (or phrase)? 'He played tag.' "

2. **The correct answer in parentheses: (3)**

3. **A note for suggested use:**

> **Note:** *Use pictured items and/or manipulatives if necessary. Use any of the following stimulus phrases or sentences and/or others you select from the story. Correct answers are in parentheses.*

4. **Ten stimulus items with correct answers in parentheses are provided for the original activities, and five stimulus items with correct answers in parentheses are provided**

for the new "From Phonological Awareness to Print" activities. For example, one of the activities at the word level is to count the number of words presented orally. Some of the items with answers from *Harry the Dirty Dog* are:

Stimulus items:
    he played dead (3)
    he slid down (3)
    Harry wagged his tail (4)
    white dog with black spots (5)

How to Use These Materials

It is recommended that materials be coordinated with corresponding activities of parents and/or teachers. For example, a unit that includes *Blueberries for Sal* might be selected and introduced, with the parent or teacher reading aloud either the version suggested for use with the *Sourcebooks* or another edition. It is recommended that the story be read to and discussed with students at least three times and that the students be able to retell the story in sequence. Younger children are not expected to retell the story with as much detail as older students. Language activities, such as flannel board presentations and hand puppet role plays, can be used to facilitate a student's use of vocabulary in the stories before introducing the corresponding phonological awareness activities.

Suggested Teaching Steps and Correction Procedures

The following suggestions are provided for use in introducing activities and in correcting student errors. These suggestions are meant as general guidelines. Users are encouraged to move through the sequence of teaching and/or correction steps in the order in which they are presented here. Please add other teaching/correction steps that you find useful with your students. The suggested teaching steps and correction procedures are only outlined here and are not repeated with the corresponding activities in the rest of this book. Users are encouraged to review this section before introducing activities.

Phonological Awareness Activities at the Word Level

1. Counting words.
What to say to the student: "We're going to count words."

> **EXAMPLE**   "How many words do you hear in this sentence (or phrase)? 'He played tag.' " (3)

Teaching Steps:

1. Place manipulatives or pictured items from the book in front of the student. For example, put one wooden block or plastic chip in front of the student and say: "This stands for a word. I'll say the word 'dog,' and you point to the block/chip and tell me how many words you hear."

2. Repeat step 1 with pictured objects from the story, such as pictures of a pail and a bear from *Blueberries for Sal*. Point to the pictured pail and say "pail." Point to the pictured bear and say "bear." Then, point to the pictured pail and say "one" and then to the pictured bear and say "two. There are two words."

3. Repeat step 2 without pictures.

4. If the student is correct, reinforce by saying: "Good. You counted the words."

5. Repeat steps 2–4 with three, four, and five words.

Correction Procedures:

1. If he or she is unable to do this activity with manipulatives or pictures from the story, the student may need more experience with counting in sequence and one-to-one correspondence. This may be achieved by providing many instances of placing one, two, and three blocks in front of the student. Ask the student to touch each block as you say "block" (using one block), or "block, block" (using two blocks), or "block, block, block" (using three blocks).

2. Ask the student to point to each block again and to count "1," or "1, 2," or "1, 2, 3." In each instance, ask the student "How many words?"

3. If the student is correct, reinforce by saying: "Good. You counted the words."

4. If the student is incorrect, provide more experiences with counting and provide the written number above the objects to help the student keep the correct number in memory while responding to your question "How many words?"

5. Repeat steps 1–3 with pictured objects.

6. Repeat steps 1–3 with four and five objects.

7. Repeat activity without manipulatives.

2. Identifying the missing word from a list.

What to say to the student: "Listen to the words I say. I'll say them again. You tell me which word I leave out."

> **EXAMPLE** "Listen to the words I say: 'tub,' 'dirty,' 'house.' I'll say them again. Tell me which one I leave out: 'tub,' house.'" (dirty)

Teaching Steps:

1. Place two pictures in front of the student (e.g., girl and wolf). Say: "I'll say two words: 'girl, wolf.'"

2. Say: "Now I'll leave one word out." Remove the pictured 'girl.' Say: "Guess which one I leave out: 'wolf.' Which word is missing?" (girl).

3. If the student is correct, reinforce by saying: "Good job. You told me which word is missing."

4. Repeat this activity without manipulatives.

Correction Procedures:

1. If he or she is unable to do this activity with manipulatives from the story, the student may need instruction on dealing with "what's missing" before this activity. This can be achieved by placing an object in front of the student. Request that the object be named. Remove the object, saying: "(object name) is missing." Immediately ask the student to name the missing object.

2. Repeat step 1 with different objects.

3. Now place one red block and one blue block in front of the student and say: "I'll say two words: 'red' and 'blue.' " Point to each block as you say each word.

4. Say: "Now I'll leave one word out." Take away the red block. Say: "Guess which one I leave out: 'blue.' Which word is missing?" (red).

5. Repeat steps 3–4 by using two different colored blocks in each example. Vary which block you remove—that is, one time take away the first block and the next time the second block.

6. If the student is correct, reinforce by saying: "Good. You told me which word is missing."

7. Repeat this activity without manipulatives (i.e., with words only).

3. Identifying the missing word in a phrase or sentence.

What to say to the student: "Listen to the sentence I read. Tell me which word is missing the second time I read the sentence."

> **EXAMPLE** " 'He felt tired.' Listen again and tell me which word I leave out. 'He felt '_____.' " (tired)

Teaching Steps:

1. Place two manipulatives (e.g., two red wooden blocks) in front of the student.

2. Point to the block on the student's left and say "red."

3. Point to the block on the student's right and say "block."

4. Point to the first block and say "red." Point to the second block and ask: "What word goes with this one?" (block)

5. If the student is correct, reinforce by saying: "OK. You told me the word I left out—the one that is missing."

6. Repeat this activity with three, four, and five blocks and words.

7. Repeat this activity without manipulatives.

Correction Procedures:

1. Place two objects in front of the student (e.g., a toy car and a toy cat).

2. Remove one object (car).

3. Point to the cat and say "The car is missing."

4. Ask the student: "Which one is missing?"

5. If the student is correct, reinforce by saying: "Right. You told me which word is missing."

6. Place one red block and one blue block in front of the student and say: "These blocks stand for words." Point to the red block and say "red"; point to the blue block as you say "blue."

7. Ask the student to point to the first block as you say "red." Ask the student to point to the second block as you say "blue."

8. Point to the first block and ask the student: "What word is this?" (red) Point to the second block and ask the student: "What word is this?" (blue)

9. Say: "I'm only going to say one of the words. You tell me the word that's missing." Point to the red block and say "red." Point to the blue block and ask: "What's this one?" (blue)

10. If the student answers correctly, reinforce by saying: "Right. You said 'blue.' You told me the missing word."

11. If the student answers incorrectly, go through steps 6–10 with additional examples of two blocks or toys.

12. Repeat this activity without manipulatives.

4. Supplying the missing word as an adult reads.

What to say to the student: "I want you to help me read the story. You fill in the words I leave out."

> **EXAMPLE**   "I've always wanted to climb a _____." (mountain)

Teaching Steps:

1. Place two objects (e.g., cup and shoe) in front of the student. Point to the cup and say "cup." Point to the shoe and say "shoe."

2. Remove the shoe. Point to the cup and say "cup." Point to where the shoe had been and say "shoe."

3. Repeat step 2, but after pointing to where the shoe was, ask: "What word was this?"

4. Repeat steps 1–3 with different sets of two objects.

5. If the student answers correctly, reinforce by saying: "Good work. You told me which word is missing."

6. Repeat this activity without manipulatives.

Correction Procedures:

1. Place two red blocks in front of the student and say: "These blocks stand for words." Point to the first block as you say "red," and point to the second block as you say "block."

2. Ask the student to point to the first block as you say "red." Ask the student to point to the second block as you say "block."

3. Point to the first block and ask the student: "What word is this?" (red) Repeat with the second block. (block)

4. Now tell the student: "I'm only going to say one of the words. You tell me the word that's missing." Point to the first block and say "red." Point to the second block and ask: "What's this one?" (block)

5. If the student answers correctly, reinforce by saying: "Right. You said 'block.' You told me the word I left out—the missing word."

6. If the student answers incorrectly, repeat steps 1–5 with two yellow blocks or toy objects, or two blue blocks or toy objects, or two green blocks or toy objects.

7. Repeat this activity without manipulatives.

5. Rearranging words.

What to say to the student: "I'll say some words out of order. You put them in the right order so they make sense."

> **EXAMPLE** " 'bank piggy.' Put those words in the right order." (piggy bank)

Teaching Steps:

1. Place two objects (e.g., a key and a book) in front of the student, with the key on the student's left and the book on the right. Point to the key and say "key"; point to the book and say "book."

2. Switch the objects so the book is to the student's left and the key to the student's right. Point to the book and say "book." Point to the key and say "key." Then, say: "I switched the words around. First, it was 'key, book'; now it's 'book, key.' "

3. Repeat steps 1–2 with different sets of two objects or pictures.

4. Repeat this activity without manipulatives.

5. If the student answers correctly, reinforce by saying: "Right. You put the words in the right order. Now they make sense."

Correction Procedures:

1. Place two objects (e.g., a key and a book) in front of the student, with the key on the student's left and the book on the right. Point to the key and say "key"; point to the book and say "book." Ask the student to name each object.

2. Ask the student to switch the objects around so the book is to the student's left and the key is to the student's right.

3. Point to the book and ask the student to name it. Point to the key and ask the student to name it. Then, say: "You switched the words around. First, it was 'key, book'; now it's 'book, key.'"

4. Repeat steps 1–4 with different sets of two objects or pictures.

5. Repeat this activity without manipulatives. Say two words of a familiar phrase (e.g., Santa Claus). Then, say: "If I switch those words around it's 'Claus Santa.' "

6. Repeat step 5 with another familiar phrase (e.g., Birthday Happy). Ask the student to "put the words in the right order."

7. If the student answers correctly, reinforce by saying: "Good. You're switching the words around so they make sense."

Phonological Awareness Activities at the Syllable Level

1. Syllable counting.

What to say to the student: "We're going to count syllables (or parts) of words."

> **EXAMPLE** "How many syllables do you hear in 'noodles'?" (2)

Teaching Steps:
1. Place one wooden block or plastic chip in front of the student.
2. Point to the block/chip and say: "This stands for a word. I'll say the word 'dog,' and you point to the block/chip and tell me how many parts you hear."
3. If the student is correct, reinforce by saying: "Yes. You told me that there is one part or syllable."
4. Place two blocks/chips in front of the student and say: "These stand for two word parts or syllables. Listen, 'dog—ee,' " pointing to the first block/chip as you say 'dog' and to the second block/chip as you say 'ee.' "There are two parts or syllables."
5. Say: "I'll say 'dog,' and you point to the block and say 'one.' Then, I'll say 'ee,' and you point to the second block and say 'two.' How many syllables in 'doggy'?"
6. If the student is correct, reinforce by saying: "Yes. You told me that there are two parts or syllables."
7. Repeat this activity without manipulatives.

Correction Procedures:
1. Show the student how some things are parts of a whole. For example, using a child's puzzle, have the student remove one piece as you say: "That is one part of the puzzle." Repeat this step several times with the puzzle. Then, explain that a syllable is a part of a word, just as a puzzle piece is part of the puzzle.
2. Place two pictures (representing the two parts of a compound word) in front of the student, such as a cup and a cake.
3. Write the number 1 below the pictured cup and the number 2 below the pictured cake. Then, say: "There are two syllables in the word 'cupcake.' " Ask the student: "How many syllables in the word 'cupcake'?"
4. If the student answers correctly, reinforce by saying: "Good. You counted the syllables."
5. Repeat steps 2–4 with additional compound words and pictures.
6. Repeat steps 2–4 with three- and four-syllable words.
7. Repeat steps 2–4 without pictured items.
8. Repeat this activity without manipulatives.

2. Initial syllable deleting.

What to say to the student: "We're going to leave out syllables (or parts of words)."

> **EXAMPLE** "Say '_____.' " (stimulus word) "Say it again without '_____.' " (stimulus syllable) (e.g., "Say 'besides.' Say it again without 'be.' ") (sides)

Teaching Steps:

1. Place two pictures, such as a cow and a boy, in front of the student. Point to the pictured cow to the student's left as you say "cow." Point to the pictured boy to the student's right as you say "boy."

2. Take the pictured cow away and say: "When I take the word 'cow' away from 'cowboy,' the part that's left is 'boy.' "

3. Repeat steps 1–2 with another compound word and two pictures (e.g., cupcake). Take away the pictured cup and say: "Say 'cupcake' without cup.' Which part is left?"

4. If the student is correct, reinforce by saying: "Good. You told me 'cake' is left; you told me which syllable is left when you take the first one away."

5. Repeat this activity without pictures.

Correction Procedures:

1. Place two colored blocks or plastic chips in front of the student (e.g., a green one and a red one). Make sure the color names have only one syllable each (e.g., red, brown, green, pink, white, etc.).

2. If you have placed the red block/chip to the left of the student and the blue block/chip to the right of the student, take away the red block and say: "Blue is left."

3. Repeat steps 1–2. Ask the student: "Which one is left?"

4. If correct, reinforce the student for naming the remaining part or syllable.

5. Repeat steps 1–4 a number of times, changing the color of the blocks/chips.

6. Repeat this activity with two small toys (e.g., a bus and a dog)—again making sure each word's name has only one syllable.

7. Repeat this activity with pictured compound or words—for example, cupcake, armchair, rainbow, baseball, and so on.

8. Ask the student to take the first part away and "Name the part that's left," such as "cake," "chair," "bow," "ball," and so on, as the student removes each.

9. If the student is correct, reinforce for naming the part or syllable that's left.

10. Repeat this activity without manipulatives.

3. Final syllable deleting.

What to say to the student: "We're going to leave out syllables (or parts of words)."

> EXAMPLE "Say '_____.' " (stimulus word) "Say it again without '_____.' "
> (stimulus syllable) (e.g., "Say 'evening' without '-ing.' ") (even)

Teaching Steps:

1. Place two pictures (e.g., a cow and a boy) in front of the student. Point to the pictured cow on the student's left as you say "cow." Point to the pictured boy to the student's right as you say "boy."

2. Take the pictured boy away and say: "When I take the word 'boy' away from 'cowboy,' the part that's left is 'cow.' "

3. Repeat steps 1–2 with another pictured compound word (e.g., horsefly). Ask the student to "Say 'horsefly' without 'fly.' Which part is left?"

4. If the student is correct, reinforce by saying: "Good. You told me which part or syllable is left."

5. Repeat this activity without manipulatives.

Correction Procedures:

1. Place two colored blocks or plastic chips in front of the student, such as a green one and a red one. Make sure the color names have one syllable each (e.g., red, brown, green, pink, white, etc.).

2. If you have placed the green block/chip to the left of the student and the red block/chip to the right of the student, take away the red block/chip and say: "When you take red away, green is left."

3. Repeat steps 1–2. Each time you take away the block/chip on the student's right, say: "You tell me which one is left."

4. Repeat steps 1–3 a number of times, changing the color of the blocks/chips.

5. Repeat steps 1–3 with two small toys, such as a bus and a dog, again making sure each word's name has only one syllable.

6. Repeat this activity with pictures of compound words (e.g., cupcake, armchair, rainbow, baseball, etc.).

7. Ask the student to take the last part away and name the syllable that's left (e.g., cup, arm, rain, base) as each is removed.

8. If correct, reinforce the student for naming the part or syllable that is left.

9. Repeat this activity without manipulatives.

4. Initial syllable adding.

What to say to the student: "Now let's add syllables (or parts) to words."

> **EXAMPLE** " Add '_____' " (stimulus syllable) "to the beginning of '_____.' "
> (stimulus syllable) (e.g., "Add 'on' to the beginning of 'to.' ") (onto)

Teaching Steps:

1. Place two pictures (e.g., a tooth and a brush) in front of the student.

2. Say: "If you add 'tooth' to the beginning of 'brush,' what new word is it?"

3. If the student is correct, reinforce by saying: "Good. You added 'tooth' to the beginning of 'brush' and made a new word, 'toothbrush.' "

4. Repeat steps 1–3 with other compound words and pictures (e.g., blue + bird).

5. Repeat this activity without manipulatives.

Correction Procedures:

1. Place three pictures in front of the student (e.g., a tooth, a brush, and a toothbrush).

2. Explain to the student that we can put two word parts (or syllables) together to make a new word.

3. Say "tooth" as you move the pictured tooth in front of the student. Say "brush" as you move the pictured brush in front of the student, making sure the tooth is on the left side of the brush.

4. Point to the toothbrush, saying: "When I add 'tooth' to the beginning of 'brush,' the new word is 'toothbrush.' "

5. Provide more pictured compound words or objects (e.g., cupcake, armchair, rainbow, baseball). In each instance, ask the student to add "_____" (first syllable) to "_____" (second syllable). Ask the student to name the new word.

6. If the student is correct, reinforce by saying: "Good. You added '_____' (first syllable) to the beginning of '_____' (second syllable) and made a new word: '_____.' "

7. Repeat this activity without manipulatives.

5. Final syllable adding.

What to say to the student: "Now let's add syllables (or parts) to words."

> **EXAMPLE** "Add '_____' " (stimulus syllable) "to the end of '_____' " (stimulus syllable) (e.g., "Add 'ment' to the end of 'depart.' ") (department).

Teaching Steps:
1. Place two pictures (e.g., butter and a fly) in front of the student.

2. Say: "If you add 'fly' to the end of 'butter,' what new word is it?"

3. If the student is correct, reinforce by saying: "Good. You added 'fly' to the end of 'butter' and made a new word: 'butterfly.' "

4. Repeat steps 1–3 with other compound words and pictures (e.g., wheel + chair).

5. Repeat steps 1–3 with three- and four-syllable words.

6. Repeat this activity without manipulatives.

Correction Procedures:
1. Place three pictures in front of the student (e.g., a dragon, a fly, and a dragonfly).

2. Explain this to the student: "We can put two word parts (or syllables) together to make a new word."

3. Say "fly" as you move the pictured fly in front of the student.

4. Say "dragon" as you move the pictured dragon in front of the student, making sure it is to the student's left.

5. Point to the pictured dragonfly, saying: "When I add 'fly' to the end of 'dragon,' the new word is 'dragonfly.' "

6. Provide more pictured compound words or objects representing them (e.g., rainbow, baseball). In each instance, ask the student to add "_____" (second syllable) to "_____" (first syllable). Ask the student to name the new word.

7. If the student is correct, reinforce by saying: "Good. You added '_____' (second syllable) to the end of '_____,' " (first syllable) "and made a new word '_____.' "

8. Repeat this activity with three- and four-syllable words.

9. Repeat this activity without manipulatives.

6. Syllable substituting.

What to say to the student: "Let's make up some new words."

> **EXAMPLE** "Say '_____.' " (stimulus word) "Instead of '_____' " (stimulus syllable) "say '_____.' " (stimulus syllable) (e.g., "Say 'buying.' Instead of '-ing' say '-er.' The new word is 'buyer.' ")

Teaching Steps:

1. Place two pictures (e.g., a tooth and a brush) next to each other (the tooth to the left of the brush) in front of the student and say "toothbrush."

2. Place a picture of "hair" (e.g., a black-and-white picture of a child where his or her hair is colored in or has an arrow pointing to it) next to the pictures of the tooth and the brush.

3. Replace the pictured tooth with the pictured hair, saying: "If I take 'tooth' away and put in 'hair,' the new word is 'hairbrush.' "

4. Repeat steps 1–3 with other compound words and pictures (e.g., black + bird). In each instance, have the student name the first compound word and then the compound word that results when you substitute one syllable with an alternative.

5. If the student is correct, reinforce by saying: "Good. You changed part of the word and made up a new word."

6. Repeat this activity without manipulatives.

Correction Procedures:

1. Place two red blocks/chips in front of the student, saying "red" as you point to the first block/chip and "red" as you point to the second block/chip.

2. Replace the second red block/chip with a blue block/chip. Say "red" as you point to the first block/chip and "blue" as you point to the second block/chip.

3. Repeat steps 1–2 several times, replacing the first *or* second block/chip with a different colored block/chip. Point to each block/chip, naming only the color.

4. Repeat steps 1–3, asking the student to name the color of the blocks/chips.

5. If the student is correct, reinforce by saying: "Good. You changed part of the word and made up a new word."

6. Repeat teaching steps 1–6 for this activity.

Phonological Awareness Activities at the Phoneme Level

1. Counting sounds.

What to say to the student: "We're going to count sounds in words."

> **EXAMPLE** "How many sounds do you hear in the word 'dog'?" (3)

Teaching Steps:

1. Place a picture from the story in front of the student (e.g., a dog). Place three wooden blocks or plastic chips below the pictured dog.

2. Point to each of the manipulatives and say: "These stand for the sounds in the word 'dog.' " Say the sounds separately as you point to each of the three blocks/chips: "/d/, /ah/, /g/—'dog.' Three sounds in the word 'dog.' "

3. Say: "I'll say the word 'dog,' and you point to the blocks/chips and tell me how many sounds you hear in the word."

4. If the student is correct, reinforce by saying: "Good. You told me how many sounds in the word."

5. Repeat this activity with additional monosyllabic words with four, five, and six sounds.

6. Repeat this activity without manipulatives.

Correction Procedures:

1. If he or she is unable to do this activity with manipulatives or pictures from the story, the student may need more experience with counting in sequence and one-to-one correspondence. This may be achieved through providing many instances of placing one, two, and three blocks/chips in front of the student. Using the pictured dog, ask the student to touch each block as you say "/d/," or "/d/ /ah/," or "/d/ /ah/ /g/."

2. Ask the student to point to each block/chip again as you count "one," or "one, two," or "one, two, three." Each time, ask: "How many sounds do you hear?"

3. If the student is correct, reinforce by saying: "Good. You counted the correct number of sounds."

4. If the student is incorrect, provide more experiences with counting and write the numeral above the objects to help the student keep each number in memory while responding to your question "How many sounds?"

5. Repeat steps 1–3, asking the student to draw lines for each sound heard as you say a word. Drawing lines replaces counting blocks/chips. You say a word (e.g., cat) and the student draws a separate line for each sound heard in the word and then the student can count the number of lines—in this case, 3.

6. Repeat this activity with additional monosyllabic words.

7. Repeat this activity without manipulatives.

2. Sound categorization or identifying rhyme oddity.

What to say to the student: "Guess which word I say does not rhyme with the other three words."

> EXAMPLE "Tell me which word does not rhyme with the other three: '_____,' '_____,' '_____,' '_____.' " (stimulus words) (e.g., "'brown,' 'down,' 'both,' 'crown.' Which word doesn't rhyme?") (both)

Teaching Steps:

1. Place four pictured items in front of the student (e.g., pictures of a blink, overalls, a sink, and a wink from *Corduroy*).

2. Name the pictures and ask the student: "Which word does not rhyme with the other three?"

3. If the student is correct, reinforce by saying: "Right. You told me the word that doesn't rhyme with the others."

4. Repeat this activity without pictures.

Correction Procedures:

1. Place two pictured items in front of the student (e.g., pictures of a blink and a wink from *Corduroy*).

2. Name the two pictures and say: "These words rhyme."

3. Repeat steps 1–2 with two additional pictured rhyming items from the story and ask: "Do these rhyme?"

4. If the student is correct, reinforce by saying: "Right. You told me the word that doesn't rhyme."

5. If the student is incorrect, place two pictured nonrhyming items in front of the student (e.g., pictures of a button and overalls from *Corduroy*).

6. Name the two pictures and say: "These words don't rhyme."

7. Place two pictured items in front of the student (e.g., pictures of a sink and overalls from *Corduroy*).

8. Name the two pictures and ask the student if these two words rhyme.

9. If the student is correct, reinforce by saying: "Good. You told me they don't rhyme."

10. Repeat this activity with two words until the student is successful at this level.

11. Repeat this activity with three words until the student is successful at this level.

12. Repeat this activity with four words until the student is successful at this level.

13. Repeat this activity without pictures.

3. Matching rhyme.

What to say to the student: "We're going to think of rhyming words."

> **EXAMPLE** "Which word rhymes with '_____'?" (stimulus word) (e.g., "Which word rhymes with 'button'? 'bed,' 'mutton,' 'quite,' 'bang.' " (mutton)

Teaching Steps:

1. Place five pictured items from the story—two of which rhyme (e.g., plum, pie, green, thumb, and sausage from *The Very Hungry Caterpillar*)—in front of the student.

2. Name one of the rhyming pictures (e.g., plum) and ask the student: "Which of these words rhymes with 'plum': 'pie,' 'green,' 'thumb,' or 'sausage'?"

3. If the student is correct, reinforce by saying: "Right. You said 'thumb' rhymes with 'plum.' "

Correction Procedures:

1. Place two rhyming pictured items from the story in front of the student (e.g., plum and thumb). Say: "These words rhyme."

2. Place the two pictured items in front of the student again and ask: "Do these words rhyme?"

3. Repeat step 2 with different sets of two pictures.

4. If the student is correct, reinforce by saying: "Right. You told me those words rhyme with each other."

5. Place two pictured items that do not rhyme in front of the student (e.g., plum and pie). Say: "These words do not rhyme."

6. Repeat step 5 and ask the student: "Do these words rhyme?"

7. Repeat steps 5–6 with different sets of two pictures.

8. If the student is correct, reinforce by saying: "Right. You told me those words don't rhyme."

9. Repeat this activity with three, four, and five words.

10. Repeat this activity without manipulatives.

4. Producing rhyme.

What to say to the student: "Now we'll say rhyming words."

> EXAMPLE "Tell me a word that rhymes with '_____.' " (stimulus word) (e.g., "Tell me a word that rhymes with 'saved.' You can make up a word if you want.") (paved)

Teaching Steps:

1. Name one word from the story (e.g., plum from *The Very Hungry Caterpillar*).

2. Say: "Tell me a word that rhymes with 'plum.' It's okay if you make up a word."

3. If the student is correct, reinforce by saying: "Yes. You told me a word that rhymes with 'plum.' "

Correction Procedures:

1. Place two pictured items in front of the student (e.g., plum and thumb) and ask: "Do these words rhyme?"

2. If the student is correct, reinforce by saying: "Right. You said 'thumb' rhymes with 'plum.' "

3. Leave the two pictures in front of the student and say: "Tell me a word that rhymes with 'plum' " and point to the picture of thumb.

4. If the student is correct, reinforce by saying: "Right. You said 'thumb' rhymes with 'plum.' "

5. Place two pictures of words that do not rhyme (e.g., plum and pie) in front of the student. Say: " 'plum,' 'pie.' These words do not rhyme."

6. Leave the pictured plum and add another pictured item from the story that does not rhyme with plum (e.g., orange). Ask: "Does 'plum' rhyme with 'orange'?"

7. If the student is correct, reinforce by saying: "Right. You told me these words do not rhyme."

8. Repeat this activity by using other words and pictured items from the story.

9. Repeat teaching steps 1–3.

5. Sound matching (initial).

What to say to the student: "Now we'll listen for the first sound in words."

> **EXAMPLE** "Listen to this sound: / /." (stimulus sound). "Guess which word I say begins with that sound: '_____,' '_____,' '_____,' '_____.' " (stimulus words) (e.g., "Listen to this sound: /w/. Guess which word I say begins with that sound: 'heard,' 'button,' 'cried,' 'wondered.' ") (wondered)

Teaching Steps:

1. Say the beginning sound of one of the words from the story (e.g., /m/).
2. Name four words from the story—one of which begins with /m/ (e.g., king, bread, meat, and fire from *Stone Soup*).
3. Say: "Tell me which word begins with /m/."
4. If the student is correct, reinforce by saying: "Okay. You said 'meat' begins with /m/."

Correction Procedures:

1. Place two pictured items in front of the student (e.g., king and meat from *Stone Soup*). Say: "The first sound in 'king' is /k/. Tell me the first sound in 'king.' "
2. If the student is correct, reinforce by saying: "Right. You said the first sound in 'king' is /k/."
3. Ask the student: "Does 'king' begin with /m/?"
4. If the student is correct, reinforce by saying: "Good. You said 'king' does not begin with /m/."
5. Repeat step 1, asking the student: "What's the first sound in 'meat'?"
6. If the student is correct, reinforce by saying: "Right. You said the first sound in 'meat' is /m/."
7. Repeat steps 1–6 with other two-word pairs from the story.
8. Repeat steps 1–6 with other three-word and four-word pairs from the story.
9. Repeat this activity without pictures.

6. Sound matching (final).

What to say to the student: "Now we'll listen for the last sound in words."

> **EXAMPLE** "Listen to this sound: / /" (stimulus sound). "Guess which word I say ends with that sound: '_____,' '_____,' '_____,' _____.' " (stimulus words) (e.g., "Listen to this sound: /r/. Guess which word I say ends with that sound: 'counted,' 'friend,' 'customer,' 'Lisa.' ") (customer)

Teaching Steps:

1. Say the final sound of one of the words from the story (e.g., /z/).
2. Name four words from the story—one of which ends with /z/ (e.g., garden, snooze, warm, red from *The Little Red Hen*).

3. Ask: "Which word ends with /z/?"

4. If the student is correct, reinforce by saying: "Good. You said 'snooze' ends with /z/."

Correction Procedures:

1. Place two pictured items in front of the student (e.g., red and snooze from *The Little Red Hen*). Say: "The last sound in 'snooze' is /z/. Tell me the last sound in 'snooze.' "

2. If the student is correct, reinforce by saying: "Right. You said the last or ending sound in 'snooze' is /z/."

3. Ask the student: "Does 'snooze' end with /t/?"

4. If the student is correct, reinforce by saying: "Right. You said 'snooze' doesn't end with /t/."

5. Repeat steps 1–4, asking: "What's the last sound in 'red'?"

6. If the student is correct, reinforce by saying: "Right. You said the last sound in 'red' is /d/."

7. Repeat steps 1–6 with other two-word pairs from the story.

8. Repeat steps 1–6 with other three-word and four-word pairs from the story.

9. Repeat this activity without pictures.

7. Identifying initial sound in words.

What to say to the student: "I'll say a word two times. Tell me what sound is missing the second time: '____,' '____.' " (stimulus words)

> **EXAMPLE** "What sound do you hear in '____' " (stimulus word) "that is missing in '____'?" (stimulus word) (e.g., "What sound do you hear in 'gate' that is missing in 'ate'?" (/g/)

Teaching Steps:

1. Choose one word from the story that can have one sound removed to form a real or non-real word (e.g., grain, rain).

2. Say "'grain,' 'rain.' What sound in 'grain' is missing in rain'?"

3. If the student is correct, reinforce by saying: "Good. You said /g/ is the missing sound in 'rain.' "

Correction Procedures:

1. Place two pictured items in front of the student (e.g., grain and rain from *The Little Red Hen*).

2. Place four wooden blocks or plastic chips under the pictured grain and three blocks/chips under the pictured rain.

3. Say "/g/ /r/ /long A/ /n/" as you point to each of the blocks/chips under "grain."

4. Say "/r / /long A/ /n/" as you point to each of the blocks under "rain."

5. Say: "Which sound in 'grain,' " pointing to the block/chip that represents /g/, "is missing in 'rain'?" as you point to the picture of rain.

6. If the student is correct, reinforce by saying: "Right. You said /g/ is the sound in 'grain' that is missing in 'rain.' "

7. Repeat this activity with other sets of two words from the story.

8. Repeat this activity without manipulatives.

8. Identifying final sound in words.

What to say to the student: "I'll say a word two times. Tell me what sound is missing the second time: '_____,' '_____.' " (stimulus words)

> **EXAMPLE**   "What sound do you hear in '_____' " (stimulus word) "that is missing in '_____'?" (stimulus word) (e.g., "What sound do you hear in 'soup' that is missing in 'Sue'?") (/p/)

Teaching Steps:

1. Choose one word from the story that can have one sound removed to form a real or non-real word (e.g., soup and Sue).

2. Say: "'soup,' 'Sue.' What sound in 'soup' is missing in 'Sue'?"

3. If the student is correct, reinforce by saying: "Good. You said /p/ is the missing sound in 'Sue.' "

Correction Procedures:

1. Place two pictured items in front of the student (e.g., brown and a brow from *Corduroy*).

2. Place four wooden blocks or plastic chips under the pictured brown and three blocks/chips under the pictured brow.

3. Say "/b/ /r/ /ow/ /n/" as you point to each of the blocks/chips under the brown picture.

4. Say "/b/ /r/ /ow/" as you point to each of the blocks/chips under the brow picture.

5. Say: "Which sound in 'brown' " (pointing to the block or chip that represents /n/) "is missing in 'brow'?" as you point to the picture of brow.

6. If the student is correct, reinforce by saying: "Right. You said /n/ is the sound in 'brown' that is missing in 'brow.' "

7. Repeat this activity without manipulatives.

9. Segmenting initial sound in words.

What to say to the student: "Listen to the word I say and tell me the first sound you hear."

> **EXAMPLE**   "What's the first sound in '_____'?" (stimulus word) (e.g., "What's the first sound in 'button'?") (/b/)

Teaching Steps:

1. Say: "Listen for the first sound in the word I say."

2. Say one word from the story (e.g., dog). Say: "What's the first sound in that word?"

3. If the student is correct, reinforce by saying: "Yes. /d/ is the first sound in 'dog.' "

Correction Procedures:

1. Place a picture of a dog in front of the student.
2. Place three wooden blocks or plastic chips beneath the pictured dog.
3. Say each sound of the word "dog" as you point to each block/chip (i.e., /d/ /ah/ /g/).
4. Point to the first block/chip again and say: "/d/ is the first sound in 'dog.' "
5. Repeat steps 1–3. Point to the first block/chip again and ask: "What's the first sound in 'dog'?"
6. If the student is correct, reinforce by saying: "Right. You said the first sound in 'dog' is /d/."
7. Repeat this activity with other pictured items from the story.
8. Repeat this activity without manipulatives.

10. Segmenting final sound in words.

What to say to the student: "Listen to the word I say and tell me the last sound you hear."

EXAMPLE "What's the last sound in the word '_____'?" (stimulus word) (e.g., "What's the last sound in the word 'lamp'?") (/p/)

Teaching Steps:

1. Say "Listen for the last sound in the word I say."
2. Say one word from the story (e.g., lamp). Say: "What's the last sound in that word?"
3. If the student is correct, reinforce by saying: "Yes. /p/ is the last sound in 'lamp.' "

Correction Procedures:

1. Place a picture of a lamp in front of the student.
2. Place four wooden blocks or plastic chips beneath the pictured lamp.
3. Say each sound of the word "lamp" as you point to each block/chip (i.e., /l/ /short A/ /m/ /p/).
4. Point to the last block/chip again and say "/p/ is the last sound in 'lamp.' "
5. Repeat steps 1–3. Point to the last block/chip again and ask: "What's the last sound in 'lamp'?"
6. If the student is correct, reinforce by saying: "Right. You said the last sound in 'lamp' is /p/."
7. Repeat this activity with other pictured items from the story.
8. Repeat this activity without manipulatives.

11. Generating words from the story beginning with a particular sound.

What to say to the student: "Let's think of words from the story that start/begin with certain sounds."

EXAMPLE "Tell me a word from the story that starts/begins with / /." (stimulus sound) (e.g., the sound /p/) (pig)

Teaching Steps:

1. Say "Listen to this sound: /p/. 'Pig' begins with that sound. Tell me another word from the story that starts with that sound."

2. If the student is correct, reinforce by saying: "Yes. 'path' begins with a /p/ sound."

Correction Procedures:

1. Place two pictures in front of the student, each beginning with /p/ (e.g., a pig and a pot from *The Three Little Pigs*).

2. Place three wooden blocks or plastic chips beneath the pictured pig.

3. Say each sound of the word "pig" as you point to each block/chip (i.e., /p/ /short I/ /g/).

4. Point to the first block/chip again and say: "The first sound in 'pig' is /p/. What's the first sound?"

5. If the student is correct, reinforce by saying: "Right. You said the first sound in 'pig' is /p/."

6. Then, ask: "What's the first sound in 'pot'?"

7. Repeat this activity with blocks/chips and other pictured items from the story.

8. Repeat this activity without manipulatives.

12. Blending sounds in monosyllabic words divided into onset/rime beginning with two consonant cluster + rime.

What to say to the student: "Now we'll put sounds together to make words."

> **EXAMPLE** "Put these sounds together to make a word: / / + / /." (stimulus sounds) "What's the word?" (e.g., "bl + ink: What's the word?") (blink)

Teaching Steps:

1. Say the first two-consonant cluster of a one-syllable word and then the rest of the one-syllable word (e.g., bl + ink).

2. Ask the student: "What word is it when you put those parts together?"

3. If the student is correct, reinforce by saying: "Right. When you put 'bl' with 'ink,' the word is 'blink.' "

Correction Procedures:

1. Select a word from the story beginning with a two-consonant blend (e.g., cheese from *The Very Hungry Caterpillar*). Copy a picture of cheese from the story and cut the picture in half.

2. Point to the left half of the pictured cheese and say /ch/. Point to the right half of the pictured cheese and say "cheese."

3. Move the two halves together and say "cheese."

4. Repeat steps 1–3 asking the student to "Say the word parts" (i.e., /ch/ and "eese").

5. Place two wooden blocks or plastic chips in front of the student.

6. Point to the block/chip on the student's left and say: "This is /ch/." Point to the block/chip on the student's right and say: "This is 'eese.' "

7. Then, move the two blocks/chips together and say: "When you put these together, the word is 'cheese.' "

8. Repeat steps 5–6, asking the student: "What do each of these say: /ch/ and 'eese?' "

9. If the student is correct, reinforce by saying: "Good. You told me this block says /ch/ and this one says 'eese.' "

10. Move the blocks/chips together and ask: "When you put the parts together, what's the word?"

11. If the student is correct, reinforce by saying: "Right. You said that when you put /ch/ and 'eese' together, the word is 'cheese.' "

12. Repeat this activity with other one-syllable words from the story beginning with two-consonant blends.

13. Repeat this activity without manipulatives.

13. Blending sounds in monosyllabic words divided into onset/rime beginning with single consonant + rime.

What to say to the student: "Let's put sounds together to make words."

> **EXAMPLE** "Put these sounds together to make a word: / / + / /." (stimulus sounds)
> "What's the word?" (e.g., "/d/ + 'og': What's the word?") (dog)

Teaching Steps:

1. Say the first single consonant of a one-syllable word and then the rest of the word (e.g., /d/ + "og").

2. Say: "When you put those sounds together, the word is 'dog.' "

3. Repeat step 1 with another word from the story beginning with a single consonant (e.g., /k/ + "at"). Ask: "What word is that?"

4. If the student is correct, reinforce by saying: "Right. When you put /k/ with 'at,' the word is 'cat.' "

Correction Procedures:

1. Select a word from the story beginning with a single consonant (e.g., dog from *Hairy the Dirty Dog*). Copy a picture of a dog from the story and cut the picture in half.

2. Point to the left half of the pictured dog and say /d/. Point to the right half of the pictured dog and say "og."

3. Move the two halves together and say "dog."

4. Repeat steps 1–3, asking the student to say the word parts (i.e., /d/ and "og").

5. Place two wooden blocks or plastic chips in front of the student.

6. Point to the block/chip on the student's left and say: "This is /d/." Point to the block/chip on the student's right and say: "This is 'og.' "

7. Then, move the two blocks/chips together and say: "When you put these together, the word is 'dog.' "

8. Repeat steps 5–6, asking the student: "What do each of these say?"

9. If the student is correct, reinforce by saying: "Good. You told me this block says /d/ and this one says 'og' " (as you point to each of the blocks/chips).

10. Point to the blocks/chips and ask: "When you put the parts together, what's the word?"

11. If the student is correct, reinforce by saying: "Right. You said when you put /d/ and 'og' together, the word is 'dog.' "

12. Repeat this activity with other one-syllable words from the story beginning with single consonant sounds.

13. Repeat this activity without manipulatives.

14. Blending sounds to form a monosyllabic word beginning with a continuant sound.

What to say to the student: "We'll put sounds together to make words."

> **EXAMPLE** "Put these sounds together to make a word: / / + / / + / /." (stimulus sounds) (e.g., /n/ /long I/ /t/) (night)

Teaching Steps:

1. Say each sound in a one-syllable word from the story (e.g., /n/ /long I/ /t/).

2. Say: "When you put those sounds together, the word is 'night.' "

3. Repeat step 1 with another word from the story beginning with a single consonant (e.g., /m/ /oo/ /n/). Ask: "What word is that?"

4. If the student is correct, reinforce by saying: "Right. When you put /m/ /oo/ /n/ together, the word is 'moon.' "

Correction Procedures:

1. Select a word from the story beginning with a continuant sound (e.g., /m/, /n/, /s/, /z/, /r/, /f/, /h/, /l/, /v/, /w/, /sh/, /voiceless th/, /voiced th/, or /j/ as in yellow—e.g., Sal from *Blueberries for Sal*). Copy a picture of Sal from the story and cut the picture in thirds.

2. Point to the left one-third of the pictured Sal and say /s/. Point to the middle one-third of the pictured Sal and say /short A/. Point to the right one-third of the pictured Sal and say /l/.

3. Move the three parts of the picture together and say "Sal."

4. Repeat steps 1–3, asking the student to say the sounds (i.e., /s/ /short A/ /l/).

5. Place three wooden blocks or plastic chips in front of the student.

6. Point to the block/chip on the student's left and say: "This is /s/." Point to the middle block/chip and say: "This is /short A/." Point to the block/chip on the student's right and say: "This is /l/."

7. Then, move the three blocks/chips together and say: "When you put these together, the word is 'Sal.' "

8. Repeat step 5 asking the student: "What do each of these say?"

9. If the student is correct, reinforce by saying: "Good. You told me what each sound is."

10. Say: "Move the blocks together and tell me the word."

11. If the student is correct, say: "Good. You told me when you put the sounds /s/ /short A/ /l/ together, the word is 'Sal.' "

12. Repeat this activity with other one-syllable words from the story beginning with continuant sounds.

13. Repeat this activity without manipulatives.

15. Blending sounds to form a monosyllabic word beginning with a noncontinuant sound.

What to say to the student: "We'll put sounds together to make words."

> **EXAMPLE** "Put these sounds together to make a word: / / + / / + / /." (stimulus sounds) (e.g., /p/ /short I/ /k/) (pick)

Teaching Steps:

1. Say each sound in a one-syllable word from the story (e.g., /p/ /short I/ /k/).

2. Say: "When you put those sounds together, the word is 'pick.' "

3. Repeat step 1 with another word from the story beginning with a single consonant (e.g., /k/ /long I/ /t/).

4. Ask: "What word is it when you put those sounds together?"

5. If the student is correct, reinforce by saying: "Right. When you put /k/ /long I/ /t/ together, the word is 'kite.' "

Correction Procedures:

1. Select a word from the story beginning with a noncontinuant sound (e.g., /p/, /b/, /t/, /d/, /k/, /g/, /ch/, /dz/ as in jelly—e.g., pig from *The Three Little Pigs*). Copy a picture of pig from the story and cut the picture in thirds.

2. Point to the left one-third of the pictured pig and say /p/. Point to the middle one-third of the pictured pig and say /short I/. Point to the right one-third of the pictured pig and say /g/.

3. Move the three parts of the picture together and say "pig."

4. Repeat steps 1–3, asking the student to say the sounds (i.e., /p/ /short I/ /g/).

5. Place three wooden blocks or plastic chips in front of the student.

6. Point to the block/chip on the student's left and say: "This is /p/." Point to the middle block/chip and say: "This is /short I/." Point to the block/chip on the student's right and say: "This is /g/."

7. Then, move the three blocks/chips together and say: "When you put these together, the word is 'pig.' "

8. Repeat step 5, asking the student: "What do each of these say?"

9. If the student is correct, reinforce by saying: "Good. You told me what each sound is."

10. Say: "Move the blocks together and tell me the word."

11. If the student is correct, say: "Good. You told me when you put the sounds /p/ /short I/ /g/ together, the word is 'pig.' "

12. Repeat this activity with other one-syllable words from the story beginning with noncontinuant sounds.

13. Repeat this activity without manipulatives.

16. Substituting the initial sound in words.

What to say to the student: "We're going to change beginning/first sounds in words."

> **EXAMPLE** "Say '_____.' " (stimulus word) "Instead of / /" (stimulus sound), "say / /." (stimulus sound) (e.g., "Say 'cat.' Instead of /k/, say /s/. What's your new word?") (sat)

Teaching Steps:

1. Place three wooden blocks or plastic chips next to each other in front of the student.

2. Say /k/ as you point to the first block/chip; say /short A/ as you point to the middle block/chip; and say /t/ as you point to the third block/chip. Motion to the blocks/chips and say: "This says 'cat.' "

3. Replace the first wooden block/chip with a different color block/chip and say: "/s/. Now this says 'sat.' "

4. Say /s/ as you point to the first block/chip; say /short A/ as you point to the middle block/chip; and say /t/ as you point to the third block/chip. Motion to the blocks and ask: "What word do these sounds make?"

5. If the student is correct, reinforce by saying: "Good. You changed the first sound in 'cat' from /k/ to /s/ and now the word is 'sat.' "

6. Repeat this activity without manipulatives.

Correction Procedures:

1. Place two red blocks/chips in front of the student and say "red" as you point to the first block/chip and "red" as you point to the second block/chip.

2. Replace the first red block/chip with a blue block/chip and say "blue" as you point to the first block and "red" as you point to the second block. Then, say: "I changed the first part."

3. Repeat step 2 several times, replacing the first colored block/chip with a different colored block/chip than the one with which you started. In each instance, have the student name the color of the first block and "red" as you point to the second block/chip.

4. If the student is correct, reinforce by saying: "Good. You changed the first part."

5. Place two blocks/chips in front of the student. Instead of saying the color of the blocks/chips, say /k/ as you point to the first block/chip and /long A/ as you point to the second block/chip.

6. Replace the first block/chip and say /d/ as you point to it and /long A/ as you point to the second block/chip. Say: "I changed the first sound of the word."

7. Repeat steps 5–6, changing the first sound as you point to the first block/chip and saying /long A/ as you point to the second block/chip. Have the student tell you what the new word is each time. Reinforce by saying: "Good. You changed the first part."

8. Repeat this activity with other one-syllable words from the story.

9. Repeat this activity without manipulatives.

17. Substituting the final sound in words.

What to say to the student: "We're going to change ending/last sounds in words."

> EXAMPLE "Say '_____.' " (stimulus word) "Instead of / /" (stimulus sound), "say / /." (stimulus sound) (e.g., "Say 'night.' Instead of /t/, say /n/. What's your new word?") (nine)

Teaching Steps:

1. Place three wooden blocks or plastic chips next to each other in front of the student.

2. Say /d/ as you point to the first block/chip; say /short O/ as you point to the middle block; and say /g/ as you point to the third block. Motion to the blocks and say: "This says 'dog.' "

3. Replace the third block/chip with a different color block/chip and say: "/k/. Now this says 'dock.' "

4. Say /d/ as you point to the first block/chip; say /short O/ as you point to the middle block/chip; and say /k/ as you point to the third block/chip. Motion to the blocks and ask: "What word do these sounds make?"

5. If the student is correct, reinforce by saying: "Good. You changed the last sound in 'dog' from /g/ to /k/ and now the word is 'dock.' "

6. Repeat this activity without manipulatives.

Correction Procedures:

1. Place two red blocks/chips in front of the student, saying "red" as you point to the first block/chip and "red" as you point to the second block/chip.

2. Replace the second block/chip with a blue block/chip, saying "red" as you point to the first block/chip and "blue" as you point to the second block/chip. Then, say: "I changed the last part."

3. Repeat step 2 several times, replacing the second colored block/chip with a different colored block/chip than the one with which you started. In each instance, have the student name the first block/chip "red" and the name of the color of the second block/chip as you point to it.

4. If the student is correct, reinforce by saying: "Good. You changed the last part."

5. Place two blocks/chips in front of the student. Instead of saying the color of the blocks/chips, say /k/ as you point to the first block/chip and say /long A/ as you point to the second block/chip.

6. Replace the second block/chip and say /k/ as you point to the first block/chip and say /long E/ as you point to the second block/chip. Say: "I changed the last sound of the word."

7. Repeat steps 5–6, changing the last (second) sound as you point to the second block/chip and saying /k/ as you point to the first block/chip. Have the student tell you what the new word is each time. Reinforce by saying: "Good. You changed the last part."

8. Repeat this activity with other one-syllable words from the story.

9. Repeat this activity without manipulatives.

18. Segmenting middle sound in monosyllabic words.

What to say to the student: "Tell me the middle sound in the word I say."

> **EXAMPLE** "What's the middle sound in the word '_____'?" (stimulus word) (e.g., "What's the middle sound in the word 'hug'?") (/short U/)

Teaching Steps:

1. Place a pictured item from the story (e.g., moon from *Happy Birthday, Moon*) and three wooden blocks or plastic chips next to each other in front of the student.

2. Say /m/ as you point to the first block/chip; say /oo/ as you point to the middle block/chip; and say /n/ as you point to the third block/chip.

3. Ask: "What's the middle sound in 'moon'?"

4. If the student is correct, reinforce by saying: "Yes. /oo/ is the middle sound in 'moon.' "

Correction Procedures:

1. Place a picture of a moon from *Happy Birthday, Moon* in front of the student.

2. Place three wooden blocks or plastic chips beneath the pictured moon.

3. Say each sound of the word as you point to each block/chip (i.e., /m/ /oo/ /n/).

4. Point to the first block/chip again and ask the student: "What's the first sound?"

5. If the student is correct, reinforce by saying: "Right. You said the first sound in 'moon' is /m/."

6. Repeat step 4, pointing to the second and third blocks and reinforcing the student by saying: "Good. You said the middle sound in 'moon' is /oo/ and the last sound in 'moon' is /n/."

7. Ask: "What's the middle sound in 'moon'?"

8. Repeat this activity with other one-syllable words and pictures from the story.

9. Repeat this activity without manipulatives.

19. Substituting middle sound in words.

What to say to the student: "We're going to change the middle sound in words."

> **EXAMPLE** "Say '_____.' " (stimulus word) "Instead of / /" (stimulus sound), "say / /." (stimulus sound) (e.g., "Say 'flop.' Instead of /ah/, say /short I/. What's your new word?") (flip)

Teaching Steps:

1. Place three wooden blocks or plastic chips next to each other in front of the student.

2. Say /d/ as you point to the first block/chip; say /ah/ as you point to the middle block/chip; and say /g/ as you point to the third block/chip. Motion to the blocks/chips and say: "This says 'dog.' "

3. Replace the middle block/chip with a different color block/chip and say /short I/.

4. Say /d/ as you point to the first block/chip; say /short I/ as you point to the middle block/chip; and say /g/ as you point to the third block/chip. Motion to the blocks and ask: "What word do these sounds make"?

5. If the student is correct, reinforce by saying: "Good. You changed the middle sound in 'dog' from /ah/ to /short I/ and now the word is 'dig.' "

6. Repeat this activity without manipulatives.

Correction Procedures:

1. Place three red blocks/chips in front of the student, saying "red" as you point to the first block/chip, "red" as you point to the second block/chip, and "red" as you point to the third block/chip.

2. Replace the second block/chip with a blue block/chip saying: "red" as you point to the first block/chip, "blue" as you point to the second block/chip, and "red" as you point to the third block/chip. Then, say: "I changed the middle part."

3. Repeat steps 1–2. In step 2, ask the student: "What do you change the middle one to?"

4. If the student is correct, reinforce by saying: "Good. You changed the middle part."

5. Place two pictures from the story in front of the student (e.g., pail and pill from *Blueberries for Sal*).

6. Place three wooden blocks or plastic chips in front of the student. Instead of saying the color of the blocks/chips, say /p/ as you point to the first block/chip, say /long A/ as you point to the second block/chip, and say /l/ as you point to the third block/chip. Point to the pictured pail and then point to the blocks/chips and say "pail."

7. Point to the pictured pill and replace the second block/chip with a different color block/chip. Say /p/ as you point to the first block/chip; say /short I/ as you point to the second block/chip; and say /l/ as you point to the third block/chip. Say: "I changed the middle sound of the word."

8. Repeat steps 5–7 several times, changing the middle (second) sound as you point to the second block/chip. Have the student tell you what the new word is each time. Reinforce by saying: "Good. You changed the middle part of the word."

9. Repeat this activity with other one-syllable words from the story.

10. Repeat this activity without manipulatives.

20. Identifying all sounds in monosyllabic words.

What to say to the student: "Now tell me all the sounds you hear in the word I say."

> EXAMPLE "What sounds do you hear in the word '_____'?" (stimulus word) (e.g., "What sounds do you hear in the word 'gave'?") (/g/ /long A/ /v/)

Teaching Steps:

1. Place three wooden blocks or plastic chips next to each other in front of the student. Say: "Each of these blocks/chips stands for one sound in a word."

2. Say "gave." Say /g/ as you point to the first block/chip; say /long A/ as you point to the middle block/chip; and say /v/ as you point to the third block/chip. Motion to the blocks/chips and say: "This says 'gave.' "

3. Place three blocks/chips in front of the student. Say another monosyllabic word from the story beginning and ending with consonants and a vowel sound in the middle.

4. Ask the student to tell you the sounds in the word you say.

5. If the student is correct, reinforce by saying: "Good. You told me what sounds are in the word."

6. Repeat this activity without manipulatives.

Correction Procedures:

1. Place a picture of a hen (from *The Little Red Hen*) in front of the student.

2. Place three wooden blocks or plastic chips beneath the pictured hen.

3. Say each sound of the word "hen" as you point to each block/chip (i.e., /h/ /short E/ /n/).

4. Then, point to the pictured hen again and ask the student: "What sounds do you hear in the word 'hen'?"

5. If the student is correct, reinforce by saying: "Yes. The sounds in 'hen' are /h/ /short E/ /n/."

6. Repeat this activity with blocks/chips and other one-syllable words and pictures from the story.

7. Repeat this activity without manipulatives.

21. Deleting sounds within words.

What to say to the student: "We're going to leave out sounds in words."

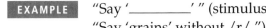 "Say '_____' " (stimulus word) "without / /." (stimulus sound) (e.g., "Say 'grains' without /r/.") (gains) Say: "The word that was left—'gains'— is a real word. Sometimes, the word won't be a real word."

Teaching Steps:

1. Place four wooden blocks or plastic chips next to each other in front of the student. Say /g/ as you point to the first block/chip; say /r/ as you point to the second block/chip; say /long A/ as you point to the next block/chip; and say /n/ as you point to the fourth block/chip. Motion to the blocks/chips and say: "This says 'grain' " (from *The Little Red Hen*) as you motion to the blocks/chips.

2. Remove the second block/chip and say: "Now this says 'gain.' "

3. Replace the second block/chip and ask: "What's the word"? (grain)

4. Remove the second block/chip and ask: "Now what's the word"?

5. If the student is correct, reinforce by saying: "Good. When you take /r/ from 'grain,' the word is 'gain.' "

6. Repeat this activity without manipulatives.

Correction Procedures:

1. Place two red blocks/chips in front of the student, saying "red" as you point to each of them.

2. Place a green block/chip between the two red blocks/chips and say "red" as you point to the first red block/chip, "green" as you point to the middle block/chip, and "red" as you point to the second red block/chip.

3. Remove the green block/chip and say: "When I take out the green block, I have 'red,' 'red' " as you point to each of the two red blocks/chips.

4. Repeat steps 1–3 several times with different colored blocks/chips—always keeping the first and third blocks/chips the same color and different from the second block/chip. In each instance, say: "Name the color of the three blocks." And each time you remove the second block/chip, say: "Name the two remaining blocks/chips."

5. Repeat this activity with four blocks/chips. Keep the first, third, and fourth blocks the same color. The second block should be a different color. Ask the student to name the colored blocks/chips (e.g., red, blue, red, red). Then, remove the blue block and have the student name the remaining blocks (e.g., red, red, red).

6. Place four blocks/chips in front of the student. Instead of saying the color of the blocks/chips, say /g/ as you point to the first block/chip, /r/ as you point to the second block/chip, /long A/ as you point to the third block/chip, and /n/ as you point to the fourth block/chip.

7. Remove the second block/chip. Ask: "What sound did I take away"? (/r/) Then, ask: "What word is this now"? (gain)

8. If the student is correct, reinforce by saying: "Good. When you take /r/ from 'grain,' the word is 'gain.' "

9. Repeat this activity with one-syllable words (four sounds each) from the story. Continue to use blocks/chips to represent the sounds of the words.

10. Repeat this activity without manipulatives.

22. Substituting a consonant in words having a two-sound cluster.

What to say to the student: "We're going to substitute sounds in words."

> **EXAMPLE** "Say '_____.' " (stimulus word) "Instead of / /" (stimulus sound), "say / /." (stimulus sound) (e.g., "Say 'climb.' Instead of /l/, say /r/.") (crime) "Sometimes, the new word won't be a word."

Teaching Steps:

1. Say one word from the story (e.g., store from *Corduroy*).

2. Draw four lines and say: "The sounds in 'store' are /s/ /t/ /long O/ /r/" as you point to each of the lines.

3. Say: "Now I'll change one of the sounds." Circle the second line and say: "/n/. I changed /t/ to /n/. The new word is 'snore.' "

4. Erase the circled line. Point to the lines and say "store." Circle the second line and say "/n/. I changed /t/ to /n/. What's the new word?"

5. If the student is correct, reinforce by saying: "Yes. When you change /t/ to /n/, the new word is 'snore.' "

6. Repeat this activity with other one-syllable words from the story.

7. Repeat this activity without drawn lines.

Correction Procedures:

1. Say two words: "store, snore."

2. Place two pictures in front of the student: store (from *Corduroy*) and snore (e.g., a picture of a person sleeping).

3. Place five wooden blocks or plastic chips in front of the student.

4. Say: "The sounds in 'store' are /s/ /t/ /long O/ /r/" as you point to each of the blocks/chips under the pictured store.

5. Replace the second block/chip with a different colored block/chip.

6. Say: "I switched /t/ to /n/. Now the word is 'snore.' " Point to the pictured snore.

7. Replace the exchanged block/chip with the original one representing /t/. Ask: "What was the first word"?

8. If the student is correct, reinforce by saying: "Right. This word is 'store' " as you point to the pictured store.

9. Reinsert the block/chip representing /n/ and ask: "What's the word now"? (snore)

10. If the student is correct, reinforce by saying: "Good. You switched /t/ to /n/. The word changed from 'store' to snore.' "

11. Repeat this activity with blocks/chips, pictures, and other one-syllable words from the story.

12. Repeat this activity without manipulatives.

23. Phoneme reversing.

What to say to the student: "We're going to say words backward."

> **EXAMPLE** "Say the word '_____' " (stimulus word) "backward." (e.g., "Say 'bed' backward.") (deb)

Teaching Steps:

1. Say one word from the story (e.g., bed). Ask: "What sounds do you hear in that word"?

2. If the student is correct, reinforce by saying: "Yes. The sounds in 'bed' are /b/ /short E/ /d/."

3. Say: "Now I'll say those same sounds in the reverse order or backward. Listen: 'deb.' "

4. Say: "I'll say another word from the story, and I want you to say the sounds in the word in the reverse order." Present another word from the story and say: "Say the sounds in the reverse order. Say the word backward."

5. If the student is correct, say: "Good. You said the word backward."

Correction Procedures:

1. Place two pictures in front of the student: a 10 and a net.

2. Place three different colored wooden blocks or plastic chips beneath the pictured 10.

3. Say each sound of the word "ten" as you point to each block/chip (i.e., as you say /t/, point to the red block/chip; as you say /short E/, point to the green block/chip; and as you say /n/, point to the blue block/chip).

4. Point to the pictured net and switch the order of the blocks/chips, putting them under the pictured net (i.e., the blue block/chip is under the /n/, the green block/chip is under the /short E/, and the red block/chip is under the /t/).

5. Say: "If you switch the sounds in 'ten' around, the new word is 'net.' "

6. Present other one-syllable words from the story with the correct number of blocks/chips under each. Ask the student to reverse the sounds and blocks/chips in each word.

7. If the student is correct, reinforce by saying: "Yes. When you reverse the sounds in the word, it makes a new word. You can say the word backward."

8. Repeat this activity without manipulatives.

24. Phoneme switching.

What to say to the student: "We're going to switch the first sounds in two words."

> EXAMPLE   "Switch the first sounds in '_____' and '_____' " (stimulus words) (e.g., "Switch the first sounds in 'her dog.' "). (der hog)

Teaching Steps:

1. Say two words from the story (e.g., her dog). Say: "What beginning sounds do you hear in those words"?

2. If the student is correct, reinforce by saying: "Yes. The first sound in 'her' is /h/ and the first sound in 'dog' is /d/."

3. Say: "When you switch the first sounds in the two words, it makes 'der hog.' "

4. Repeat steps 1–2 with two more words (e.g., red hen). Tell the student to: "Switch the first sounds. What are the words now"? (head ren)

5. If the student is correct, reinforce by saying: "Great. You switched the first sounds so 'red hen' became 'head ren.' "

Correction Procedures:

1. Place two pictures in front of the student (e.g., a bear and a hat from *Happy Birthday, Moon*).

2. Place three wooden blocks or plastic chips beneath each picture. The first block/chip under the picture is different from the others (e.g., a black block/chip under the bear and an orange block/chip under the hat). The next two blocks/chips under each picture should be the same in color but not black or orange (e.g., under the bear is one black block/chip and two red blocks/chips; under the hat is one orange block/chip and two red blocks/chips).

3. Say each sound of the word "bear" (i.e., /b/ /long A/ /r/) as you point to each block/chip under the pictured bear, and say each sound of the word "hat" (i.e., /h/ /short A/ /t/) as you point to the pictured hat.

4. Say: "If you reverse the first sounds in 'bear' and 'hat' " (as you switch the black and orange blocks/chips), "the new words are 'hair' and 'bat.' "

5. Repeat steps 2–4. Ask the student what the new words are when you reverse the first sounds.

6. If the student is correct, reinforce by saying: "Yes, when you reverse the first sounds in the words, the new words are 'hair' and 'bat.' "

7. Repeat this activity with other sets of two one-syllable words.

8. Repeat this activity without manipulatives.

25. Pig Latin.

What to say to the student: "We're going to speak a secret language by using words from the story. In pig Latin, you take off the first sound of a word, put it at the end of the word, and add a /long A/ sound."

EXAMPLE "Say chest in pig Latin." (estchay)

Teaching Steps:

1. Say one word from the story (e.g., rice).
2. Say: "When you take the first sound off the word 'rice,' the new word is 'ice.' "
3. Say: "If you put the /r/ at the end of 'ice,' the word is 'icer.' "
4. Say: "Now if you add a /long A/ sound to the end of 'icer,' the word is 'iceray.' This is how we speak pig Latin."
5. Say: "Say 'rice' in pig Latin."
6. If the student is correct, reinforce by saying: "Good work. You can speak pig Latin."

Correction Procedures:

1. Place three wooden blocks or plastic chips in front of the student.
2. Place a picture of a cat in front of the student and move two of the blocks/chips under the pictured cat, saying: "This is /k/" as you point to the block/chip on the student's left. Say: "This is 'at' " as you point to the block/chip on the student's right.
3. Move the first block/chip to the right of the second block/chip and say: "Now this says 'atk.' "
4. Move the third block/chip to the right of the block representing /k/ and say: "/long A/. Now this says 'atkay.' "
5. Repeat step 2 asking the student to tell you what the two blocks stand for. (/k/ and "at")
6. Repeat step 3, asking the student to tell you what the new word is when you move the first block/chip to the right of the second block/chip. ("atk")
7. Repeat step 4, asking the student to say what the new word is.
8. If the student is correct, reinforce by saying: "Great. You said the new word is 'atkay.' You can speak pig Latin."
9. Repeat this activity with other pictured one-syllable words from the story and colored blocks/chips.
10. Repeat this activity without manipulatives.

From Phonological Awareness into Print

NOTE: *Only six examples per activity are included in this resource due to space. You are encouraged to add many more words into this section that you feel your student(s) is(are) ready to write.*

1. **Substituting the initial sound/letter in words.** See "Teaching Steps" and "Correction Procedures" for activity 16 under "Phonological Awareness Activities at the Phoneme Level."

2. **Substituting the final sound or letter in words.** See "Teaching Steps" and "Correction Procedures" for activity 17 under "Phonological Awareness Activities at the Phoneme Level."

3. **Substituting the middle sound or letter in words.** See "Teaching Steps" and "Correction Procedures" for activity 18 under "Phonological Awareness Activities at the Phoneme Level."

4. **Supplying the initial sound or letter in words.** See "Teaching Steps" and "Correction Procedures" for activity 7 under "Phonological Awareness Activities at the Phoneme Level."

5. **Supplying the final sound or letter in words.** See "Teaching Steps" and "Correction Procedures" for activity 8 under "Phonological Awareness Activities at the Phoneme Level."

6. **Switching the first sound and letter in words (ADVANCED).** See "Teaching Steps" and "Correction Procedures" for activity 24 under "Phonological Awareness Activities at the Phoneme Level."

Some Specific Suggestions for Use with Materials

Begin at the level where your student performs below the 80% to 100% accuracy level. If your student can already correctly perform activities at the word level, begin activities at the syllable level. Or if the student demonstrates errors on some of the syllable level activities, begin with them and move into phonemic level activities.

It is extremely important for the user of these materials to give the sound the letters make rather than giving the letter names when presenting all the activities. The sound system of our language is what phonological awareness training is about, not teaching students names of alphabet letters. For example, when asking the student to provide words from the story beginning with /b/, be sure to give the sound /b/ and not the alphabet letter name [B]. With the exception of /dz/ (as in jelly), alphabetic letters were used rather than the phonetic symbols typically employed by speech-language specialists. Likewise, the descriptors "long" and "short" instead of phonetic symbols indicate vowel sounds. In many instances, the way a word sounds is presented for ease of presentation instead of the correct spelling—for example, "Add 'possess' to the ending 'shun' " (rather than "sion").

If your student is not yet able to count objects, select other activities at the word level to increase phonological awareness abilities as the student is learning counting and one-to-one correspondence.

If your student uses another word instead of the one listed or the one you are thinking of in the "fill in the missing word" activities, you can suggest that the student think of a word from the story. For example, one item under activity 2 at the word level ("Supplying Words as an Adult Reads") included under *Stone Soup*: "Came back with big _____ of meat." The correct answer is "chunks." If the student answers "bites," ask the student to think about the words from the story. Pictured items from the book may be used to assist the student in recalling the specific vocabulary item intended. If additional prompting does not cue the student to provide the intended response, the response "bites" should be considered correct. The purpose of the activity is to increase the student's ability to supply a missing word, not correctly recalling specific vocabulary items. If the student's response is totally incorrect, then additional readings of the story and exposure to the vocabulary should be undertaken prior to specific work on phonological awareness activities.

If your student cannot add syllables (e.g., "add 'boy' to the end of 'cow'") or delete syllables (e.g., say "cowboy" without "boy"), use two pictures (e.g., a cow and a boy) to help illustrate the example. In training the student to add pictures, show the picture of a cow and have the student name the picture. Then, add the picture of the boy to the right of cow and ask your student to put the two words together to make a new word—for example, "cowboy." In training your student to delete a syllable, show both pictures, with the pictured boy to the right of the pictured cow. Then, take away one of the pictures—for example, the boy—and ask your student to tell you "What's left"?

If your student cannot correctly respond to an item involving counting words, syllables, or phonemes, add in manipulatives (e.g., plastic or wooden blocks or square pieces of paper) so the student has something concrete to count. Or have the student draw lines (_____ _____ _____) or slash marks (/ / /) to represent each word, syllable, or phoneme in the stimulus word you say. Only use such manipulatives when necessary. If the student can perform the activity without the use of manipulatives, then present the activity stimulus items without them.

If your student is having trouble with blending syllables (e.g., cow + boy) *or phonemes* (/k/ /ae/ /t/) *to form a word,* use plastic or wooden blocks or plastic cubes that snap together as you add a syllable or sounds together to form words.

If your student adds voicing to sounds when saying them after you—for example, /kuh/ (with voice) rather than /k/ (voiceless)—tell him or her to "turn voice off" or "no voice." It is important that our students play with the sounds in isolation as much as possible.

If your student's memory is a factor in following directions during phonological awareness activities, simplify the direction. For example, FIRST DIRECTION: "We're going to leave out syllables or parts of words. Say 'cowboy.' Now say it again without 'cow.' What's left"? SECOND DIRECTION: "Let's drop syllables. Say 'cowboy' without 'cow.'"

If you need to increase or decrease the number of items for any given activity, do so. Use the vocabulary listed for the story or any other vocabulary from the story version you use. Add or delete items depending on students' memory.

Always begin each activity with training on words not included in the stimulus items listed for the activity if you are using those stimulus items to count for a student's performance level.

Phonological Awareness Activities to Use with *Benny's Pennies*

Text version used for selection of stimulus items:
Brisson, P., and Barner, B. (Illustrator). (1993). *Benny's Pennies.* New York: Random House.

Phonological Awareness Activities at the Word Level

1. Counting words.

What to say to the student: "We're going to count words."

> **EXAMPLE** "How many words do you hear in this sentence (or phrase): 'What should I buy?'" (4)

NOTE: *Use pictured items and/or manipulatives if necessary. Use any of the following stimulus phrases or sentences and/or others you select from the story. The correct answers are in parentheses.*

Stimulus items:

a penny (2)

Michael Bess (2)

five new pennies (3)

quite a shopper (3)

sell me a cookie (4)

a fine paper hat (4)

a girl was baking cookies (5)

her name was Mrs. Rose (5)

will you sell me a rose? (6)

strolled home in the morning sun (6)

2. Identifying the missing word from a list.

What to say to the student: "Listen to the words I say. I'll say them again. You tell me which word I leave out."

EXAMPLE "Listen to the words I say: 'nice,' 'me,' 'Benny.' I'll say them again. Tell me which one I leave out: 'nice,' 'Benny.'" (me)

NOTE: *Use pictured items and/or manipulatives if necessary. Use any of the following stimulus words and/or others you select from the story. The correct answers are in parentheses.*

Stimulus set #1	Stimulus set #2
cat, meaty	meaty (cat)
butcher, four	four (butcher)
floppy, Hill, rose	floppy, rose (Hill)
you're, woof, Beal	woof, Beal (you're)
Hopper, buy, strolled	Hopper, buy (strolled)
Benny, sun, thank	sun, thank (Benny)
sister, good, meow, Michael	sister, meow, Michael (good)
bought, McBride, name, fish	bought, McBride, fish (name)
hat, welcome, Lucy, penny	hat, welcome, Lucy (penny)
cookie, beautiful, deal, sweet	beautiful, deal, sweet (cookie)

3. Identifying the missing word in a phrase or sentence.

What to say to the student: "Listen to the sentence I read. Tell me which word is missing the second time I read the sentence."

EXAMPLE "'sell a cookie.' Listen again and tell me which word I leave out: 'a cookie.'" (sell)

NOTE: *Use pictured items and/or manipulatives if necessary. Use any of the following stimulus sentences and/or others you select from the story. The correct answers are in parentheses.*

Stimulus items:

Morning sun. Morning _____. (sun)

Cutting roses. Cutting _____. (roses)

Buy something beautiful. Buy _____ beautiful. (something)

Soft, warm cookie. _____, warm cookie. (soft)

It's a deal. It's a _____. (deal)

What should I buy? What _____ I buy? (should)

A fine paper hat. A _____ paper hat. (fine)

You're quite a shopper. _____ quite a shopper. (you're)

A boy was making hats. A boy was _____ hats. (making)

Her name was Lucy May. Her name was _____ May. (Lucy)

4. Supplying the missing word as an adult reads.

What to say to the student: "I want you to help me read the story. You fill in the words I leave out."

> **EXAMPLE**   "Benny _____." (McBride)

> **NOTE:** *Use pictured items and/or manipulatives if necessary. Use any of the following stimulus sentences and/or others you select from the story. The correct answers are in parentheses.*

Stimulus items:

What should I _____ ? (buy)

Will you _____ me a fish? (sell)

"Woof! Woof!" said his _____. (dog)

A _____ was catching fish. (man)

A soft, warm _____. (cookie)

A butcher was cutting _____. (meat)

"You're quite a _____," said Mr. Hopper. (shopper)

Then Benny McBride with three _____ pennies. (new)

Strolled on in the _____ sun. (morning)

A sweet-_____ rose. (smelling)

5. Rearranging words.

What to say to the student: "I'll say some words out of order. You put them in the right order so they make sense."

> **EXAMPLE**   "'eat to good.' Put those words in the right order." (good to eat)

> **NOTE:** *Use pictured items and/or manipulatives if necessary. Use any of the following stimulus words and/or others you select from the story. The correct answers are in parentheses. This word-level activity can be more difficult than some of the syllable- or phoneme-level activities because of the memory load. If your students are only able to deal with two or three words to be rearranged, add more two- and three-word samples from the story and omit the four-word level items.*

Stimulus items:

McBride Benny (Benny McBride)

Her name was Hill Mrs. (Her name was Mrs. Hill.)

What buy I should? (What should I buy?)

a rose sweet-smelling (a sweet-smelling rose)

Buy beautiful something. (Buy something beautiful.)

"Will you me a cookie sell?" ("Will you sell me a cookie?")

A fish was catching man. (A man was catching fish.)

"Welcome you're," said Benny McBride. ("You're welcome," said Benny McBride.)

strolled home in sun the morning (strolled home in the morning sun)

"Yes, oh yes," Michael said Bess. ("Yes, oh yes," said Michael Bess.)

Phonological Awareness Activities at the Syllable Level

1. Syllable counting.

What to say to the student: "We're going to count syllables (or parts) of words."

> EXAMPLE "How many syllables do you hear in '_____'?" (stimulus word)
> (e.g., "How many syllables do you hear in 'hat'?") (1)

> **NOTE:** *Use pictured items and/or manipulatives if necessary. Use any of the following stimulus words and/or others you select from the story. Use any group of 10 stimulus items you select per teaching set.*

Stimulus items:

One-syllable words: boy, had, new, buy, what, should, mom, good, eat, nice, wear, woof, dog, cat, so, five, out, sun, he, stroll, Hill, sell, rose, yes, soft, four, sweet, May, girl, Bess, name, three, two, warm, hat, fine, bone, meat, one, big, man, Beal, fish, wet, bought

Two-syllable words: Benny, McBride, penny, something, brother, meow, morning, sister, woman, butcher, cutting, baking, roses, Lucy, cookie, making, Michael, paper, shopper, meaty, catching, Hopper, floppy, welcome

Three-syllable words: beautiful, together

2. Initial syllable deleting.

What to say to the student: "We're going to leave out syllables (or parts of words)."

> EXAMPLE "Say '_____.'" (stimulus word) "Say it again without '_____.'"
> (stimulus syllable) (e.g., "Say 'catching.' Say it again without 'catch.'") (ing)

> **NOTE:** *Use pictured items and/or manipulatives if necessary. Use any of the following stimulus words and/or others you select from the story. The correct answers are in parentheses.*

Stimulus items:

"Say 'something' without 'some.'" (thing)

"Say 'sister' without 'sis.'" (ter)

"Say 'cutting' without 'cut.'" (ing)

"Say 'shopper' without 'shop.'" (er)

"Say 'baking' without 'bake.'" (ing)

"Say 'Hopper' without 'hop.'" (er)

"Say 'morning' without 'morn.'" (ing)

"Say 'roses' without 'rose.'" (ez)

"Say 'paper' without 'pay.'" (per)

"Say 'meow' without 'me.'" (ow)

3. Final syllable deleting.

What to say to the student: "We're going to leave out syllables (or parts of words)."

> **EXAMPLE** "Say '_____.'" (stimulus word) "Say it again without '_____.'" (stimulus syllable) (e.g., "Say 'baking' without 'ing.'") (bake)

> **NOTE:** *Use pictured items and/or manipulatives if necessary. Use any of the following stimulus words and/or others you select from the story. The correct answers are in parentheses.*

Stimulus items:

"Say 'beautiful' without 'full.'" (beauty)

"Say 'something' without 'thing.'" (some)

"Say 'cutting' without 'ing.'" (cut)

"Say 'Benny' without 'ee.'" (Ben)

"Say 'Lucy' without 'see.'" (lew)

"Say 'welcome' without 'come.'" (well)

"Say 'meow' without 'ow.'" (me)

"Say 'brother' without 'er.'" (bruth)

"Say 'sister' without 'ter.'" (sis)

"Say 'catching' without 'ing.'" (catch)

4. Initial syllable adding.

What to say to the student: "Now let's add syllables (or parts) to words."

> **EXAMPLE** "Add '_____'" (stimulus syllable) "to the beginning of '_____.'" (stimulus syllable) (e.g., "Add 'bake' to the beginning of 'ing.'") (baking)

> **NOTE:** *Use pictured items and/or manipulatives if necessary. Use any of the following stimulus words and/or others you select from the story. The correct answers are in parentheses.*

Stimulus items:

"Add 'some' to the beginning of 'thing.'" (something)

"Add 'catch' to the beginning of 'ing.'" (catching)

"Add 'shop' to the beginning of 'er.'" (shopper)

"Add 'cut' to the beginning of 'ing.'" (cutting)

"Add 'hop' to the beginning of 'er.'" (Hopper)

"Add 'Ben' to the beginning of 'ee.'" (Benny)

"Add 'lew' to the beginning of 'see.'" (Lucy)

"Add 'meat' to the beginning of 'ee.'" (meaty)

"Add 'be' to the beginning of 'gan.'" (began)

"Add 'row' to the beginning of 'zez.'" (roses)

5. Final syllable adding.

What to say to the student: "Now let's add syllables (or parts) to words."

> **EXAMPLE** "Add '_____'" (stimulus syllable) "to the end of '_____.'" (stimulus syllable) (e.g., "Add 'ing' to the end of 'cut.'") (cutting)

> **NOTE:** *Use pictured items and/or manipulatives if necessary. Use any of the following stimulus words and/or others you select from the story. The correct answers are in parentheses.*

Stimulus items:

"Add 'thing' to the end of 'some.'" (something)

"Add 'ing' to the end of 'catch.'" (catching)

"Add '-er' to the end of 'hop.'" (Hopper)

"Add '-ee' to the end of 'Ben.'" (Benny)

"Add '-er' to the end of 'bruth.'" (brother)

"Add '-ee' to the end of 'flop.'" (floppy)

"Add '-er to the end of 'shop.'" (shopper)

"Add 'ease' to the end of 'cook.'" (cookies)

"Add '-ul' to the end of 'Mike.'" (Michael)

"Add '-er' to the end of 'butch.'" (butcher)

6. Syllable substituting.

What to say to the student: "Let's make up some new words."

> **EXAMPLE** "Say '_____.'" (stimulus word) "Instead of '_____'" (stimulus syllable), "say '_____.'" (stimulus syllable) (e.g., "Say 'cutting.' Instead of 'cut,' say 'bake.' The new word is 'baking.'")

> **NOTE:** *Use pictured items and/or manipulatives if necessary. Use of the following stimulus words and/or others you select from the story. The correct answers are in parentheses.*

Stimulus items:

"Say 'Benny.' Instead of 'Ben,' say 'pen.'" (penny)

"Say 'shopper.' Instead of 'shop,' say 'hop.'" (Hopper)

"Say 'catching.' Instead of 'ing,' say 'er.'" (catcher)

"Say 'making.' Instead of 'make,' say 'bake.'" (baking)

"Say 'something.' Instead of 'thing,' say 'where.'" (somewhere)

"Say 'McBride.' Instead of 'Bride,' say 'Beal.'" (McBeal)

"Say 'welcome.' Instead of 'wel,' say 'be.'" (become)

"Say 'Hopper.' Instead of 'er,' say 'ing.'" (hopping)

"Say 'morning.' Instead of 'morn,' say 'make.'" (making)

"Say 'cutting.' Instead of 'ing,' say 'er.'" (cutter)

Phonological Awareness Activities at the Phoneme Level

1. Counting sounds.

What to say to the student: "We're going to count sounds in words."

> **EXAMPLE** "How many sounds do you hear in this word? 'dog.'" (3)

> **NOTE:** *Use pictured items and/or manipulatives if necessary. Use any of the following stimulus words and/or others you select from the story. Be sure to give the letter sound and not the letter name. Use any group of 10 stimulus items you select per teaching set.*

Stimulus items:

Stimulus words with two sounds: boy, new, eat, so, out, he, May, two

Stimulus words with three sounds: had, should, mom, good, nice, woof, dog, cat, five, sun, Hill, sell, rose, yes, Bess, name, three, hat, fine, bone, meat, big, man, Beal, fish, wet, bought

Stimulus words with four sounds: soft, sweet, Benny, penny, Lucy, paper, shopper, Hopper, meaty

Stimulus words with five sounds: stroll, sister, roses, floppy

2. Sound categorization or identifying a rhyme oddity.

What to say to the student: "Guess which word I say doesn't rhyme with the other three words."

> **EXAMPLE** "Tell me which word doesn't rhyme with the other three words: '_____,' '_____,' '_____,' '_____.'" (stimulus words) (e.g., "'Bess,' 'dress,' 'less,' 'meow.' Which word doesn't rhyme?") (meow)

> **NOTE:** *Use pictured items if necessary. Use any of the following stimulus words and/or others you select from the story. The correct answers are in parentheses.*

Stimulus items:

Hopper, shopper, Lucy, bopper (Lucy)

floppy, paper, taper, caper (floppy)

baking, cookie, making, taking (cookie)

bone, cone, Beal, zone (Beal)

sister, blister, twister, McBride (McBride)

meat, bone, feet, tweet (bone)

Benny, penny, brother, Lenny (brother)

bought, warm, caught, jot (warm)

Bess, mess, Michael, guess (Michael)

Lucy, bone, tone, cone (Lucy)

3. Matching rhyme.

What to say to the student: "We're going to think of rhyming words."

> **EXAMPLE** "Which word rhymes with '_____'?" (stimulus word) (e.g., "Which word rhymes with 'dog': 'cookie,' 'fog,' 'cat,' 'Lucy'?") (fog)

NOTE: *Use pictured items if necessary. Use any of the following stimulus words and/or others you select from the story. The correct answers are in parentheses.*

Stimulus items:

Bess: guess, feet, Beal, paper (guess)

brother: sell, Lucy, sister, mother (mother)

rose: morning, toes, three, meow (toes)

stroll: troll, should, Hill, wet (troll)

fish: meat, McBride, morning, dish (dish)

Benny: warm, Kay, penny, caught (penny)

buy: cookie, guy, rose, girl (guy)

floppy: Michael, something, hat, choppy (choppy)

meat: tweet, baking, Bess, morning (tweet)

sun: welcome, Hopper, bought, fun (fun)

4. Producing rhyme.

What to say to the student: "Now we'll say rhyming words."

> **EXAMPLE** "Tell me a word that rhymes with '_____.'" (stimulus word) (e.g., "Tell me a word that rhymes with 'penny.' You can make up a word if you want.") (Jenny or Benny)

NOTE: *Use pictured items if necessary. Use any of the following stimulus words and/or others you select from the story (i.e., you say a word from the list below and the student should think of a rhyming word). Use any group of 10 stimulus items you select per teaching set.*

Stimulus items:

/p/: pennies, penny, paper

/b/: Benny, buy, beautiful, brother, baking, boy, Bess, butcher, bone, big, Beal, back, bought

/t/: two, together

/d/: dog, deal

/k/: cat, cutting, cookie, quite, catching, called

/g/: good, girl

/m/: McBride, mom, meow, morning, me, May, making, Michael, meat, meaty, man, Mister

/n/: new, nice, name

/s/: something, sister, strolled, sun, sell, sweet, smelling, soft, said

/f/: five, four, fine, fish, floppy

/h/: Hill, hats, hat, Hopper, his, home

/r/: rose, roses

/l/: Lucy, like

/w/, /wh/: wear, woof, will, woman, with, was, warm, one, wet, welcome

/sh/: should, shopper

/voiceless th/: three, thank

/voiced th/: then, they

/y/ (as in yellow): you, yes, you're

vowels: asked, and, eat, I'm, I, all

5. Sound matching (initial).

What to say to the student: "Now we'll listen for the first sound in words."

EXAMPLE "Listen to this sound: / /." (stimulus sound). "Guess which word I say begins with that sound: '_____,' '_____,' '_____,' '_____.'" (stimulus words) (e.g., "Listen to this sound: /d/. Guess which word I say begins with that sound: 'woman,' 'dog,' 'Benny,' 'Lucy.'") (dog)

NOTE: *Give the letter sound, not the letter name. Use pictured items if necessary. Use any of the following stimulus words and/or others you select from the story. The correct answers are in parentheses.*

Stimulus items:

/m/: name, strolled, McBride, Benny (McBride)

/s/: fish, Hopper, Mister, soft (soft)

/f/: fine, good, paper, brother (fine)

/h/: cutting, Hill, together, butcher (Hill)

/sh/: thank, cookie, war, shopper (shopper)

/l/: Lucy, three, rose, beautiful (Lucy)

/k/: good, cookies, meow, floppy (cookies)

/b/: Benny, Michael, paper, pennies (Benny)

/r/: Beal, catching, meaty, rose (rose)

/t/: something, together, fish, penny (together)

6. Sound matching (final).

What to say to the student: "Now we'll listen for the last sound in words."

EXAMPLE "Listen to this sound: / /." (stimulus sound) "Guess which word I say ends with that sound: '_____,' '_____,' '_____,' '_____.'" (stimulus words) (e.g., "Listen to this sound: /g/. Guess which word I say ends with that sound: 'fish,' 'beautiful,' 'dog,' 'Beal.'") (dog)

NOTE: *Give the letter sound, not the letter name. Use pictured items and/or manipulatives if necessary. Use any of the following stimulus words and/or others you select from the story. The correct answers are in parentheses.*

Stimulus items:

/t/: baking, mom, Benny, sweet (sweet)

/sh/: Bess, butcher, fish, wonderful (fish)

/z/: pennies, cookie, home, Beal (pennies)

/ng/: beautiful, smelling, strolled, cat (smelling)

/v/: cutting, sun, juice, five (five)

/long E/: deal, hats, floppy, meat (floppy)

/s/: something, paper, juice, cookies (juice)

/d/: fine, McBride, butcher, cutting (McBride)

/n/: Benny, fine, name, Hopper (fine)

/l/: morning, strolled, pennies, Michael (Michael)

7. Identifying the initial sound in words.

What to say to the student: "I'll say a word two times. Tell me what sound is missing the second time: '_____,' '_____.'" (stimulus words)

> **EXAMPLE** "What sound do you hear in '_____'" (stimulus word) "that is missing in '_____'?" (stimulus word) (e.g., "What sound do you hear in 'his' that is missing in 'is'?") (/h/)

> **NOTE:** *Give the letter sound, not the letter name. Use pictured items and/or manipulatives if necessary. Use any of the following stimulus words and/or others you select from the story. The correct answers are in parentheses.*

Stimulus items:

"quite, white. What sound do you hear in 'quite' that is missing in 'white'?" (/k/)

"deal, eel. What sound do you hear in 'deal' that is missing in 'eel'?" (/d/)

"cat, at. What sound do you hear in 'cat' that is missing in 'at'?" (/k/)

"nice, ice. What sound do you hear in 'nice' that is missing in 'ice'?" (/n/)

"meat, eat. What sound do you hear in 'meat' that is missing in 'eat'?" (/m/)

"stroll, troll. What sound do you hear in 'stroll' that is missing in 'troll'?" (/s/)

"sweet, wheat. What sound do you hear in 'sweet' that is missing in 'wheat'?" (/s/)

"bone, own. What sound do you hear in 'bone' that is missing in 'own'?" (/b/)

"call, all. What sound do you hear in 'call' that is missing in 'all'?" (/k/)

"man, an. What sound do you hear in 'man' that is missing in 'an'?" (/m/)

8. Identifying the final sound in words.

What to say to the student: "I'll say a word two times. Tell me what sound is missing the second time. '_____,' '_____.'" (stimulus words)

> **EXAMPLE** "What sound do you hear in '_____'" (stimulus word) " that is missing in '_____'?" (stimulus word) (e.g., "What sound do you hear in 'meat' that is missing in 'me'?") (/t/)

NOTE: *Give the letter sound, not the letter name. Use pictured items and/or manipulatives if necessary. Use any of the following stimulus words and/or others you select from the story. The correct answers are in parentheses.*

Stimulus items:

"strolled, stroll. What sound do you hear in 'strolled' that is missing in 'stroll'?" (/d/)

"meaty, meat. What sound do you hear in 'meaty' that is missing in 'meat'?" (/long E/)

"hats, hat. What sound do you hear in 'hats' that is missing in 'hat'?" (/s/)

"home, hoe. What sound do you hear in 'home' that is missing in 'hoe'?" (/m/)

"Benny's, Benny. What sound do you hear in 'Benny's' that is missing in 'Benny'?" (/z/)

"Hopper, hop. What sound do you hear in 'Hopper' that is missing in 'hop'?" (/r/)

"penny, pen. What sound do you hear in 'penny' that is missing in 'pen'?" (/long E/)

"bone, bow. What sound do you hear in 'bone' that is missing in 'bow'?" (/n/)

"cookies, cookie. What sound do you hear in 'cookies' that is missing in 'cookie'?" (/z/)

"Lucy, loose. What sound do you hear in 'Lucy' that is missing in 'loose'?" (/long E/)

9. Segmenting the initial sound in words.

What to say to the student: "Listen to the word I say and tell me the first sound you hear."

> **EXAMPLE** "What's the first sound in '_____'?" (stimulus word) (e.g., "What's the first sound in 'dog'?") (/d/)

NOTE: *Give the letter sound, not the letter name. Use pictured items and/or manipulatives if necessary. Use any of the following stimulus words and/or others you select from the story. Use any group of 10 stimulus items you select per teaching set.*

Stimulus items:

/p/: pennies, penny, paper

/b/: Benny, buy, beautiful, brother, baking, boy, Bess, butcher, bone, big, Beal, back, bought

/t/: two, together

/d/: dog, deal

/k/: cat, cutting, cookie, quite, catching, called

/g/: good, girl

/m/: McBride, mom, meow, morning, me, May, making, Michael, meat, meaty, man, Mister

/n/: new, nice, name

/s/: something, sister, strolled, sun, sell, sweet, smelling, soft, said

/f/: five, four, fine, fish, floppy

/h/: Hill, hats, hat, Hopper, his, home

/r/: rose, roses

/l/: Lucy, like

/w/, /wh/: wear, woof, will, woman, with, was, warm, one, wet, welcome

/sh/: should, shopper

/voiceless th/: three, thank

/voiced th/: then, they

/y/ (as in yellow): you, yes, you're

/short A/: asked, and

/long E/: eat

/long I/: I'm, I

/ah/: all

10. Segmenting the final sound in words.

What to say to the student: "Listen to the word I say and tell me the last sound you hear."

> **EXAMPLE** "What's the last sound in the word '_____'?" (stimulus word)
> (e.g., "What's the last sound in the word 'cat'?") (/t/)

NOTE: *Give the letter sound, not the letter name. Use pictured items and/or manipulatives if necessary. Use any of the following stimulus words and/or others you select from the story. Use any group of 10 stimulus items you select per teaching set.*

Stimulus items:

/t/: bought, cat, quite, meat, sweet, soft, hat

/d/: good, McBride, strolled, said

/k/: back

/g/: dog

/m/: mom, name, home

/n/: bone, fine, man, sun

/ng/: baking, cutting, morning, making, something, smelling

/s/: Bess, juice, hats

/z/: his, pennies, Benny's, cookies

/v/: five

/r/: paper, brother, butcher, together, Mister, sister, four, Hopper

/l/: beautiful, Beal, deal, girl, Michael, sell, Hill

/sh/: fish

/long A/: May

/long E/: penny, Benny, cookie, me, meaty, floppy

/oo/: two

11. Generating words from the story beginning with a particular sound.

What to say to the student: "Let's think of words from the story that start with certain sounds."

> **EXAMPLE** "Tell me a word from the story that starts with / /." (stimulus sound)
> (e.g., the sound /b/) (Benny)

NOTE: *Give the letter sound, not the letter name. Use pictured items if necessary. Use any of the following stimulus words and/or others you select from the story. You say the sound (e.g., a voiceless /p/ sound) and the student is to say a word from the story that begins with that sound. Use any group of 10 stimulus items you select per teaching set.*

Stimulus items:

/p/: pennies, penny, paper

/b/: Benny, buy, beautiful, brother, baking, boy, Bess, butcher, bone, big, Beal, back, bought

/t/: two, together

/d/: dog, deal

/k/: cat, cutting, cookie, quite, catching, called

/g/: good, girl

/m/: McBride, mom, meow, morning, me, May, making, Michael, meat, meaty, man, Mister

/n/: new, nice, name

/s/: something, sister, strolled, sun, sell, sweet, smelling, soft, said

/f/: five, four, fine, fish, floppy

/h/: Hill, hats, hat, Hopper, his, home

/r/: rose, roses

/l/: Lucy, like

/w/, /wh/: wear, woof, will, woman, with, was, warm, one, wet, welcome

/sh/: should, shopper

/voiceless th/: three, thank

/voiced th/: then, they

/y/ (as in yellow): you, yes, you're

/short A/: asked, and

/long E/: eat

/long I/: I'm, I

/ah/: all

12. Blending sounds in monosyllabic words divided into onset/rime beginning with a two-consonant cluster + rime.

What to say to the student: "Now we'll put sounds together to make words."

> **EXAMPLE** "Put these sounds together to make a word: / / + / /." (stimulus sounds)
> "What's the word?" (e.g., "fl + ip: What's the word?") (flip)

NOTE: *Give the letter sound, not the letter name. Use pictured items and/or manipulatives if necessary. Use any of the following stimulus words and/or others you select from the story. The correct answers are in parentheses.*

Stimulus items:

br+ ide (bride)

sm + ell (smell)

fl + op (flop)

st + roll (stroll)

voiceless /th/ + ree (three)

sp + ots (spots)

kw+ ite (quite)

sw + eat (sweet)

Sourcebook users are encouraged to add stimulus items into this activity from curriculum materials they may be using with *Benny's Pennies.*

13. Blending sounds in monosyllabic words divided into onset/rime beginning with a single consonant + rime.

What to say to the student: "Let's put sounds together to make words."

> **EXAMPLE** "Put these sounds together to make a word: / / + / /." (stimulus sounds) "What's the word?" (e.g., "/g/ + ood: What's the word?") (good)

NOTE: *Give the letter sound, not the letter name. Use pictured items and/or manipulatives if necessary. Use any of the following stimulus words and/or others you select from the story. The correct answers are in parentheses.*

Stimulus items:

/d/ + og (dog)

/b/ + own (bone)

/n/ + ice (nice)

/h/ + ill (Hill)

/k/ + at (cat)

/b/ + ess (Bess)

/d/ + eel (deal)

/g/ + earl (girl)

/n/ + aim (name)

/s/ + oft (soft)

14. Blending sounds to form a monosyllabic word beginning with a continuant sound.

What to say to the student: "We'll put sounds together to make words."

> **EXAMPLE** "Put these sounds together to make a word: / / + / / + / /." (stimulus sounds) (e.g., "/m/ /ah/ /m/") (mom)

NOTE: *Give the letter sound, not the letter name. Use pictured items and/or manipulatives if necessary. Use any of the following stimulus words and/or others you select from the story. The correct answers are in parentheses.*

Stimulus items:

/n/ /long I/ /s/ (nice)

/s/ /ah/ /f/ /t/ (soft)

/f/ /long I/ /v/ (five)

/h/ /long O/ /m/ (home)

/f/ /short I/ /sh/ (fish)

/m/ /long E/ /t/ (meat)

/w/ /short I/ /th/ (with)

/r/ /long O/ /z/ (rose)

/n/ /long A/ /m/ (name)

/s/ /w/ /long E/ /t/ (sweet)

15. Blending sounds to form a monosyllabic word beginning with a noncontinuant sound.

What to say to the student: "We'll put sounds together to make words."

> **EXAMPLE** "Put these sounds together to make a word: / / + / / + / /." (stimulus sounds) (e.g., /d/ /ah/ /g/) (dog)

NOTE: *Give the letter sound, not the letter name. Use pictured items and/or manipulatives if necessary. Use any of the following stimulus words and/or others you select from the story. The correct answers are in parentheses.*

Stimulus items:

/b/ /long E/ /l/ (Beal)

/t/ /oo/ (two)

/n/ /long I/ /s/ (nice)

/b/ /long O/ /n/ (bone)

/k/ /ah/ /l/ /d (called)

/b/ /short E/ /s/ (Bess)

/k/ /w/ /long I/ /t/ (quite)

/b/ /short A/ /k/ (back)

/b/ /long I/ (buy)

/b/ /long A/ /k/ (bake)

16. Substituting the initial sound in words.

What to say to the student: "We're going to change beginning/first sounds in words."

> **EXAMPLE** "Say '_____.'" (stimulus word) "Instead of / /" (stimulus sound), "say / /." (stimulus sound) (e.g., "Say 'fine.' Instead of /f/, say /p/. What's your new word?") (pine)

NOTE: *Give the letter sound, not the letter name. Use pictured items and/or manipulatives if necessary. Use any of the following stimulus words and/or others you select from the story. The correct answers are in parentheses.*

Stimulus items:

"Say 'penny.' Instead of /p/, say /b/." (Benny)

"Say 'fish.' Instead of /f/, say /d/." (dish)

"Say 'Hopper.' Instead of /h/, say /p/." (popper)

"Say 'wet.' Instead of /w/, say /p/." (pet)

"Say 'should.' Instead of /sh/, say /k/." (could)

"Say 'deal.' Instead of /d/, say /b/." (Beal)

"Say 'boy.' Instead of /b/, say /t/." (toy)

"Say 'meat.' Instead of /m/, say /b/." (beat)

"Say 'nice.' Instead of /n/, say /r/." (rice)

"Say 'Bess.' Instead of /b/, say /m/." (mess)

17. Substituting the final sound in words.

What to say to the student: "We're going to change ending/last sounds in words."

> **EXAMPLE** "Say '_____.'" (stimulus word) "Instead of / /" (stimulus sound), "say / /." (stimulus sound) (e.g., "Say 'back.' Instead of /k/, say /t/. What's your new word?") (bat)

NOTE: *Give the letter sound, not the letter name. Use pictured items and/or manipulatives if necessary. Use any of the following stimulus words and/or others you select from the story. The correct answers are in parentheses.*

Stimulus items:

"Say 'dog.' Instead of /g/, say /t/." (dot)

"Say 'fine.' Instead of /n/, say /v/." (five)

"Say 'Bess.' Instead of /s/, say /t/." (bet)

"Say 'said.' Instead of /d/, say /z/." (says)

"Say 'fish.' Instead of /sh/, say /t/." (fit)

"Say 'his.' Instead of /z/, say /m/." (him)

"Say 'strolled.' Instead of /d/, say /z/." (strolls)

"Say 'sweet.' Instead of /t/, say /p/." (sweep)

"Say 'floppy.' Instead of /long E/, say /t/." (flopped)

"Say 'home.' Instead of /m/, say /p/." (hope)

18. Segmenting the middle sound in monosyllabic words.

What to say to the student: "Tell me the middle sound in the word I say."

> **EXAMPLE** "What's the middle sound in the word '_____'?" (stimulus word) (e.g., "What's the middle sound in the word 'back'?") (/short A/)

NOTE: *Give the letter sound, not the letter name. Use pictured items and/or manipulatives if necessary. Use any of the following stimulus words and/or others you select from the story. The correct answers are in parentheses.*

Stimulus items:

name (/long A/)

fish (/short I/)

dog (/ah/)

said (/short E/)

juice (/oo/)

Bess (/short E/)

bought (/ah/)

home (/long O/)

meat (/long E/)

sun (/short U/)

19. Substituting the middle sound in words.

What to say to the student: "We're going to change the middle sound in words."

EXAMPLE "Say '_____.'" (stimulus word) "Instead of / /" (stimulus sound), "say / /." (stimulus sound) (e.g., "Say 'flop.' Instead of /ah/, say /short I/. What's your new word?") (flip)

NOTE: *Give the letter sound, not the letter name. Use pictured items and/or manipulatives if necessary. Use any of the following stimulus words and/or others you select from the story. The correct answers are in parentheses.*

Stimulus items:

"Say 'cat.' Instead of /short A/, say /ah/." (cot)

"Say 'deal.' Instead of /long E/, say /short I/." (dill)

"Say 'mom.' Instead of /ah/, say /long I/." (mime)

"Say 'soft.' Instead of /ah/, say /short I/." (sift)

"Say 'bought.' Instead of /ah/, say /long I/." (bite)

"Say 'back.' Instead of /short A/, say /long I/." (bike)

"Say 'Bess.' Instead of /short E/, say /ah/." (boss)

"Say 'fine.' Instead of /long I/, say /short U/." (fun)

"Say 'said.' Instead of /short E/, say /short A/." (sad)

"Say 'dog.' Instead of /ah/, say /short U/." (dug)

20. Identifying all sounds in monosyllabic words.

What to say to the student: "Now tell me all the sounds you hear in the word I say."

EXAMPLE "What sounds do you hear in the word '_____'?" (stimulus word) (e.g., "What sounds do you hear in the word 'dog'?") (/d/ /ah/ /g/)

NOTE: *Give the letter sound, not the letter name. Use pictured items and/or manipulatives if necessary. Use any of the following stimulus words and/or others you select from the story. The correct answers are in parentheses.*

Stimulus items:

deal (/d/ /long E/ /l/)

said (/s/ /short E/ /d/)

mom (/m/ /ah/ /m/)

back (/b/ /short A/ /k/)

fine (/f/ /long I/ /n/)

soft (/s/ /ah/ /f/ /t/)

five (/f/ /long I/ /v/)

cat (/k/ /short A/ /t/)

meat (/m/ /long E/ /t/)

home (/h/ /long O/ /m/)

21. Deleting sounds within words.

What to say to the student: "We're going to leave out sounds in words."

> EXAMPLE "Say '_____' " (stimulus word) "without / /." (stimulus sound) (e.g., "Say 'slid' without /l/.") (sid) Say: "The word that is left—'sid'—is a real word. Sometimes, the word won't be a real word."

NOTE: *Give the letter sound, not the letter name. Use pictured items and/or manipulatives if necessary. Use any of the following stimulus words and/or others you select from the story. The correct answers are in parentheses.*

Stimulus items:

"Say 'bride' without /r/." (bide)

"Say 'smell' without /m/." (sell)

"Say 'sweet' without /w/." (seat)

"Say 'floppy' without /l/." (foppy)

"Say 'stroll' without /r/." (stole)

"Say 'rose' without /z/." (row)

"Say 'and' without /d/." (an)

"Say 'quite' without /w/." (kite)

"Say 'and' without /n/." (ad)

"Say 'ask' without /s/." (aak)

22. Substituting consonants in words that have a two-sound cluster.

What to say to the student: "We're going to substitute sounds in words."

EXAMPLE "Say '_____.'" (stimulus word) "Instead of / /" (stimulus sound), "say / /." (stimulus sound) (e.g., "Say 'stop.' Instead of /t/, say /l/.") (slop) Say: "Sometimes, the new word won't be a real word."

NOTE: *Give the letter sound, not the letter name. Use pictured items and/or manipulatives if necessary. Use any of the following stimulus words and/or others you select from the story. The correct answers are in parentheses.*

Stimulus items:

"Say 'ask.' Instead of /k/, say /p/." (asp)

"Say 'sweet.' Instead of /w/, say /l/." (sleet)

"Say 'bride.' Instead of /b/, say /p/." (pride)

"Say 'smell.' Instead of /m/, say /p/." (spell)

"Say 'and.' Instead of /d/, say /t/." (ant)

"Say 'three.' Instead of /voiceless th/, say /f/." (free)

"Say 'stroll.' Instead of /t/, say /k/." (scroll)

"Say 'floppy.' Instead of /l/, say /r/." (froppy)

"Say 'soft.' Instead of /f/, say /p/." (sopped)

"Say 'bride.' Instead of /b/, say /k/." (cried)

23. Phoneme reversing.

What to say to the student: "We're going to say words backward."

EXAMPLE "Say the word '_____'" (stimulus word) "backward." (e.g., "Say 'bone' backward.") (nobe)

NOTE: *This is a difficult phoneme-level task and should only be done with older students. Give the letter sound, not the letter name. Use pictured items and/or manipulatives if necessary. Use any of the following stimulus words and/or others you select from the story. The correct answers are in parentheses.*

Stimulus items:

back (cab)

Bess (seb)

cat (tack)

Beal (leeb)

nice (sign)

deal (lead)

fine (knife)

name (mane)

eat (tea)

shop (posh)

24. Phoneme switching.

What to say to the student: "We're going to switch the first sounds in two words."

> EXAMPLE "Switch the first sounds in '_____' and '_____.'" (stimulus words)
> (e.g., "Switch the first sounds in 'sell' and 'me.'") (mell see)

NOTE: *This is a difficult phoneme-level task and should only be done with older students. Give the letter sound, not the letter name. Use pictured items and/or manipulatives if necessary. Use any of the following stimulus words and/or others you select from the story. The correct answers are in parentheses.*

Stimulus items:

Benny penny (penny Benny)

Mr. Hopper (hister mopper)

paper hat (haper pat)

meaty bone (beaty moan)

making hats (haking mats)

Michael Bess (Bichael Mess)

cutting roses (rutting koses)

morning sun (sorning mun)

thank you (yank thoo)

Mrs. Hill (hissus mill)

25. Pig Latin.

What to say to the student: "We're going to speak a secret language by using words from the story. In pig Latin, you take off the first sound of a word, put it at the end of the word, and add an 'ay' sound."

> EXAMPLE "Say 'dog' in pig Latin." (ogday)

NOTE: *This is a difficult phoneme-level task and should only be done with older students. Use pictured items and/or manipulatives if necessary. Use any of the following stimulus words and/or others you select from the story. The correct answers are in parentheses.*

Stimulus items:

fish (ishfay)

rose (oseray)

Benny (ennybay)

Hill (illhay)

sister (istersay)

penny (ennypay)

fine (inefay)

cookie (ookiekay)

beautiful (eautifulbay)

butcher (ootcherbay)

From Phonological Awareness into Print

NOTE: *Only five examples per activity are included in this resource due to space. You are encouraged to add many more words into this section that you feel your student(s) is (are) ready to write.*

1. Substituting the initial sound or letter in words.

NOTE: *Use lined paper or copy the sheet of lined paper included in the back of this book.*

Stimulus items:

1.1 hat/cat

Task a. "Say 'hat.' Instead of /h/, say /k/. What's your new word?" (cat) "Write/copy 'hat' and 'cat.'"

Task b. "Circle the **letters** that make the words different." ([h], [c])

Task c. "What **sounds** do these letters make?" (/h/, /k/)

1.2 rose/pose

Task a. "Say 'rose.' Instead of /r/, say /p/. What's your new word?" (pose) "Write/copy 'rose' and 'pose.'"

Task b. "Circle the **letters** that make the words different." ([r], [p])

Task c. "What **sounds** do these letters make?" (/r/, /p/)

1.3 Benny/penny

Task a. "Say 'Benny.' Instead of /b/, say /p/. What's your new word?" (penny) "Write/copy 'Benny' and 'penny.'"

Task b. "Circle the **letters** that make the words different." ([B], [p])

Task c. "What **sounds** do these letters make?" (/b/, /p/)

1.4 cookie/lookie

Task a. "Say 'cookie.' Instead of the first /k/, say /l/. What's your new word?" (lookie) "Write/copy 'cookie' and 'lookie.'"

Task b. "Circle the **letters** that make the words different." ([c], [l])

Task c. "What **sounds** do these letters make?" (/k/, /l/)

1.5 Hopper/shopper

Task a. "Say 'Hopper.' Instead of /h/, say /sh/. What's your new word?" (shopper) "Write/copy 'Hopper' and 'shopper.'"

Task b. "Circle the **letters** that make the words different." ([H], [s], [h])

Task c. "What **sounds** do these letters make?" (/h/, /sh/)

2. Substituting the final sound or letter in words.

NOTE: *Use lined paper or copy the sheet of lined paper included in the back of this book.*

Stimulus items:

2.1 dog/dot

Task a. "Say 'dog.' Instead of /g/, say /t/. What's your new word?" (dot) "Write/copy 'dog' and 'dot.'"

Task b. Say "Circle the **letters** that make the words different." ([g], [t])

Task c. Say "What **sounds** do these letters make?" (/g/, /t/)

2.2 cat/cap

Task a. "Say 'cat.' Instead of /t/, say /p/. What's your new word?" (cap) "Write/copy 'cat' and 'cap.'"

Task b. "Circle the **letters** that make the words different." ([t], [p])

Task c. "What **sounds** do these letters make?" (/t/, /p/)

2.3 hat/has

Task a. "Say 'hat.' Instead of /t/, say /z/. What's your new word?" (has) "Write/copy 'hat' and 'has.'"

Task b. "Circle the **letters** that make the words different." ([t], [s])

Task c. "What **sounds** do these letters make?" (/t/, /z/)

2.4 me/my

Task a. "Say 'me.' Instead of /long E/, say /long I/. What's your new word?" (my) "Write/copy 'me' and 'my.'"

Task b. "Circle the **letters** that make the words different." ([e], [y])

Task c. "What **sounds** do these letters make?" (/long E/, /long I/)

2.5 meat/mean

Task a. "Say 'meat.' Instead of /t/, say /n/. What's your new word?" (mean) "Write/copy 'meat' and 'mean.'"

Task b. "Circle the **letters** that make the words different." ([t], [n])

Task c. "What **sounds** do these letters make?" (/t/, /n/)

3. Substituting the middle sound or letter in words.

NOTE: *Use lined paper or copy the sheet of lined paper included in the back of this book.*

Stimulus items:

3.1 cat/cut

Task a. "Say 'cat.' Instead of /short A/, say /short U/. What's your new word?" (cut) "Write/copy 'cat' and 'cut.'"

Task b. "Circle the **letters** that make the words different." ([a], [u])

Task c. "What **sounds** do these letters make?" (/short A/, /uh/)

3.2 hat/hit

Task a. "Say 'hat.' Instead of /short A/, say /short I/. What's your new word?" (hit) "Write/copy 'hat' and 'hit.'"

Task b. "Circle the **letters** that make the words different." ([a], [i])

Task c. "What **sounds** do these letters make?" (/short A/, /short I/)

3.3 rose/rise

Task a. "Say 'rose.' Instead of /long O/, say /long I/. What's your new word?" (rise) "Write/copy 'rose' and 'rise.'"

Task b. "Circle the **letters** that make the words different." ([o], [i])

Task c. "What **sounds** do these letters make?" (/long O/, /long I/)

3.4 will/well

Task a. "Say 'will.' Instead of /short I/, say /short E/. What's your new word?" (well) "Write/copy 'will' and 'well.'"

Task b. "Circle the **letters** that make the words different." ([i], [e])

Task c. "What **sounds** do these letters make?" (/short I/, /short E/)

3.5 Lucy/lacy

Task a. "Say 'Lucy.' Instead of /oo/, say /long A/. What's your new word?" (lacy) "Write/copy 'Lucy' and 'lacy.'"

Task b. "Circle the **letters** that make the words different." ([u], [a])

Task c. "What **sounds** do these letters make?" (/oo/, /long A/)

4. Supplying the initial sound or letter in words.

NOTE: *Use lined paper or copy the sheet of lined paper included in the back of this book.*

Stimulus items:

4.1 cat/at

Task a. "Say 'cat,' say 'at.' What sound did you hear in 'cat' that is missing in 'at'?" (/k/) "Now we'll change the **letter**. Write/copy 'cat' and 'at.'"

Task b. "Circle the beginning **letter** that makes the words different." ([c])

Task c. "What **sound** does this letter make?" (/k/)

4.2 man/an

Task a. "Say 'man,' say 'an.' What sound did you hear in 'man' that is missing in 'an'?" (/m/) "Now we'll change the **letter**. Write/copy 'man' and 'an.'"

Task b. "Circle the beginning **letter** that makes the words different." ([m])

Task c. "What **sound** does this letter make?" (/m/)

4.3 nice/ice

Task a. "Say 'nice,' say 'ice.' What sound did you hear in 'nice' that is missing in 'ice'?" (/n/) "Now we'll change the **letter**. Write/copy 'nice' and 'ice.'"

Task b. "Circle the beginning **letter** that makes the words different." ([n])

Task c. "What **sound** do these letters make?" (/n/)

4.4 meat/eat

Task a. "Say 'meat,' say 'eat.' What sound did you hear in 'meat' that is missing in 'eat'?" (/m/) "Now we'll change the **letter**. Write/copy 'meat' and 'eat.'"

Task b. "Circle the beginning **letter** that makes the words different." ([m])

Task c. "What **sound** does this letter make?" (/m/)

4.5 stroll/troll

Task a. "Say 'stroll,' say 'troll.' What sound did you hear in 'stroll' that is missing in 'troll'?" (/s/) "Now we'll change the **letter**. Write/copy 'stroll' and 'troll.'"

Task b. "Circle the beginning **letter** that makes the words different." ([s])

Task c. "What **sound** does this letter make?" (/s/)

5. Supplying the final sound or letter in words.

NOTE: *Use lined paper or copy the sheet of lined paper included in the back of this book.*

Stimulus items:

5.1 and/an

Task a. "Say 'and,' say 'an.' What sound did you hear in 'and' that is missing in 'an'?" (/d/) "Now we'll change the **letter.** Write/copy 'and' and 'an.'"

Task b. "Circle the ending/last **letter** that makes the words different." ([d])

Task c. "What **sound** does this letter make?" (/d/)

5.2 hats/hat

Task a. "Say 'hats,' say 'hat.' What sound did you hear in 'hats' that is missing in 'hat'?" (/s/) "Now we'll change the **letter.** Write/copy 'hats' and 'hat.'"

Task b. "Circle the ending/last **letter** that makes the words different." ([s])

Task c. "What **sound** does this letter make?" (/s/)

5.3 called/call

Task a. "Say 'called,' say 'call.' What sound did you hear in 'called' that is missing in 'call'?" (/d/) "Now we'll change the **letters.** Write/copy 'called' and 'call.'"

Task b. "Circle the ending/last **letters** that make the words different." ([e], [d])

Task c. "What **sound** do these letters make?" (/d/)

5.4 cookies/cookie

Task a. "Say 'cookies,' say 'cookie.' What sound did you hear in 'cookies' that is missing in 'cookie'?" (/z/) "Now we'll change the **letter.** Write/copy 'cookies' and 'cookie.'"

Task b. "Circle the ending/last **letter** that makes the word different." ([s])

Task c. "What **sound** does this letter make?" (/z/)

5.5 dirty/dirt

Task a. "Say 'dirty,' say 'dirt.' What sound did you hear in 'dirty' that is missing in 'dirt'?" (/long E/) "Now we'll change the **letter.** Write/copy 'dirty' and 'dirt.'"

Task b. "Circle the ending/last **letter** that makes the words different." ([y])

Task c. "What **sound** does this letter make?" (/long E/)

6. Switching the first sound and letter in words (ADVANCED).

NOTE: *Use lined paper or copy the sheet of lined paper included in the back of this book.*

Stimulus items:

6.1 Benny penny

Task a. "Say 'Benny,' say 'penny.' What sound do you hear in the beginning of 'Benny'?" (/b/) "What sound do you hear in the beginning of 'penny'?" (/p/) "Switch the first sounds in those words." (penny Benny) "Now we'll change the **letters.** Write/copy 'Benny penny' and 'penny Benny.'"

Task b. "Circle the beginning **letters** that change the words." ([B], [p])

Task c. "What **sounds** do those letters make?" (/b/, /p/)

6.2 big meaty

Task a. "Say 'big,' say 'meaty.' What sound do you hear in the beginning of 'big'?" (/b/) "What sound do you hear in the beginning of 'meaty'?" (/m/) "Switch the first sounds in those words." (mig beaty) "Now we'll change the **letters.** Write/copy 'big meaty' and 'mig beaty.'"

Task b. "Circle the beginning **letters** that change the words." ([b], [m])

Task c. "What **sounds** do those letters make?" (/b/, /m/)

6.3 making hats

Task a. "Say 'making,' say 'hats.' What sound do you hear in the beginning of 'making'?" (/m/) "What sound do you hear in the beginning of 'hats'?" (/h/) "Switch the first sounds in those words." (haking mats) "Now we'll change the **letters.** Write/copy 'making hats' and 'haking mats.'"

Task b. "Circle the beginning **letters** that change the words." ([m], [h])

Task c. "What **sounds** do those letters make?" (/m/, /h/)

6.4 Michael Bess

Task a. "Say 'Michael,' say 'Bess.' What sound do you hear in the beginning of 'Michael'?" (/m/) "What sound do you hear in the beginning of 'Bess'?" (/b/) "Switch the first sounds in those words." (Bichael Mess) "Now we'll change the **letters.** Write/copy 'Michael Bess' and 'Bichael Mess.'"

Task b. "Circle the beginning **letters** that change the words." ([M], [B])

Task c. "What **sounds** do those letters make?" (/m/, /b/)

6.5 morning sun

Task a. "Say 'morning,' say 'sun.' What sound do you hear in the beginning of 'morning'?" (/m/) "What sound do you hear in the beginning of 'sun'?" (/s/) "Switch the first sounds in those words." (sorning mun) "Now we'll change the **letters.** Write/copy 'morning sun' and 'sorning mun.'"

Task b. "Circle the beginning **letters** that change the words." ([m], [s])

Task c. "What **sounds** do those letters make?" (/m/, /s/)

CHAPTER 4

Phonological Awareness Activities to Use with *Bunny Cakes*

Text version used for selection of stimulus items:

Wells, R. (1997). *Bunny Cakes.* New York: Puffin Books.

Phonological Awareness Activities at the Word Level

1. Counting words.

What to say to the student: "We're going to count words."

EXAMPLE "How many words do you hear in this sentence (or phrase): 'But it was too late'?" (5)

NOTE: *Use pictured items and/or manipulatives if necessary. Use any of the following stimulus phrases or sentences and/or others you select from the story. The correct answers are in parentheses.*

Stimulus items:

no Max (2)

what's this? (2)

his earthworm cake (3)

don't touch anything (3)

over went the flour (4)

it was Grandma's birthday (4)

red hot marshmallow squirters (4)

Ruby got out her pencil (5)

a sign on the kitchen door (6)

but Max crossed the line anyway (6)

2. Identifying the missing word from a list.

What to say to the student: "Listen to the words I say. I'll say them again. You tell me which word I leave out."

> **EXAMPLE** "Listen to the words I say: 'late,' 'Max,' 'list.' I'll say them again. Tell me which one I leave out: 'late,' 'Max.'" (list)

> **NOTE:** *Use pictured items and/or manipulatives if necessary. Use any of the following stimulus words and/or others you select from the story. The correct answers are in parentheses.*

Stimulus set #1	Stimulus set #2
cake, eggs	cake (eggs)
bump, floor	floor (bump)
raspberry, silver, roses	raspberry, silver (roses)
sugar, marshmallow, fluff	marshmallow, fluff (sugar)
squirters, milk, stars	squirters, stars (milk)
hearts, candles, hot	hearts, hot (candles)
sister, cakes, taste, caterpillar	sister, cakes, taste (caterpillar)
Ruby, yellow, sister, door	yellow, sister, door (Ruby)
flour, Grandma's, pencil, gave	flour, Grandma's, gave (pencil)
anyway, frosting, angel, you	anyway, angel, you (frosting)

3. Identifying the missing word in a phrase or sentence.

What to say to the student: "Listen to the sentence I read. Tell me which word is missing the second time I read the sentence."

> **EXAMPLE** "'on the floor.' Listen again and tell me which word I leave out: 'the floor.'" (on)

> **NOTE:** *Use pictured items and/or manipulatives if necessary. Use any of the following stimulus sentences and/or others you select from the story. The correct answers are in parentheses.*

Stimulus items:

Silver stars. Silver_____. (stars)

Buttercream roses. _____ roses. (buttercream)

To the grocer. To _____ grocer. (the)

She didn't know. _____ didn't know. (She)

His earthworm cake. His _____ cake. (earthworm)

Max hoped and hoped. Max hoped and _____. (hoped)

He gave Max eggs. He _____ Max eggs. (gave)

He could not wait. He could _____ wait. (not)

It needs something else. It _____ something else. (needs)

Ruby's cake looked just beautiful. Ruby's cake _____ just beautiful. (looked)

4. Supplying the missing word as an adult reads.

What to say to the student: "I want you to help me read the story. You fill in the words I leave out."

> EXAMPLE   "Marshmallow _____." (squirters)

> **NOTE:** *Use pictured items and/or manipulatives if necessary. Use any of the following stimulus sentences and/or others you select from the story. The correct answers are in parentheses.*

Stimulus items:

Angel surprise _____. (cake)

But it was _____ late. (too)

Max wanted to _____. (help)

Ruby sent _____ to the store. (Max)

Don't touch _____, Max. (anything)

You can't _____ over that line. (step)

But Max crossed the line _____. (anyway)

Max hoped and hoped for his _____. (squirters)

Max could almost taste the _____ squirters. (marshmallow)

A sign on the _____ door. (kitchen)

5. Rearranging words.

What to say to the student: "I'll say some words out of order. You put them in the right order so they make sense."

> EXAMPLE   "'home Max got.' Put those words in the right order." (Max got home)

> **NOTE:** *Use pictured items and/or manipulatives if necessary. Use any of the following stimulus words and/or others you select from the story. The correct answers are in parentheses. This word-level activity can be more difficult than some of the syllable- or phoneme-level activities because of the memory load. If your students are only able to deal with two or three words to be rearranged, add more two- and three-word samples from the story and omit the four-word level items.*

Stimulus items:

stars silver (silver stars)

grocer the to (to the grocer)

needs something it else (it needs something else)

a idea new brand (a brand-new idea)

on earthworm cake his (on his earthworm cake)

he picture drew a (he drew a picture)

the writing beautiful most (the most beautiful writing)

Ruby Max store the to sent. (Ruby sent Max to the store.)

Grandma's birthday was it (it was Grandma's birthday)

sign a kitchen door the on (a sign on the kitchen door)

Phonological Awareness Activities at the Syllable Level

1. Syllable counting.

What to say to the student: "We're going to count syllables (or parts) of words."

> **EXAMPLE** "How many syllables do you hear in '_____'?" (stimulus word) (e.g., "How many syllables do you hear in 'hat'?") (1)

> **NOTE:** *Use pictured items and/or manipulatives if necessary. Use any of the following stimulus words and/or others you select from the story. Use any group of 10 stimulus items you select per teaching set.*

Stimulus items:

One-syllable words: place, put, but, bump, back, be, by, brand, don't, door, drew, cakes, cake, could, can't, crossed, cooled, know, gave, got, Max, made, make, milk, must, no, not, knew, needs, new, said, sent, store, still, step, sign, so, red, wrote, read, ran, fluff, for, floor, first, her, help, hot, his, he, home, hoped, hearts, had, late, list, line, looked, was, we, with, way, went, when, wait, what's, why, which, she, thrilled, the, that, this, there's, there, you, it, an, are, a, eggs, on, and, in, out, is, up, iced, else, eat, too

Two-syllable words: pencil, picture, bunny, birthday, table, didn't, couldn't, kitchen, candles, Grandma, Grandma's, going, grocer, Max's, meanwhile, sister, surprise, squirters, something, silver, Ruby, writing, roses, Ruby's, finished, frosting, wanted, sugar, yellow, earthworm, angel, icing, almost

Three-syllable words: beautiful, buttercream, marshmallow, raspberry, Rosemary, anything, anyway

Four-syllable words: caterpillar

2. Initial syllable deleting.

What to say to the student: "We're going to leave out syllables (or parts of words)."

> **EXAMPLE** "Say '_____.'" (stimulus word) "Say it again without '_____.'" (stimulus syllable) (e.g., "Say 'birthday.' Say it again without 'birth.'") (day)

> **NOTE:** *Use pictured items and/or manipulatives if necessary. Use any of the following stimulus words and/or others you select from the story. The correct answers are in parentheses.*

Stimulus items:

"Say 'pencil' without 'pen.'" (sull)

"Say 'Max's' without 'Max.'" (iz)

"Say 'meanwhile' without 'mean.'" (while)

"Say 'silver' without 'sil.'" (ver)

"Say 'marshmallow' without 'marsh.'" (mallow)

"Say 'squirters' without 'squir.'" (ters)

"Say 'sister' without 'sis.'" (ter)

"Say 'Rosemary' without 'Rose.'" (mary)

"Say 'wanted' without 'wan.'" (ted)

"Say 'frosting' without 'fros.'" (ting)

3. Final syllable deleting.

What to say to the student: "We're going to leave out syllables (or parts of words)."

> **EXAMPLE** "Say '_____.'" (stimulus word) "Say it again without '_____.'"
> (stimulus syllable) (e.g., "Say 'something' without 'thing.'") (some)

> **NOTE:** *Use pictured items and/or manipulatives if necessary. Use any of the following stimulus words and/or others you select from the story. The correct answers are in parentheses.*

Stimulus items:

"Say 'beautiful' without 'full.'" (beauti)

"Say 'something' without 'thing.'" (some)

"Say 'frosting' without 'ting.'" (fros)

"Say 'Ruby' without 'bee.'" (rue)

"Say 'marshmallow' without 'oh.'" (marshmall)

"Say 'birthday' without 'day.'" (birth)

"Say 'surprise' without 'prize.'" (sir)

"Say 'icing' without 'ing.'" (ice)

"Say 'writing' without 'ing.'" (write)

"Say 'raspberry' without 'ee.'" (raspber)

4. Initial syllable adding.

What to say to the student: "Now let's add syllables (or parts) to words."

> **EXAMPLE** "Add '_____'" (stimulus syllable) "to the beginning of '_____.'"
> (stimulus syllable) (e.g., "Add 'birth' to the beginning of 'day.'") (birthday)

> **NOTE:** *Use pictured items and/or manipulatives if necessary. Use any of the following stimulus words and/or others you select from the story. The correct answers are in parentheses.*

Stimulus items:

"Add 'some' to the beginning of 'thing.'" (something)

"Add 'sis' to the beginning of 'ter.'" (sister)

"Add 'rose' to the beginning of 'mary.'" (Rosemary)

"Add 'can' to the beginning of 'dulls.'" (candles)

"Add 'any' to the beginning of 'thing.'" (anything)

"Add 'earth' to the beginning of 'worm.'" (earthworm)

"Add 'rue' to the beginning of 'bee.'" (Ruby)

"Add 'any' to the beginning of 'way.'" (anyway)

"Add 'all' to the beginning of 'most.'" (almost)

"Add 'tay' to the beginning of 'bull.'" (table)

5. Final syllable adding.

What to say to the student: "Now let's add syllables (or parts) to words."

> **EXAMPLE** "Add '_____'" (stimulus syllable) "to the end of '_____.'" (stimulus syllable) (e.g., "Add 'day' to the end of 'birth.'") (birthday)

> **NOTE:** *Use pictured items and/or manipulatives if necessary. Use any of the following stimulus words and/or others you select from the story. The correct answers are in parentheses.*

Stimulus items:

"Add 'prize' to the end of 'sir.'" (surprise)

"Add 'ing' to the end of 'go.'" (going)

"Add 'oh' to the end of 'yell.'" (yellow)

"Add 'way' to the end of 'any.'" (anyway)

"Add 'sull' to the end of 'pen.'" (pencil)

"Add 'thing' to the end of 'any.'" (anything)

"Add 'ing to the end of 'frost.'" (frosting)

"Add 'bee' to the end of 'rue.'" (Ruby)

"Add 'while' to the end of 'mean.'" (meanwhile)

"Add 'ma's' to the end of 'grand.'" (grandma's)

6. Syllable substituting.

What to say to the student: "Let's make up some new words."

> **EXAMPLE** "Say '_____.'" (stimulus word) "Instead of '_____'" (stimulus syllable), "say '_____.'" (stimulus syllable) (e.g., "Say 'baking.' Instead of 'bake,' say 'cut.' The new word is 'cutting.'")

> **NOTE:** *Use pictured items and/or manipulatives if necessary. Use of the following stimulus words and/or others you select from the story. The correct answers are in parentheses.*

Stimulus items:

"Say 'meanwhile.' Instead of 'while,' say 'time.'" (meantime)

"Say 'anyway.' Instead of 'way,' say 'thing.'" (anything)

"Say 'something.' Instead of 'some,' say 'any.'" (anything)

"Say 'grandma's.' Instead of 'ma's,' say 'pa's.'" (grandpa's)

"Say 'writing.' Instead of 'ting,' say 'zing.'" (rising)

"Say 'candles.' Instead of 'dulls,' say 'dees.'" (candies)

"Say 'surprise.' Instead of 'prize,' say 'viss.'" (service)

"Say 'buttercream.' Instead of 'cream,' say 'milk.'" (buttermilk)

"Say 'frosting.' Instead of 'ting,' say 'tud.'" (frosted)

"Say 'baking.' Instead of 'bake,' say 'rake.'" (raking)

Phonological Awareness Activities at the Phoneme Level

1. Counting sounds.

What to say to the student: "We're going to count sounds in words."

EXAMPLE "How many sounds do you hear in this word? 'cake.'" (3)

NOTE: *Use pictured items and/or manipulatives if necessary. Use any of the following stimulus words and/or others you select from the story. Be sure to give the letter sound and not the letter name. Use any group of 10 stimulus items you select per teaching set.*

Stimulus words with one sound: *a*

Stimulus words with two sounds: be, by, to, know, no, knew, new, so, her, he, we, way, why, she, the, you, it, an, are, on, in, is, up, eat

Stimulus words with three sounds: put, but, back, touch, time, door, drew, cake, could, gave, got, made, make, not, said, sign, red, wrote, read, ran, hot, his, home, had, late, line, time, touch, that, there, was, with, wrote, when, wait, which, this, eggs, and, over, iced, else

Stimulus words with four sounds: bunny, cakes, place, brought, bump, baked, table, taste, don't, can't, cooled, just, Max, milk, most, must, needs, sent, still, step, Ruby, fluff, first, help, hoped, list, looked, went, what's, sugar, there's, yellow, idea

Stimulus words with five sounds: picture, birthday, brand, didn't, crossed, grocer, Max's, sister, silver, stars, Ruby's, thrilled, earthworm, anyway

Stimulus words with six sounds: candles, meanwhile, surprise, finished, almost

Stimulus words with seven sounds: squirters, raspberry

Stimulus words with eight sounds: buttercream, caterpillar

2. Sound categorization or identifying a rhyme oddity.

What to say to the student: "Guess which word I say does not rhyme with the other three words."

EXAMPLE "Tell me which word does not rhyme with the other three: '_____,' '_____,' '_____,' '_____.'" (stimulus words) (e.g., "'bunny,' 'honey,' 'money,' 'cake.' Which word doesn't rhyme?") (cake)

NOTE: *Use pictured items if necessary. Use any of the following stimulus words and/or others you select from the story. The correct answers are in parentheses.*

Stimulus items:

    roses, poses, Ruby, noses (Ruby)

    fluff, sister, blister, mister (fluff)

    stars, surprise, cars, Mars (surprise)

    bump, jump, Max, lump (Max)

    looked, cooked, booked, yellow (yellow)

    eggs, read, legs, begs (read)

    hearts, carts, earthworm, darts (earthworm)

    iced, floor, diced, sliced (floor)

    wait, gate, raspberry, late (raspberry)

    touch, Max, fax, lax (touch)

3. Matching rhyme.

What to say to the student: "We're going to think of rhyming words."

> **EXAMPLE** "Which word rhymes with '_____'?" (stimulus word) (e.g., "Which word rhymes with 'cake': 'bake,' 'just,' 'made,' 'Ruby'?") (bake)

NOTE: *Use pictured items if necessary. Use any of the following stimulus words and/or others you select from the story. The correct answers are in parentheses.*

Stimulus items:

    roses: Grandma's, different, candles, poses (poses)

    sister: going, couldn't, kitchen, blister (blister)

    thrilled: time, grilled, eggs, step (grilled)

    hearts: smarts, wrote, floor, cakes (smarts)

    Max: fluff, roses, sacks, stars (sacks)

    candles: going, handles, angel, sugar (handles)

    for: home, locked, yellow, bore (bore)

    table: label, marshmallow, surprise, knew (label)

    icing: almost, something, Ruby, slicing (slicing)

    cooled: raspberry, pooled, milk, different (pooled)

4. Producing rhyme.

What to say to the student: "Now we'll say rhyming words."

> **EXAMPLE** "Tell me a word that rhymes with '_____.'" (stimulus word) (e.g., "Tell me a word that rhymes with 'bunny.' You can make up a word if you want.") (funny, money, honey)

NOTE: *Use pictured items if necessary. Use any of the following stimulus words and/or others you select from the story (i.e., you say a word from the list below and the student is to think of a rhyming word). Use any group of 10 stimulus items you select per teaching set.*

Stimulus items:

/p/: place, put

/b/: bunny, but, brought, bump, back, baked, buttercream, brand, be, by

/t/: to, touch, table, time, taste

/d/: don't, door, drew

/k/: cakes, cake, could, can't, crossed, kitchen, cooled, candles

/g/: Grandma's, going, gave, got

/dz/ (as the first sound in jelly): just

/m/: Max, made, make, marshmallow, must, meanwhile

/n/: no, not, knew, needs, new

/s/: said, sister, sent, store, squirters, so, still, step, sign, something, silver, stars, so

/f/: fluff, for, floor, finished, frosting, first

/h/: her, hot, his, he, home, hoped, had

/r/: Ruby, raspberry, red, wrote, read, writing, roses, ran

/l/: late, list, line, looked

/w/, /wh/: was, we, wanted, wrote, way, went, when, wait, what's, why

/sh/: she, sugar

/voiceless th/: thrilled

/voiced th/: the, that, this, there's, there

/y/ (as the first sound in yellow): yellow, you

vowels: it, an, are, angel, icing, a, eggs, on, and, in, over, anyway, almost, is, up, iced, eat

5. Sound matching (initial).

What to say to the student: "Now we'll listen for the first sound in words."

EXAMPLE "Listen to this sound: / /." (stimulus sound). "Guess which word I say begins with that sound. '_____,' '_____,' _____,' '_____.'" (stimulus words) (e.g., "Listen to this sound: /d/. Guess which word I say begins with that sound: 'bunny,' 'door,' 'cakes,' 'place.'") (door)

NOTE: *Give the letter sound, not the letter name. Use pictured items if necessary. Use any of the following stimulus words and/or others you select from the story. The correct answers are in parentheses.*

Stimulus items:

/m/: cakes, grandma, needs, Max (Max)

/t/: Ruby, taste, marshmallow, squirters (taste)

/f/: help, grocer, fluff, caterpillar (fluff)

/h/: late, hearts, yellow, buttercream (hearts)

/p/: picture, milk, earthworm, which (picture)

/l/: frosting, different, raspberry, list (list)

/k/: grandma's, silver, kitchen, bump (kitchen)

/b/: buttercream, Max, going, sugar (buttercream)

/r/: baked, Rosemary, meanwhile, first (Rosemary)

/s/: stars, time, picture, fluff (stars)

6. Sound matching (final).

What to say to the student: "Now we'll listen for the last sound in words."

> **EXAMPLE** "Listen to this sound: / /." (stimulus sound) "Guess which word I say ends with that sound: '_____,' '_____,' '_____,' '_____.'" (stimulus words) (e.g., "Listen to this sound: /k/. Guess which word I say ends with that sound: 'milk,' 'stars,' 'sign,' 'Max.'") (milk)

NOTE: *Give the letter sound, not the letter name. Use pictured items and/or manipulatives if necessary. Use any of the following stimulus words and/or others you select from the story. The correct answers are in parentheses.*

Stimulus items:

/ch/: fluff, touch, raspberry, brought (touch)

/p/: touch, sugar, time, bump (bump)

/z/: Grandma's, red, cake, angel (Grandma's)

/ng/: thrilled, icing, hot, bump (icing)

/r/: frosting, candles, silver, kitchen (silver)

/long E/: pencil, with, milk, Ruby (Ruby)

/s/: Max, back, gave, candles (Max)

/m/: ran, earthworm, of, anything (earthworm)

/n/: knew, door, sign, table (sign)

/f/: fluff, buttercream, raspberry, this (fluff)

7. Identifying the initial sound in words.

What to say to the student: "I'll say a word two times. Tell me what sound is missing the second time: '_____,' '_____.'" (stimulus words)

> **EXAMPLE** "What sound do you hear in '_____'" (stimulus word) "that is missing in '_____'?" (stimulus word) (e.g., "What sound do you hear in 'red' that is missing in 'Ed'?") (/r/)

NOTE: *Give the letter sound, not the letter name. Use pictured items and/or manipulatives if necessary. Use any of the following stimulus words and/or others you select from the story. The correct answers are in parentheses.*

Stimulus items:

"cakes, aches. What sound do you hear in 'cakes' that is missing in 'aches'?" (/k/)

"door, or. What sound do you hear in 'door' that is missing in 'or'?" (/d/)

"Max, axe. What sound do you hear in 'Max' that is missing in 'axe'?" (/m/)

"no, owe. What sound do you hear in 'no' that is missing in 'owe'?" (/n/)

"late, ate. What sound do you hear in 'late' that is missing in 'ate'?" (/l/)

"stars, tars. What sound do you hear in 'stars' that is missing in 'tars'?" (/s/)

"hearts, arts. What sound do you hear in 'hearts' that is missing in 'arts'?" (/h/)

"by, eye. What sound do you hear in 'by' that is missing in 'eye'?" (/b/)

"there's, airs. What sound do you hear in 'there's' that is missing in 'airs'?" (/voiced th/)

"floor, lore. What sound do you hear in 'floor' that is missing in 'lore'?" (/f/)

8. Identifying the final sound in words.

What to say to the student: "I'll say a word two times. Tell me what sound is missing the second time: '_____,' '_____.'" (stimulus words)

> EXAMPLE "What sound do you hear in '_____'" (stimulus word) "that is missing in '_____'?" (stimulus word) (e.g., "What sound do you hear in 'time' that is missing in 'tie'?") (/m/)

NOTE: *Give the letter sound, not the letter name. Use pictured items and/or manipulatives if necessary. Use any of the following stimulus words and/or others you select from the story. The correct answers are in parentheses.*

Stimulus items:

"Max, Mack. What sound do you hear in 'Max' that is missing in 'Mack'?" (/s/)

"Ruby, Rube. What sound do you hear in 'Ruby' that is missing in 'Rube'?" (/long E/)

"needs, need. What sound do you hear in 'needs' that is missing in 'need'?" (/z/)

"hearts, heart. What sound do you hear in 'hearts' that is missing in 'heart'?" (/s/)

"grocer, gross. What sound do you hear in 'grocer' that is missing in 'gross'?" (/r/)

"yellow, yell. What sound do you hear in 'yellow' that is missing in 'yell'?" (/long O/)

"sign, sigh. What sound do you hear in 'sign' that is missing in 'sigh'?" (/n/)

"home, hoe. What sound do you hear in 'home' that is missing in 'hoe'?" (/m/)

"bump, bum. What sound do you hear in 'bump' that is missing in 'bum'?" (/p/)

"Grandma's, Grandma. What sound do you hear in 'Grandma's' that is missing in 'Grandma'?" (/z/)

9. Segmenting the initial sound in words.

What to say to the student: "Listen to the word I say and tell me the first sound you hear."

> EXAMPLE "What's the first sound in '_____'?" (stimulus word) (e.g., "What's the first sound in 'bunny'?") (/b/)

NOTE: *Give the letter sound, not the letter name. Use pictured items and/or manipulatives if necessary. Use any of the following stimulus words and/or others you select from the story. Use any group of 10 stimulus items you select per teaching set.*

Stimulus items:

/p/: pencil, place, picture, put

/b/: bunny, birthday, but, brought, bump, back, beautiful, baked, buttercream, brand, be, by

/t/: to, touch, too, table, time, taste

/d/: don't, different, door, drew, didn't

/k/: cakes, cake, could, couldn't, can't, crossed, kitchen, cooled, candles, caterpillar

/g/: Grandma's, going, Grandma, grocer, gave, got

/dz/ (as the first sound in jelly): just

/m/: Max, made, make, marshmallow, Max's, milk, must, meanwhile

/n/: no, not, knew, needs, new

/s/: said, sister, surprise, sent, store, squirters, so, still, step, sign, something, silver, stars

/f/: fluff, for, floor, finished, frosting, first

/h/: her, help, hot, his, he, home, hoped, hearts, had

/r/: Ruby, raspberry, red, wrote, read, writing, roses, Ruby's, ran

/l/: late, list, line, looked

/w/, /wh/: was, we, with, wanted, wrote, way, went, when, wait, what's, why, which

/sh/: she, sugar

/voiceless th/: thrilled

/voiced th/: the, that, this, there's, there

/y/ (as the first sound in yellow): yellow, you

vowels: it, an, angel, icing, anything, eggs, on, and, in, over, anyway, almost, is, up, iced, else, idea, eat

10. Segmenting the final sound in words.

What to say to the student: "Listen to the word I say and tell me the last sound you hear."

> **EXAMPLE** "What's the last sound in the word '_____'?" (stimulus word)
> (e.g., "What's the last sound in the word 'up'?") (/p/)

NOTE: *Give the letter sound, not the letter name. Use pictured items and/or manipulatives if necessary. Use any of the following stimulus words and/or others you select from the story. Use any group of 10 stimulus items you select per teaching set.*

Stimulus items:

/p/: help, bump, step, up

/t/: it, don't, but, late, sent, list, that, hot, wrote, must, looked, just, didn't, first, put, eat, not, brought, don't, different, hoped, couldn't, can't, crossed, went, got, out, most, almost, taste, finished, baked, iced, wait

/d/: made, said, wanted, red, could, read, and, could, cooled, had, brand, thrilled

/k/: cake, make, back, milk

/ch/: touch, which

/m/: earthworm, home, time, buttercream

/n/: an, on, in, line, when, sign, kitchen, ran

/ng/: going, icing, anything, writing, frosting, something

/s/: Max, this, place, else, hearts, what's

/z/: was, Grandma's, Max's, surprise, eggs, squirters, his, there's, is, needs, candles, stars, roses, Ruby's

/f/: fluff

/v/: gave, of

/r/: her, sister, are, store, for, grocer, floor, over, flour, there, door, silver, sugar, picture, caterpillar

/l/: angel, table, still, pencil, beautiful, meanwhile

/voiceless th/: with

/long A/: birthday, way, anyway

/long E/: Ruby, we, raspberry, be, he, she

/long I/: why

/long O/: no, so, yellow, marshmallow

/oo/: too

11. Generating words from the story beginning with a particular sound.

What to say to the student: "Let's think of words from the story that start with certain sounds."

EXAMPLE "Tell me a word from the story that starts with / /." (stimulus sound) (e.g., the sound /m/) (Max)

NOTE: *Give the letter sound, not the letter name. Use pictured items if necessary. Use any of the following stimulus words and/or others you select from the story. You say the sound (e.g., a voiceless /p/ sound) and the student is to say a word from the story that begins with that sound. Use any group of 10 stimulus items you select per teaching set.*

Stimulus items:

/p/: pencil, place, picture, put

/b/: bunny, birthday, but, brought, bump, back, beautiful, baked, buttercream, brand, be, by

/t/: to, touch, too, table, time, taste

/d/: don't, different, door, drew, didn't

/k/: cakes, cake, could, couldn't, can't, crossed, kitchen, cooled, candles, caterpillar

/g/: Grandma's, going, Grandma, grocer, gave, got

/dz/ (as the first sound in jelly): just

/m/: Max, made, make, marshmallow, Max's, milk, must, meanwhile

/n/: no, not, knew, needs, new

/s/: said, sister, surprise, sent, store, squirters, so, still, step, sign, something, silver, stars

/f/: fluff, for, floor, finished, frosting, first

/h/: her, help, hot, his, he, home, hoped, hearts, had

/r/: Ruby, raspberry, red, wrote, read, writing, roses, Ruby's, ran

/l/: late, list, line, looked

/w/, /wh/: was, we, with, wanted, wrote, way, went, when, wait, what's, why, which

/sh/: she, sugar

/voiceless th/: thrilled

/voiced th/: the, that, this, there's, there

/y/ (as the first sound in yellow): yellow, you

vowels: it, an, angel, icing, anything, eggs, on, and, in, over, anyway, almost, is, up, iced, else, idea, eat

12. Blending sounds in monosyllabic words divided into onset–rime beginning with a two-consonant cluster + rime.

What to say to the student: "Now we'll put sounds together to make words."

> EXAMPLE   "Put these sounds together to make a word: / / + / /." (stimulus sounds)
> "What's the word?" (e.g., "st + ep: What's the word?") (step)

> **NOTE:** *Give the letter sound, not the letter name. Use pictured items and/or manipulatives if necessary. Use any of the following stimulus words and/or others you select from the story. The correct answers are in parentheses.*

Stimulus items:

st + ars (stars)

br + ought (brought)

br + and (brand)

dr + ew (drew)

cr + ossed (crossed)

fl + uff (fluff)

st+ ore (store)

pl + ace (place)

fl + oor (floor)

st + ep (step)

13. Blending sounds in monosyllabic words divided into onset–rime beginning with a single consonant + rime.

What to say to the student: "Let's put sounds together to make words."

> EXAMPLE   "Put these sounds together to make a word: / / + / /." (stimulus sounds)
> "What's the word?" (e.g., "/m/ + ax: What's the word?") (Max)

NOTE: *Give the letter sound, not the letter name. Use pictured items and/or manipulatives if necessary. Use any of the following stimulus words and/or others you select from the story. The correct answers are in parentheses.*

Stimulus items:

/b/ + ump (bump)

/t/ + ime (time)

/dz/ (as the first sound in jelly) + ust (just)

/s/ + ign (sign)

/r/ + an (ran)

/h/ + ome (home)

/d/ + ont (don't)

/l/ + ate (late)

/n/ + ot (not)

/g/ + ave (gave)

14. Blending sounds to form a monosyllabic word beginning with a continuant sound.

What to say to the student: "We'll put sounds together to make words."

EXAMPLE   "Put these sounds together to make a word: / / + / / + / /." (stimulus sounds) (e.g., /r/ /short E/ /d/) (red)

NOTE: *Give the letter sound, not the letter name. Use pictured items and/or manipulatives if necessary. Use any of the following stimulus words and/or others you select from the story. The correct answers are in parentheses.*

Stimulus items:

/l/ /long A/ /t/ (late)

/s/ /t/ /ah/ /r/ /z/ (stars)

/r/ /short A/ /n/ (ran)

/h/ /long O/ /m/ (home)

/w/ /long A/ /t/ (wait)

/y/ (as in yellow) /oo/ (you)

/m/ /short I/ /l/ /k/ (milk)

/n/ /ah/ /t/ (not)

/f/ /l/ /short U/ /f/ (fluff)

/s/ /long I/ /n/ (sign)

15. Blending sounds to form a monosyllabic word beginning with a noncontinuant sound.

What to say to the student: "We'll put sounds together to make words."

EXAMPLE "Put these sounds together to make a word: / / + / / + / /." (stimulus sounds) (e.g., /p/ /l/ /long A/ /s/) (place)

NOTE: *Give the letter sound, not the letter name. Use pictured items and/or manipulatives if necessary. Use any of the following stimulus words and/or others you select from the story. The correct answers are in parentheses.*

Stimulus items:

/b/ /r/ /short A/ /n/ /d/ (brand)

/t/ /long I/ /m/ (time)

/g/ /ah/ /t/ (got)

/b/ /long I/ (by)

/k/ /long A/ /k/ /s/ (cakes)

/g/ /long A/ /v/ (gave)

/dz/ (as the first sound in jelly) /short U/ /s/ /t/ (just)

/d/ /r/ /oo/ (drew)

/b/ /short U/ /m/ /p/ (bump)

/k/ /oo/ /l/ /d/ (cooled)

16. Substituting the initial sound in words.

What to say to the student: "We're going to change beginning/first sounds in words."

EXAMPLE "Say '_____.'" (stimulus word) "Instead of / /" (stimulus sound), "say / /." (stimulus sound) (e.g., "Say 'Max.' Instead of /m/, say /f/. What's your new word?") (fax)

NOTE: *Give the letter sound, not the letter name. Use pictured items and/or manipulatives if necessary. Use any of the following stimulus words and/or others you select from the story. The correct answers are in parentheses.*

Stimulus items:

"Say 'bunny.' Instead of /b/, say /s/." (sunny)

"Say 'cakes.' Instead of /k/, say /l/." (lakes)

"Say 'list.' Instead of /l/, say /f/." (fist)

"Say 'sign.' Instead of /s/, say /l/." (line)

"Say 'she.' Instead of /sh/, say /h/." (he)

"Say 'fluff.' Instead of /f/, say /b/." (bluff)

"Say 'that.' Instead of /voiced th/, say /k/." (cat)

"Say 'make.' Instead of /m/, say /l/." (lake)

"Say 'needs.' Instead of /n/, say /b/." (beads)

"Say 'baked.' Instead of /b/, say /f/." (faked)

17. Substituting the final sound in words.

What to say to the student: "We're going to change ending/last sounds in words."

> **EXAMPLE** "Say '_____.'" (stimulus word) "Instead of / /" (stimulus sound), "say / /." (stimulus sound) (e.g., "Say 'back.' Instead of /k/, say /t/. What's your new word?") (bat)

> **NOTE:** *Give the letter sound, not the letter name. Use pictured items and/or manipulatives if necessary. Use any of the following stimulus words and/or others you select from the story. The correct answers are in parentheses.*

Stimulus items:

"Say 'make.' Instead of /k/, say /n/." (main)

"Say 'sign.' Instead of /n/, say /t/." (sight)

"Say 'home.' Instead of /m/, say /p/." (hope)

"Say 'which.' Instead of /ch/, say /t/." (wit)

"Say 'was.' Instead of /z/, say /n/." (one)

"Say 'cooled.' Instead of /d/, say /z/." (cools)

"Say 'still.' Instead of /l/, say /f/." (stiff)

"Say 'ran.' Instead of /n/, say /t/." (rat)

"Say 'place.' Instead of /s/, say /t/." (plate)

"Say 'stars.' Instead of /z/, say /t/." (start)

"Say 'help.' Instead of /p/, say /long O/." (hello)

18. Segmenting the middle sound in monosyllabic words.

What to say to the student: "Tell me the middle sound in the word I say."

> **EXAMPLE** "What's the middle sound in the word '_____'?" (stimulus word) (e.g., "What's the middle sound in the word 'his'?") (/short I/)

> **NOTE:** *Give the letter sound, not the letter name. Use pictured items and/or manipulatives if necessary. Use any of the following stimulus words and/or others you select from the story. The correct answers are in parentheses.*

Stimulus items:

made (/long A/)

said (/short E/)

hot (/ah/)

had (/short A/)

wrote (/long O/)

sign (/long I/)

back (/short A/)

home (/long O/)

ran (/short A/)

gave (/long A/)

19. Substituting the middle sound in words.

What to say to the student: "We're going to change the middle sound in words."

> **EXAMPLE** "Say '_____.'" (stimulus word) "Instead of / /" (stimulus sound), "say //."
> (stimulus sound) (e.g., "Say 'make.' Instead of /long A/, say /long I/.
> What's your new word?") (Mike)

> **NOTE:** *Give the letter sound, not the letter name. Use pictured items and/or manipulatives if necessary. Use any of the following stimulus words and/or others you select from the story. The correct answers are in parentheses.*

Stimulus items:

"Say 'back.' Instead of /short A/, say /long E/." (beak)

"Say 'time.' Instead of /long I/, say /long E/." (team)

"Say 'made.' Instead of /long A/, say /short I/." (mid)

"Say 'got.' Instead of /ah/, say /short E/." (get)

"Say 'not.' Instead of /ah/, say /short U/." (nut)

"Say 'hot.' Instead of /ah/, say /long E/." (heat)

"Say 'read.' Instead of /short E/, say /long O/." (road)

"Say 'sign.' Instead of /long I/, say /short U/." (sun)

"Say 'stars.' Instead of /ah/ say, /long E/." (steers)

"Say 'brand.' Instead of /short A/, say /long I/." (brined)

20. Identifying all sounds in monosyllabic words.

What to say to the student: "Now tell me all the sounds you hear in the word I say."

> **EXAMPLE** "What sounds do you hear in the word '_____'?" (stimulus word)
> (e.g., "What sounds do you hear in the word 'time'?") (/t/ /long I/ /m/)

> **NOTE:** *Give the letter sound, not the letter name. Use pictured items and/or manipulatives if necessary. Use any of the following stimulus words and/or others you select from the story. The correct answers are in parentheses.*

Stimulus items:

touch (/t/ /short U/ /ch/)

cake (/k/ /long A/ /k/)

got (/g/ /ah/ /t/)

said (/s/ /short E/ /d/)

fluff (/f/ /l/ /short U/ /f/)

still (/s/ /t/ /short I/ /l/)

wrote (/r/ /long O/ /t/)

help (/h/ /short E/ /l/ /p/)

needs (/n/ /long E/ /d/ /z/)

Max (/m/ /short A/ /k/ /s/)

21. Deleting sounds within words.

What to say to the student: "We're going to leave out sounds in words."

EXAMPLE "Say '_____'" (stimulus word) "without / /." (stimulus sound) (e.g., "Say 'brand' without /r/.") (band) Say: "The word that is left— 'band'—is a real word. Sometimes, the word won't be a real word."

NOTE: *Give the letter sound, not the letter name. Use pictured items and/or manipulatives if necessary. Use any of the following stimulus words and/or others you select from the story. The correct answers are in parentheses.*

Stimulus items:

"Say 'place' without /l/." (pace)

"Say 'store' without /t/." (sore)

"Say 'must' without /s/." (mutt)

"Say 'floor' without /l/." (four)

"Say 'Ruby's' without /long E/." (Rube's)

"Say 'can't' without /n/." (cat)

"Say 'sent' without /n/." (set)

"Say 'Max' without /k/." (mass)

"Say 'don't' without /n/." (dote)

"Say 'just' without /s/." (jut)

22. Substituting consonants in words having a two-sound cluster.

What to say to the student: "We're going to substitute sounds in words."

EXAMPLE "Say '_____.'" (stimulus word) "Instead of / /" (stimulus sound), "say / /." (stimulus sound) (e.g., "Say 'store.' Instead of /t/, say /k/.") (score) Say: "Sometimes, the new word will be a made-up word."

NOTE: *Give the letter sound, not the letter name. Use pictured items and/or manipulatives if necessary. Use any of the following stimulus words and/or others you select from the story. The correct answers are in parentheses.*

Stimulus items:

"Say 'brand.' Instead of /r/, say /l/." (bland)

"Say 'brought.' Instead of /b/, say /f/." (fraught)

"Say 'fluff.' Instead of /f/, say /s/." (sluff)

"Say 'stars.' Instead of /t/, say /p/." (spars)

"Say 'and.' Instead of /d/, say /t/." (ant)

"Say 'thrilled.' Instead of /voiceless th/, say /g/." (grilled)

"Say 'Max.' Instead of /k/, say /t/." (mats)

"Say 'frosting.' Instead of /r/, say /l/." (flosting)

"Say 'hoped.' Instead of /t/, say /s/." (hopes)

"Say 'place.' Instead of /p/, say /f/." (flace)

23. Phoneme reversing.

What to say to the student: "We're going to say words backward."

> **EXAMPLE** "Say the word '_____'" (stimulus word) "backward." (e.g., "Say 'back' backward.") (cab)

NOTE: *This is a difficult phoneme-level task and should only be done with older students. Give the letter sound, not the letter name. Use pictured items and/or manipulatives if necessary. Use any of the following stimulus words and/or others you select from the story. The correct answers are in parentheses.*

Stimulus items:

time (might)

make (came)

late (tail)

line (Nile)

got (tog)

but (tub)

too (oot)

cakes (skake)

still (lits)

step (pets)

24. Phoneme switching.

What to say to the student: "We're going to switch the first sounds in two words."

> **EXAMPLE** "Switch the first sounds in '_____' and '_____.'" (stimulus words) (e.g., "Switch the first sounds in 'to' and 'Ruby.'") (roo toobie)

NOTE: *This is a difficult phoneme-level task and should only be done with older students. Give the letter sound, not the letter name. Use pictured items and/or manipulatives if necessary. Use any of the following stimulus words and/or others you select from the story. The correct answers are in parentheses.*

Stimulus items:

no Max (mo nax)

too late (loo tate)

red hot (hed rot)

Max hoped (hax moped)

that line (lat thine)

birthday candles (kirthday bandles)

buttercream roses (ruttercream boses)

just beautiful (bust jeautiful)

Max's writing (rax's miting)

Grandma's birthday (brandma's girthday)

25. Pig Latin.

What to say to the student: "We're going to speak a secret language by using words from the story. In pig Latin, you take off the first sound of a word, put it at the end of the word, and add an 'ay' sound."

> EXAMPLE "Say 'put' in pig Latin." (utpay)

NOTE: *This is a difficult phoneme-level task and should only be done with older students. Use pictured items and/or manipulatives if necessary. Use any of the following stimulus words and/or others you select from the story. The correct answers are in parentheses.*

Stimulus items:

cakes (akescay)

roses (osesray)

Max (axmay)

sister (istersay)

Ruby (ubyray)

silver (ilversay)

kitchen (itchenkay)

something (omethingsay)

marshmallow (arshmallowmay)

raspberry (aspberryray)

From Phonological Awareness into Print

NOTE: *Only five examples per activity are included in this resource due to space. You are encouraged to add many more words into this section that you feel your student(s) is(are) ready to write.*

1. Substituting the initial sound or letter in words.

NOTE: *Use lined paper or copy the sheet of lined paper included in the back of this book.*

Stimulus items:

1.1 got/tot

Task a. "Say 'got.' Instead of /g/, say /t/. What's your new word?" (tot) "Write/copy 'got' and 'tot.'"

Task b. "Circle the **letters** that make the words different." ([g], [t])

Task c. "What **sounds** do these letters make?" (/g/, /t/)

1.2 roses/poses

Task a. "Say 'roses.' Instead of /r/, say /p/. What's your new word?" (poses) "Write/copy 'roses' and 'poses.'"

Task b. "Circle the **letters** that make the words different." ([r], [p])

Task c. "What **sounds** do these letters make?" (/r/, /p/)

1.3 bunny/funny

Task a. "Say 'bunny.' Instead of /b/, say /f/. What's your new word?" (funny) "Write/copy 'bunny' and 'funny.'"

Task b. "Circle the **letters** that make the words different." ([b], [f])

Task c. "What **sounds** do these letters make?" (/b/, /f/)

1.4 cakes/lakes

Task a. "Say 'cakes.' Instead of /k/, say /l/. What's your new word?" (lakes) "Write/copy 'cakes' and 'lakes.'"

Task b. "Circle the **letters** that make the words different." ([c], [l])

Task c. "What **sounds** do these letters make?" (/k/, /l/)

1.5 milk/silk

Task a. "Say 'milk.' Instead of /m/, say /s/. What's your new word?" (silk) "Write/copy 'milk' and 'silk.'"

Task b. "Circle the **letters** that make the words different." ([m], [s])

Task c. "What **sounds** do these letters make?" (/m/, /s/)

2. Substituting the final sound or letter in words.

NOTE: *Use lined paper or copy the sheet of lined paper included in the back of this book.*

Stimulus items:

2.1 hot/hop

Task a. "Say 'hot.' Instead of /t/, say /p/. What's your new word?" (hop) "Write/copy 'hot' and 'hop.' "

Task b. "Circle the **letters** that make the words different." ([t], [p])

Task c. "What **sounds** do these letters make?" (/t/, /p/)

2.2 it/if

Task a. "Say 'it.' Instead of /t/, say /f/. What's your new word?" (if) "Write/copy 'it' and 'if.' "

Task b. "Circle the **letters** that make the words different." ([t], [f])

Task c. "What **sounds** do these letters make?" (/t/, /f/)

2.3 ran/rap

Task a. "Say 'ran.' Instead of /n/, say /p/. What's your new word?" (rap) "Write/copy 'ran' and 'rap.' "

Task b. "Circle the **letters** that make the words different." ([n], [p])

Task c. "What **sounds** do these letters make?" (/n/, /p/)

2.4 she/shy

Task a. "Say 'she.' Instead of /long E/, say /long I/. What's your new word?" (shy) "Write/copy 'she' and 'shy.' "

Task b. "Circle the **letters** that make the words different." ([e], [y])

Task c. "What **sounds** do these letters make?" (/long E/, /long I/)

2.5 line/live

Task a. "Say 'line.' Instead of /n/, say /v/. What's your new word?" (live) "Write/copy 'line' and 'live.' "

Task b. "Circle the **letters** that make the words different." ([n], [v])

Task c. "What **sounds** do these letters make?" (/n/, /v/)

3. Substituting the middle sound or letter in words.

NOTE: *Use lined paper or copy the sheet of lined paper included in the back of this book.*

Stimulus items:

3.1 but/bit

Task a. "Say 'but' Instead of /short U/, say /short I/. What's your new word?" (bit) "Write/copy 'but' and 'bit.' "

Task b. "Circle the **letters** that make the words different." ([u], [i])

Task c. "What **sounds** do these letters make?" (/short U/, /short I/)

3.2 his/has

Task a. "Say 'his.' Instead of /short I/, say /short A/. What's your new word?" (has) "Write/copy 'his' and 'has.' "

Task b. "Circle the **letters** that make the words different." ([i], [a])

Task c. "What **sounds** do these letters make?" (/short I/, /short A/)

3.3 ran/run

Task a. "Say 'ran.' Instead of /short A/, say /short U/. What's your new word?" (run) "Write/copy 'ran' and 'run.'"

Task b. "Circle the **letters** that make the words different." ([a], [u])

Task c. "What **sounds** do these letters make?" (/short A/, /short U/)

3.4 time/tame

Task a. "Say 'time.' Instead of /long I/, say /long A/. What's your new word?" (tame) "Write/copy 'time' and 'tame.'"

Task b. "Circle the **letters** that make the words different." ([i], [a])

Task c. "What **sounds** do these letters make?" (/long I/, /long A/)

3.5 had/hid

Task a. "Say 'had.' Instead of /short A/, say /short I/. What's your new word?" (hid) "Write/copy 'had' and 'hid.'"

Task b. "Circle the **letters** that make the words different." ([a], [i])

Task c. "What **sounds** do these letters make?" (/short A/, /short I/)

4. Supplying the initial sound or letter in words.

NOTE: *Use lined paper or copy the sheet of lined paper included in the back of this book.*

Stimulus items:

4.1 Max/ax

Task a. "Say 'Max,' say 'ax.' What sound did you hear in 'Max' that is missing in 'ax'?" (/m/) "Now we'll change the **letter.** Write/copy 'Max' and 'ax.'"

Task b. "Circle the beginning **letter** that makes the words different." ([m])

Task c. "What **sound** does this letter make?" (/m/)

4.2 stars/tars

Task a. "Say 'stars,' say 'tars.' What sound did you hear in 'stars' that is missing in 'tars'?" (/s/) "Now we'll change the **letter.** Write/copy 'stars' and 'tars.'"

Task b. "Circle the beginning **letter** that makes the words different." ([s])

Task c. "What **sound** does this letter make?" (/s/)

4.3 his/is

Task a. "Say 'his,' say 'is.' What sound did you hear in 'his' that is missing in 'is'?" (/h/) "Now we'll change the **letter.** Write/copy 'his' and 'is.'"

Task b. "Circle the beginning **letter** that makes the words different." ([h])

Task c. "What **sound** does this letter make?" (/h/)

4.4 late/ate

Task a. "Say 'late,' say 'ate.' What sound did you hear in 'late' that is missing in 'ate'?" (/l/) "Now we'll change the **letter.** Write/copy 'late' and 'ate.'"

Task b. "Circle the beginning **letter** that makes the words different." ([l])

Task c. "What **sound** does this letter make?" (/l/)

4.5 table/able

Task a. "Say 'table,' say 'able.' What sound did you hear in 'table' that is missing in 'able'?" (/t/) "Now we'll change the **letter**. Write/copy 'table' and 'able.'"

Task b. "Circle the beginning **letter** that makes the words different." ([t])

Task c. "What **sound** does this letter make?" (/t/)

5. Supplying the final sound or letter in words.

NOTE: *Use lined paper or copy the sheet of lined paper included in the back of this book.*

Stimulus items:

5.1 stars/star

Task a. "Say 'stars,' say 'star.' What sound did you hear in 'stars' that is missing in 'star'?" (/z/) "Now we'll change the **letter**. Write/copy 'stars' and 'star.'"

Task b. "Circle the ending/last **letter** that makes the words different." ([s])

Task c. "What **sound** does this letter make?" (/z/)

5.2 hearts/heart

Task a. "Say 'hearts,' say 'heart.' What sound did you hear in 'hearts' that is missing in 'heart'?" (/s/) "Now we'll change the **letter**. Write/copy 'hearts' and 'heart.'"

Task b. "Circle the ending/last **letter** that makes the words different." ([s])

Task c. "What **sound** does this letter make?" (/s/)

5.3 cooled/cool

Task a. "Say 'cooled,' say 'cool.' What sound did you hear in 'cooled' that is missing in 'cool'?" (/d/) "Now we'll change the **letters**. Write/copy 'cooled' and 'cool.'"

Task b. "Circle the ending/last **letters** that make the words different." ([e], [d])

Task c. "What **sound** do these letters make?" (/d/)

5.4 roses/rose

Task a. "Say 'roses,' say 'rose.' What sound did you hear in 'roses' that is missing in 'rose'?" (/z/) "Now we'll change the **letter**. Write/copy 'roses' and 'rose.'"

Task b. "Circle the ending/last **letter** that makes the word different." ([s])

Task c. "What **sound** does this letter make?" (/z/)

5.5 yellow/yell

Task a. "Say 'yellow,' say 'yell.' What sound did you hear in 'yellow' that is missing in 'yell'?" (/long O/) "Now we'll change the **letters**. Write/copy 'yellow' and 'yell.'"

Task b. "Circle the ending/last **letters** that make the words different." ([o], [w])

Task c. "What **sound** do these letters make?" (/long O/)

6. Switching the first sound and letter in words (ADVANCED).

NOTE: *Use lined paper or copy the sheet of lined paper included in the back of this book.*

Stimulus items:

6.1 no Max

> **Task a.** "Say 'no,' say 'Max.' What sound do you hear in the beginning of 'no'?" (/n/) "What sound do you hear in the beginning of 'Max'?" (/m/) "Switch the first sounds in those words." (mo nax) "Now we'll change the **letters.** Write/copy 'no Max' and 'Mo nax.'"
>
> **Task b.** "Circle the beginning **letters** that change the words." ([n], [M])
>
> **Task c.** "What **sounds** do those letters make?" (/n/, /m/)

6.2 that line

> **Task a.** "Say 'that,' say 'line.' What sound do you hear in the beginning of 'that'?" (/voiced th/) "What sound do you hear in the beginning of 'line'?" (/l/) "Switch the first sounds in those words." (lat thine) "Now we'll change the **letters.** Write/copy 'that line' and 'lat thine.'"
>
> **Task b.** "Circle the beginning **letters** that change the words." ([t], [h], [l])
>
> **Task c.** "What **sounds** do those letters make?" (/voiced th/, /l/)

6.3 too late

> **Task a.** "Say 'too,' say 'late.' What sound do you hear in the beginning of 'too'?" (/t/) "What sound do you hear in the beginning of 'late'?" (/l/) "Switch the first sounds in those words." (loo tate) "Now we'll change the **letters.** Write/copy 'too late' and 'loo tate.'"
>
> **Task b.** "Circle the beginning **letters** that change the words." ([t], [l])
>
> **Task c.** "What **sounds** do those letters make?" (/t/, /l/)

6.4 Max hoped

> **Task a.** "Say 'Max,' say 'hoped.' What sound do you hear in the beginning of 'Max'?" (/m/) "What sound do you hear in the beginning of 'hoped'?" (/h/) "Switch the first sounds in those words." (hax Moped) "Now we'll change the **letters.** Write/copy 'Max hoped' and 'hax Moped.'"
>
> **Task b.** "Circle the beginning **letters** that change the words." ([M], [h])
>
> **Task c.** "What **sounds** do those letters make?" (/m/, /h/)

6.5 red hot

> **Task a.** "Say 'red,' say 'hot.' What sound do you hear in the beginning of 'red'?" (/r/) "What sound do you hear in the beginning of 'hot'?" (/h/) "Switch the first sounds in those words." (hed rot) "Now we'll change the **letters.** Write/copy 'red hot' and 'hed rot.'"
>
> **Task b.** "Circle the beginning **letters** that change the words." ([r], [h])
>
> **Task c.** "What **sounds** do those letters make?" (/r/, /h/)

CHAPTER

5

Phonological Awareness Activities to Use with *Chicken Soup with Rice*

Text version used for selection of stimulus items:

Sendak, M., and Barner, B. (Illustrator). (1990). *Chicken Soup with Rice*. New York: Harper Trophy/HarperCollins Publishers Inc.

Phonological Awareness Activities at the Word Level

1. Counting words.

What to say to the student: "We're going to count words."

> **EXAMPLE** "How many words do you hear in this sentence (or phrase)? 'sipping chicken soup'" (3)

> **NOTE:** *Use pictured items and/or manipulatives if necessary. Use any of the following stimulus phrases or sentences and/or others you select from the story. The correct answers are in parentheses.*

Stimulus items:

in March (2)

chicken soup (2)

I will ride (3)

I'll serve them (3)

whoopy once whoopy twice (4)

merry chicken soup (3)

paddle chicken soup with rice (5)

her name was Mrs. Rose (5)

dream about hot soup all day (6)

I will become a cooking pot (6)

2. Identifying the missing word from a list.

What to say to the student: "Listen to the words I say. I'll say them again. You tell me which word I leave out."

> **EXAMPLE** "Listen to the words I say: 'floor,' 'Nile,' 'March.' I'll say them again. Tell me which one I leave out: 'Nile,' 'March.'" (floor)

NOTE: *Use pictured items and/or manipulatives if necessary. Use any of the following stimulus words and/or others you select from the story. The correct answers are in parentheses.*

Stimulus set #1	Stimulus set #2
robin, whoopy	whoopy (robin)
January, droop	droop (January)
charming, whale	charming (whale)
hot, tree, Bombay	hot, tree (Bombay)
October, gale, mix	October, mix (gale)
toast, baubled, roars	toast, roars (baubled)
once, flippy, dressed	flippy, dressed (once)
soup, April, chicken, group	soup, chicken, group (April)
July, fishy, think, cool	July, fishy, cool (think)
crocodile, bangled, wind, door	bangled, wind, door (crocodile)

3. Identifying the missing word in a phrase or sentence.

What to say to the student: "Listen to the sentence I read. Tell me which word is missing the second time I read the sentence."

> **EXAMPLE** "'with chicken soup.' Listen again and tell me which word I leave out: 'with _____ soup.'" (chicken)

NOTE: *Use pictured items and/or manipulatives if necessary. Use any of the following stimulus sentences and/or others you select from the story. The correct answers are in parentheses.*

Stimulus items:

sliding ice. sliding _____. (ice)

sprinkle once. _____ once. (sprinkle)

hot chicken soup. hot _____ soup. (chicken)

Mix it twice. _____ it twice. (mix)

chicken soup with rice. chicken _____ with rice. (soup)

to be a robin. to be a _____. (robin)

I'll take a peep. I'll take a _____. (peep)

a bangled Christmas tree. a bangled Christmas _____. (tree)

I pepped them up. I _____ them up. (pepped)

paddle chicken soup with rice. paddle _____ soup with rice. (chicken)

4. Supplying the missing word as an adult reads.

What to say to the student: "I want you to help me read the story. You fill in the words I leave out."

> EXAMPLE   "chicken _____." (soup)

> **NOTE:** *Use pictured items and/or manipulatives if necessary. Use any of the following stimulus sentences and/or others you select from the story. The correct answers are in parentheses.*

Stimulus items:

sprinkle _____. (once, twice)

sipping _____ soup. (chicken)

I will ride a _____. (crocodile)

slipping on the sliding _____. (ice)

paddle once, paddle _____. (twice)

A butcher was cutting _____. (meat)

March wind blows _____ the door. (down)

I pepped them _____. (up)

witches, _____, and a ghost. (goblins)

concocting soup inside my _____. (nest)

5. Rearranging words.

What to say to the student: "I'll say some words out of order. You put them in the right order so they make sense."

> EXAMPLE   " 'soup chicken.' Put those words in the right order." (chicken soup)

> **NOTE:** *Use pictured items and/or manipulatives if necessary. Use any of the following stimulus words and/or others you select from the story. The correct answers are in parentheses. This word-level activity can be more difficult than some of the syllable- or phoneme-level activities because of the memory load. If your students are only able to deal with two or three words to be rearranged, add more two- and three-word samples from the story and omit the four-word level items.*

Stimulus items:

once sipping (sipping once)

tree Christmas (Christmas tree)

September in (in September)

with bowls soup (with soup bowls)

nest inside my (inside my nest)

rice with soup (soup with rice)

I twice told you (I told you twice)

I up pepped them (I pepped them up)

It up it laps (It laps it up)

while slipping on the ice sliding (while slipping on the sliding ice)

Phonological Awareness Activities at the Syllable Level

1. Syllable counting.

What to say to the student: "We're going to count syllables (or parts) of words."

> **EXAMPLE** "How many syllables do you hear in '_____'?" (stimulus word) (e.g., "How many syllables in 'ice'?") (1)

> **NOTE:** *Use pictured items and/or manipulatives if necessary. Use any of the following stimulus words and/or others you select from the story. Use any group of 10 stimulus items you select per teaching set.*

Stimulus items:

One-syllable words: peep, pot, be, blows, bowl, to, twice, take, toast, tail, tree, told, down, door, dream, day, dress, droop, deep, down, drape, cake, cool, course, go, group, gale, cheep, June, my, me, March, more, may, mix, nest, not, nice, soup, so, sip, spill, Spain, saw, spout, for, floor, far, flop, hot, him, host, rice, roars, ride, laps, with, while, once, will, wind, where, whale, think, then, year, and, it, up, off, old, oh, ice, all

Two-syllable words: paddle, blowing, Bombay, begin, become, baubled, bangled, truly, cooking, goblins, chicken, charming, gusty, July, merry, Nile, sliding, sipping, snowman, sprinkle, selling, soupy, spouting, season, fishy, flippy, happy, robin, roses, lightly, witches, whoopy, upon, away, about, inside, April, eating, over, August,

Three-syllable words: December, concocting, crocodile, November, slippery, September, October

Four-syllable words: January, February

Five-syllable word: anniversary

2. Initial syllable deleting.

What to say to the student: "We're going to leave out syllables (or parts of words)."

> **EXAMPLE** "Say '_____.'" (stimulus word) "Say it again without '_____.'" (stimulus syllable) (e.g., "Say 'cooking.' Say it again without 'cook.'") (ing)

> **NOTE:** *Use pictured items and/or manipulatives if necessary. Use any of the following stimulus words and/or others you select from the story. The correct answers are in parentheses.*

Stimulus items:

"Say 'robin' without 'rob.'" (in)

"Say 'snowman' without 'snow.'" (man)

"Say 'upon' without 'up.'" (on)

"Say 'spouting' without 'spout.'" (ing)

"Say 'goblins' without 'gob.'" (lins)

"Say 'December' without 'De-.'" (cember)

"Say 'inside' without 'in.'" (side)

"Say 'crocodile' without 'croc.'" (odile)

"Say 'October' without 'oct.'" (ober)

"Say 'lightly' without 'light.'" (lee)

3. Final syllable deleting.

What to say to the student: "We're going to leave out syllables (or parts of words)."

> **EXAMPLE** "Say '_____.'" (stimulus word) "Say it again without '_____.'" (stimulus syllable) (e.g., "Say 'blowing' without 'ing.'") (blow)

> **NOTE:** *Use pictured items and/or manipulatives if necessary. Use any of the following stimulus words and/or others you select from the story. The correct answers are in parentheses.*

Stimulus items:

"Say 'snowman' without 'man.'" (snow)

"Say 'robin' without 'in.'" (rob)

"Say 'Bombay' without 'bay.'" (Bom)

"Say 'lightly' without 'lee.'" (light)

"Say 'inside' without 'side.'" (in)

"Say 'charming' without 'ing.'" (charm)

"Say 'upon' without 'on.'" (up)

"Say 'concocting' without 'ing.'" (concoct)

"Say 'August' without 'ust.'" (Aug)

"Say 'crocodile' without 'dile.'" (croco)

4. Initial syllable adding.

What to say to the student: "Now let's add syllables (or parts) to words."

> **EXAMPLE** "Add '_____'" (stimulus syllable) "to the beginning of '_____.'" (stimulus syllable) (e.g., "Add 'charm' to the beginning of 'ing.'") (charming)

> **NOTE:** *Use pictured items and/or manipulatives if necessary. Use any of the following stimulus words and/or others you select from the story. The correct answers are in parentheses.*

Stimulus items:

"Add 'in' to the beginning of 'side.'" (inside)

"Add 'sip' to the beginning of '-ing.'" (sipping)

"Add 'Bom' to the beginning of 'bay.'" (Bombay)

"Add 'snow' to the beginning of 'man.'" (snowman)

"Add 'eat' to the beginning of 'ing.'" (eating)

"Add 'gob' to the beginning of 'lins.'" (goblins)

"Add 'rob' to the beginning of 'in.'" (robin)

"Add 'No' to the beginning of 'vember.'" (November)

"Add 'light' to the beginning of 'lee.'" (lightly)

"Add 'seize' to the beginning of '-uns.'" (seasons)

5. Final syllable adding.

What to say to the student: "Now let's add syllables (or parts) to words."

> **EXAMPLE** "Add '_____'" (stimulus syllable) "to the end of '_____.'" (stimulus syllable) (e.g., "Add 'ing' to the end of 'cook.'") (cooking)

> **NOTE:** *Use pictured items and/or manipulatives if necessary. Use any of the following stimulus words and/or others you select from the story. The correct answers are in parentheses.*

Stimulus items:

"Add 'in' to the end of 'rob.'" (robin)

"Add 'man' to the end of 'snow.'" (snowman)

"Add 'ber' to the end of 'Novem.'" (November)

"Add '-ing' to the end of 'sip.'" (sipping)

"Add '-ee' to the end of 'whoop.'" (whoopy)

"Add '-ing' to the end of 'eat.'" (eating)

"Add 'on' to the end of 'up.'" (upon)

"Add 'way' to the end of 'a.'" (away)

"Add 'lins' to the end of 'gob.'" (goblins)

"Add 'dile' to the end of croco-" (crocodile)

6. Syllable substituting.

What to say to the student: "Let's make up some new words."

> **EXAMPLE** "Say '_____.'" (stimulus word) "Instead of '_____'" (stimulus syllable), "say '_____.'" (stimulus syllable) (e.g., "Say 'cutting.' Instead of 'cut,' say 'bake.' The new word is 'baking.'")

> **NOTE:** *Use pictured items and/or manipulatives if necessary. Use of the following stimulus words and/or others you select from the story. The correct answers are in parentheses.*

Stimulus items:

"Say 'snowman.' Instead of 'snow,' say 'door.'" (doorman)

"Say 'cooking.' Instead of 'cook,' say 'charm.'" (charming)

"Say 'slipping.' Instead of '-ing,' say '-er.'" (slipper)

"Say 'witches.' Instead of 'witch,' say 'rose.'" (roses)

"Say 'selling.' Instead of '-ing,' say '-er.'" (seller)

"Say 'baubled.' Instead of 'baub,' say 'bang.'" (bangled)

"Say 'inside.' Instead of 'side,' say 'put.'" (input)

"Say 'blowing.' Instead of '-ing,' say '-er.'" (blower)

"Say 'truly.' Instead of 'true,' say 'light.'" (lightly)

"Say 'begin.' Instead of 'be,' say 'rob.'" (robin)

Phonological Awareness Activities at the Phoneme Level

1. Counting sounds.

What to say to the student: "We're going to count sounds in words."

> **EXAMPLE**   "How many sounds do you hear in this word: 'not'?" (3)

> **NOTE:** *Use pictured items and/or manipulatives if necessary. Use any of the following stimulus words and/or others you select from the story. Be sure to give the letter sound, not the letter name. Use any group of 10 stimulus items you select per teaching set.*

Stimulus words with two sounds: be, to, day, go, my, me, may, so, saw, it, up, off, all, ice

Stimulus words with three sounds: take, tail, tree, deep, down, cake, cool, gale, cheep, June, March, not, Nile, nice, soup, sip, hot, him, rice, ride, with, will, whale, then, its, and, old, away

Stimulus words with four sounds: pepped, paddle, twice, toast, told, dream, dressed, droop, group, July, mix, nest, Spain, soupy, spout, fishy, happy, host, laps, whoopy, upon, about

Stimulus words with five sounds: chicken, draped, gusty, spills, flippy, robin, roses, lightly, inside, April

2. Sound categorization or identifying a rhyme oddity.

What to say to the student: "Guess which word I say doesn't rhyme with the other three words."

> **EXAMPLE**   "Tell me which word doesn't rhyme with the other three words: '_____,' '_____,' '_____,' '_____.'" (stimulus words) (e.g., "'cool,' 'pool,' 'gusty,' 'tool.' Which word doesn't rhyme with the other three words?") (gusty)

> **NOTE:** *Use pictured items if necessary. Use any of the following stimulus words and/or others you select from the story. The correct answers are in parentheses.*

Stimulus items:

ice, group, rice, nice (group)

toast, roast, boast, March (March)

cheep, leap, floor, Jeep (floor)

robin, gale, bale, whale (robin)

June, dune, soon, whale (whale)

dream, beam, whoopy, seem (whoopy)

gusty, rusty, fishy, dusty (fishy)

floppy, fishy, mishy, wishy (floppy)

soup, chicken, hoop, loop (chicken)

witches, twitches, itches, goblins (goblins)

3. Matching rhyme.

What to say to the student: "We're going to think of rhyming words."

> **EXAMPLE** "Which word rhymes with '_____'?" (stimulus word) (e.g., "Which word rhymes with 'take': 'chicken,' 'host,' 'cake,' 'group'?") (cake)

> **NOTE:** *Use pictured items if necessary. Use any of the following stimulus words and/or others you select from the story. The correct answers are in parentheses.*

Stimulus items:

flop: merry, goblins, cop, door (cop)

chicken: licken, rice, witches, go (licken)

rose: whoopy, toes, bangled, flop (toes)

dream: happy, think, group, seem (seem)

Nile: pile, fishy, Christmas, soupy (pile)

rice: January, cake, ice, think (ice)

sipping: crocodile, wind, robin, dripping (dripping)

witches: whale, riches, February, soup (riches)

charming: goblins, October, March, farming (farming)

merry: cheep, July, berry, ride (berry)

4. Producing rhyme.

What to say to the student: "Now we'll say rhyming words."

> **EXAMPLE** "Tell me a word that rhymes with '_____.'" (stimulus word) (e.g., "Tell me a word that rhymes with 'day.' You can make up a word if you want.") (say)

> **NOTE:** *Use pictured items if necessary. Use any of the following stimulus words and/or others you select from the story (i.e., you say a word from the list below and the student is to think of a rhyming word). Use any group of 10 stimulus items you select per teaching set.*

Stimulus items:

/p/: pepped, peep, pot, paddle

/b/: be, blows, blowing, Bombay, begin, become, baubled, bangled, bowls

/t/: to, twice, truly, take, toast, tail, tree, told

/d/: down, door, dream, day, dressed, droop, deep, down, December, draped

/k/: cake, concocting, cool, cooking, crocodile, Christmas

/g/: go, group, goblins, gusty, gale

/ch/: chicken, charming, cheep

/dz/ (as in gem): January, June, July

/m/: my, me, March, more, may, mix, merry

/n/: nest, not, Nile, November, nice

/s/: soup, so, slippery, sliding, sip, sipping, snowman's, spills, Spain, saw, sprinkle, selling, September, soupy, spout, spouting, seasons

/f/: February, for, floor, far, fishy, flop, flippy

/h/: hot, him, happy, host

/r/: rice, roars, robin, roses, ride

/l/: laps, lightly

/w/: with, while, once, will, wind, where, witches, whoopy, whale

/voiceless th/: think

/voiced th/: then

/y/ (as in yellow): year

/short I/: in, its, it, inside

/short A/: anniversary, and

/short U/: about, upon, up

/short O/: off, August, all, October

/long A/: April

/long E/: eating

/long I/: ice

/long O/: over, old

5. Sound matching (initial).

What to say to the student: "Now we'll listen for the first sound in words."

> **EXAMPLE** "Listen to this sound: / /." (stimulus sound). "Guess which word I say begins with that sound: '_____,' '_____,' '_____,' '_____.'" (stimulus words) (e.g., "Listen to this sound: /f/. Guess which word I say begins with that sound: 'merry,' 'far,' 'roses,' 'once.'") (far)

NOTE: *Give the letter sound, not the letter name. Use pictured items if necessary. Use any of the following stimulus words and/or others you select from the story. The correct answers are in parentheses.*

Stimulus items:

/ch/: floor, think, chicken, once (chicken)

/s/: gusty, soup, bangled, tree (soup)

/r/: baubled, draped, sip, rice (rice)

/h/: February, hot, roars, become (hot)

/f/: Nile, flippy, cooking, blowing (flippy)

/w/: tail, mix, witches, dream (witches)

/k/: Christmas, gusty, begin, lightly (Christmas)

/long A/: chicken, toast, April, blows (April)

/g/: rest, goblins, witches, door (goblins)

/long E/: bowl, crocodile, host, eating (eating)

6. Sound matching (final).

What to say to the student: "Now we'll listen for the last sound in words."

> **EXAMPLE** "Listen to this sound: / /" (stimulus sound). "Guess which word I say ends with that sound: '_____,' '_____,' '_____,' '_____.'" (stimulus words) (e.g., "Listen to this sound: /t/. Guess which word I say ends with that sound: 'cool,' 'host,' 'July,' 'nice.'") (host)

> **NOTE:** *Give the letter sound, not the letter name. Use pictured items and/or manipulatives if necessary. Use any of the following stimulus words and/or others you select from the story. The correct answers are in parentheses.*

Stimulus items:

/s/: March, rice, gusty, told (rice)

/t/: roses, bowls, draped, where (draped)

/z/: seasons, June, paddle, twice (seasons)

/ng/: nice, sprinkle, cooking, snowman (cooking)

/n/: blowing, chicken, baubled, ghost (chicken)

/long E/: sip, eating, spills, February (February)

/v/: April, serve, March, papped (serve)

/d/: about, bangled, whoopy, three (bangled)

/r/: off, Spain, September, inside (September)

/long A/: over, sprinkle, Bombay, far (Bombay)

7. Identifying the initial sound in words.

What to say to the student: "I'll say a word two times. Tell me what sound is missing the second time: '_____,' '_____.'" (stimulus words)

> **EXAMPLE** "What sound do you hear in '_____'" (stimulus word) "that is missing in '_____'?" (stimulus word) (e.g., "What sound do you hear in 'laps' that is missing in 'aps'?") (/l/)

> **NOTE:** *Give the letter sound, not the letter name. Use pictured items and/or manipulatives if necessary. Use any of the following stimulus words and/or others you select from the story. The correct answers are in parentheses.*

Stimulus items:

"rice, ice. What sound do you hear in 'rice' that is missing in 'ice'?" (/r/)

"gale, ale. What sound do you hear in 'gale' that is missing in 'ale'?" (/g/)

"more, ore. What sound do you hear in 'more' that is missing in 'ore'?" (/m/)

"nice, ice. What sound do you hear in 'nice' that is missing in 'ice'?" (/n/)

"Spain, pain. What sound do you hear in 'Spain' that is missing in 'pain'?" (/s/)

"flop, lop. What sound do you hear in 'flop' that is missing in 'lop'?" (/f/)

"think, ink. What sound do you hear in 'think' that is missing in 'ink'?" (/th/)

"year, ear. What sound do you hear in 'year' that is missing in 'ear'?" (/y/)

"charm, arm. What sound do you hear in 'charm' that is missing in 'arm'?" (/ch/)

"witches, itches. What sound do you hear in 'witches' that is missing in 'itches'?" (/w/)

8. Identifying the final sound in words.

What to say to the student: "I'll say a word two times. Tell me what sound is missing the second time: '_____,' '_____.'" (stimulus words)

> **EXAMPLE** "What sound do you hear in '_____'" (stimulus word) "that is missing in '_____'?" (stimulus word) (e.g., "What sound do you hear in 'laps' that is missing in 'lap'?") (/s/)

> **NOTE:** *Give the letter sound, not the letter name. Use pictured items and/or manipulatives if necessary. Use any of the following stimulus words and/or others you select from the story. The correct answers are in parentheses.*

Stimulus items:

"rice, rye. What sound do you hear in 'rice' that is missing in 'rye'?" (/s/)

"soupy, soup. What sound do you hear in 'soupy' that is missing in 'soup'?" (/long E/)

"once, one. What sound do you hear in 'once' that is missing in 'one'?" (/s/)

"gusty, gust. What sound do you hear in 'gusty' that is missing in 'gust'?" (/long E/)

"bangled, bangle. What sound do you hear in 'bangled' that is missing in 'bangle'?" (/d/)

"group, grew.' What sound do you hear in 'group' that is missing in 'grew'?" (/p/)

"mix, Mick. What sound do you hear in 'mix' that is missing in 'Mick'?" (/s/)

"wind, win. What sound do you hear in 'wind' that is missing in 'win'?" (/d/)

"whoopy, whoop. What sound do you hear in 'whoopy' that is missing in 'whoop'?" (/long E/)

"goblins, goblin. What sound do you hear in 'goblins' that is missing in 'goblin'?" (/z/)

9. Segmenting the initial sound in words.

What to say to the student: "Listen to the word I say and tell me the first sound you hear."

> **EXAMPLE** "What's the first sound in '_____'?" (stimulus word) (e.g., "What's the first sound in 'soup'?") (/s/)

> **NOTE:** *Give the letter sound, not the letter name. Use pictured items and/or manipulatives if necessary. Use any of the following stimulus words and/or others you select from the story. Use any group of 10 stimulus items you select per teaching set.*

Stimulus items:

/p/: pepped, peep, pot, paddle

/b/: be, blows, blowing, Bombay, begin, become, baubled, bangled, bowls

/t/: to, twice, truly, take, toast, tail, tree, told

/d/: down, door, dream, day, dressed, droop, deep, down, December, draped

/k/: cake, concocting, cool, cooking, crocodile, Christmas

/g/: go, group, goblins, gusty, gale

/ch/: chicken, charming, cheep

/dz/ (as in gem) January, June, July

/m/: my, me, March, more, may, mix, merry

/n/: nest, not, Nile, November, nice

/s/: soup, so, slippery, sliding, sip, sipping, snowman's, spills, Spain, saw, sprinkle, selling, September, soupy, spout, spouting, seasons

/f/: February, for, floor, far, fishy, flop, flippy

/h/: hot, him, happy, host

/r/: rice, roars, robin, roses, ride

/l/: laps, lightly

/w/: with, while, once, will, wind, where, witches, whoopy, whale

/voiceless th/: think

/voiced th/: then

/y/ (as in yellow): year

/short I/: in, its, it, inside

/short A/: anniversary, and

/short U/: about, upon, up

/short O/: off, August, all, October

/long A/: April

/long E/: eating

/long I/: ice

/long O/: over, old

10. Segmenting the final sound in words.

What to say to the student: "Listen to the word I say and tell me the last sound you hear."

> **EXAMPLE** "What's the last sound in the word '_____'?" (stimulus word) (e.g., "What's the last sound in the word 'host'?") (/t/)

NOTE: *Give the letter sound, not the letter name. Use pictured items and/or manipulatives if necessary. Use any of the following stimulus words and/or others you select from the story. Use any group of 10 stimulus items you select per teaching set.*

Stimulus items:

/p/: soup, sip, up, group, droop, pep, peep, deep, cheap, flop

/t/: hot, it, about, best, dressed, nest, pepped, August, not, host, ghost, toast, draped, that

/d/: wind, and, old, inside, ride, baubled, bangled, told

/k/: cake, think, take

/m/: him, dream, them

/n/: chicken, in, upon, Spain, robin, June, begin

/ng/: slipping, sliding, sipping, blowing, concocting, charming, selling, cooking, spouting, eating

/s/: rice, it's, nice, ice, once, twice, laps, mix

/z/: seasons, snowman's, blows, spills, roars, is, roses, bowls

/f/: off

/v/: serve

/r/: year, are, for, door, over, floor, more, far, where, September, October, November, December

/l/: all, while, April, will, sprinkle, Nile, paddle, I'll, gale, tail

/long A/: away, Bombay, day, May

/long E/: be, lightly, fishy, soupy, whoopy, gusty, flippy, three, me, January, February, anniversary, happy, truly

/long I/: my, July, why

/long O/: so, go

11. Generating words from the story beginning with a particular sound.

What to say to the student: "Let's think of words **from the story** that start with certain sounds."

> EXAMPLE "Tell me a word from the story that starts with / /." (stimulus sound) (e.g., "the sound /b/.") (Bombay)

NOTE: *Give the letter sound, not the letter name. Use pictured items if necessary. Use any of the following stimulus words and/or others you select from the story. You say the sound (e.g., a voiceless /p/ sound), and the student is to say a word from the story that begins with that sound. Use any group of 10 stimulus items you select per teaching set.*

Stimulus items:

/p/: pepped, peep, pot, paddle

/b/: be, blows, blowing, Bombay, begin, become, baubled, bangled, bowls

/t/: to, twice, truly, take, toast, tail, tree, told

/d/: down, door, dream, day, dressed, droop, deep, down, December, draped

/k/: cake, concocting, cool, cooking, crocodile, Christmas

/g/: go, group, goblins, gusty, gale

/ch/: chicken, charming, cheep

/dz/ (as in gem): January, June, July

/m/: my, me, March, more, may, mix, merry

/n/: nest, not, Nile, November, nice

/s/: soup, so, slippery, sliding, sip, sipping, snowman's, spills, Spain, saw, sprinkle, selling, September, soupy, spout, spouting, seasons

/f/: February, for, floor, far, fishy, flop, flippy

/h/: hot, him, happy, host

/r/: rice, roars, robin, roses, ride

/l/: laps, lightly

/w/: with, while, once, will, wind, where, witches, whoopy, whale

/voiceless th/: think

/voiced th/: then

/y/ (as in yellow): year

/short I/: in, its, it, inside

/short A/: anniversary, and

/short U/: about, upon, up

/short O/: off, August, all, October

/long A/: April

/long E/: eating

/long I/: ice

/long O/: over, old

12. Blending sounds in monosyllabic words divided into onset/rime beginning with a two-consonant cluster + rime.

What to say to the student: "Now we'll put sounds together to make words."

> **EXAMPLE** "Put these sounds together to make a word: / / + / /." (stimulus sounds)
> "What's the word?" (e.g., "fl + ip: What's the word?") (flip)

NOTE: *Give the letter sound, not the letter name. Use pictured items and/or manipulatives if necessary. Use any of the following stimulus words and/or others you select from the story. The correct answers are in parentheses.*

Stimulus items:

dr + eem (dream)

fl + or (floor)

fl + op (flop)

gr + oop (group)

sl + ide (slide)

sn + oh (snow)

sp + ain (Spain)

dr + ess (dress)

sl + ip (slip)

dr + oop (droop)

13. Blending sounds in monosyllabic words divided into onset/rime beginning with a single consonant + rime.

What to say to the student: "Let's put sounds together to make words."

EXAMPLE "Put these sounds together to make a word: (/ / + / /)." (stimulus sounds) "What's the word?" (e.g., "/g/ + ale: What's the word?") (gale)

NOTE: *Give the letter sound, not the letter name. Use pictured items and/or manipulatives if necessary. Use any of the following stimulus words and/or others you select from the story. The correct answers are in parentheses.*

Stimulus items:

/f/ + ish (fish)

/g/ + ust (gust)

/s/ + oop (soup)

/r/ + ice (rice)

/p/ + eep (peep)

/m/ + icks (mix)

/k/ + ache (cake)

/t/ + oast (toast)

/p/ + ot (pot)

/w/ + ith (with)

14. Blending sounds to form a monosyllabic word beginning with a continuant sound.

What to say to the student: "We'll put sounds together to make words."

EXAMPLE "Put these sounds together to make a word (/ / + / / + / /)." (stimulus sounds) (e.g., "/s/ /short I/ /p/.") (sip)

NOTE: *Give the letter sound, not the letter name. Use pictured items and/or manipulatives if necessary. Use any of the following stimulus words and/or others you select from the story. The correct answers are in parentheses.*

Stimulus items:

/m/ /long E/ (me)

/s/ /oo/ /p/ (soup)

/m/ /long A/ (may)

/w/ /short I/ /n/ /d/ (wind)

/f/ /short I/ /sh/ (fish)

/r/ /long I/ /s/ (rice)

/w/ /long A/ /l/ (whale)

/r/ /long O/ /z/ (rose)

/n/ /short E/ /s/ /t/ (nest)

/r/ /long I/ /d/ (ride)

15. Blending sounds to form a monosyllabic word beginning with a noncontinuant sound.

What to say to the student: "We'll put sounds together to make words."

> EXAMPLE "Put these sounds together to make a word (/ / + / / + / /)." (stimulus sounds) (e.g., "/g/ /long O/.") (go)

> **NOTE:** *Give the letter sound, not the letter name. Use pictured items and/or manipulatives if necessary. Use any of the following stimulus words and/or others you select from the story. The correct answers are in parentheses.*

Stimulus items:

/p/ /long E/ /p/ (peep)

/t/ /long A/ /k/ (take)

/p/ /ah/ /t/ (pot)

/d/ /long A/ (day)

/k/ /long A/ /k/ (cake)

/t/ /long O/ /l/ /d/ (told)

/d/ /long E/ /p/ (deep)

/dz/ (as in gem) /oo/ /n/ (June)

/g/ /long A/ /l/ (gale)

/ch/ /long E/ /p/ (cheep)

16. Substituting the initial sound in words.

What to say to the student: "We're going to change beginning/first sounds in words."

> EXAMPLE "Say '_____.'" (stimulus word) "Instead of / /" (stimulus sound), "say / /." (stimulus sound) (e.g., "Say 'fish.' Instead of /f/, say /d/. What's your new word?") (dish)

> **NOTE:** *Give the letter sound, not the letter name. Use pictured items and/or manipulatives if necessary. Use any of the following stimulus words and/or others you select from the story. The correct answers are in parentheses.*

Stimulus items:

"Say 'cheep.' Instead of /ch/, say /p/." (peep)

 "Say 'took.' Instead of /t/, say /k/." (cook)

"Say 'hot.' Instead of /h/, say /p/." (pot)

"Say 'tail.' Instead of /t/, say /f/." (fail)

"Say 'soup.' Instead of /s/, say /g/." (goop)

"Say 'nile.' Instead of /n/, say /f/." (file)

"Say 'gust.' Instead of /g/, say /r/." (rust)

"Say 'door.' Instead of /d/, say /m/." (more)

"Say 'rice.' Instead of /r/, say /n/." (nice)

"Say 'mix.' Instead of /m/, say /f/." (fix)

17. Substituting the final sound in words.

What to say to the student: "We're going to change ending/last sounds in words."

> **EXAMPLE** "Say '_____.'" (stimulus word) "Instead of / /" (stimulus sound), "say / /." (stimulus sound) (e.g., "Say 'in.' Instead of /n/, say /t/. What's your new word?") (it)

> **NOTE:** *Give the letter sound, not the letter name. Use pictured items and/or manipulatives if necessary. Use any of the following stimulus words and/or others you select from the story. The correct answers are in parentheses.*

Stimulus items:

"Say 'hot.' Instead of /t/, say /p/." (hop)

"Say 'march.' Instead of /ch/, say /k/." (mark)

"Say 'rice.' Instead of /s/, say /p/." (ripe)

"Say 'him.' Instead of /m/, say /t/." (hit)

"Say 'rose.' Instead of /z/, say /p/." (rope)

"Say 'soup.' Instead of /p/, say /t/." (suit)

"Say 'serve.' Instead of /v/, say /ch/." (search)

"Say 'draped.' Instead of /t/, say /s/." (drapes)

"Say 'floppy.' Instead of /long E/, say /t/." (flopped)

"Say 'home.' Instead of /m/, say /p/." (hope)

18. Segmenting the middle sound in monosyllabic words.

What to say to the student: "Tell me the middle sound in the word I say."

> **EXAMPLE** "What's the middle sound in the word '_____'?" (stimulus word) (e.g., "What's the middle sound in the word 'back'?") (/short A/)

> **NOTE:** *Give the letter sound, not the letter name. Use pictured items and/or manipulatives if necessary. Use any of the following stimulus words and/or others you select from the story. The correct answers are in parentheses.*

Stimulus items:

hot (/ah/)

fish (/short I/)

June (/oo/)

rice (/long I/)

soup (/oo/)

tree (/r/)

deep (/long E/)

rose (/long O/)

whale (/long A/)

cake (/long A/)

19. Substituting the middle sound in words.

What to say to the student: "We're going to change the middle sound in words."

> **EXAMPLE** "Say '_____.'" (stimulus word) "Instead of / /" (stimulus sound), "say / /." (stimulus sound) (e.g., "Say 'flop.' Instead of /ah/, say /short I/. What's your new word?") (flip)

> **NOTE:** *Give the letter sound, not the letter name. Use pictured items and/or manipulatives if necessary. Use any of the following stimulus words and/or others you select from the story. The correct answers are in parentheses.*

Stimulus items:

"Say 'soup.' Instead of /oo/, say /short I/." (sip)

"Say 'host.' Instead of /long O/, say /long A/." (haste)

"Say 'rice.' Instead of /long I/, say /long A/." (race)

"Say 'gale.' Instead of /long A/, say /long O/." (goal)

"Say 'dream.' Instead of /long E/, say /short U/." (drum)

"Say 'nice.' Instead of /long I/, say /long E/." (niece)

"Say 'whale.' Instead of /long A/, say /long I/." (while)

"Say 'not.' Instead of /ah/, say /short E/." (net)

"Say 'tail.' Instead of /long A/, say /long I/." (tile)

"Say 'paddle.' Instead of /short A/, say /short U/." (puddle)

20. Identifying all sounds in monosyllabic words.

What to say to the student: "Now tell me all the sounds you hear in the word I say."

> **EXAMPLE** "What sounds do you hear in the word '_____'?" (stimulus word) (e.g., "What sounds do you hear in the word 'hot'?") (/h/ /ah/ /t/)

> **NOTE:** *Give the letter sound, not the letter name. Use pictured items and/or manipulatives if necessary. Use any of the following stimulus words and/or others you select from the story. The correct answers are in parentheses.*

Stimulus items:

tail (/t/ /long A/ /l/)

rice (/r/ /long I/ /s/)

gale (/g/ /long A/ /l/)

sip (/s/ /short I/ /p/)

cool (/k/ /oo/ /l/)

tree (/t/ /r/ /long E/)

soup (/s/ /oo/ /p/)

cake (/k/ /long A/ /k/)

rose (/r/ /long O/ /z/)

flop (/f/ /l/ /ah/ /p/)

21. Deleting sounds within words.

What to say to the student: "We're going to leave out sounds in words."

> **EXAMPLE** "Say '_____'" (stimulus word) "without / /." (stimulus sound) (e.g., "Say 'flip' without /l/.") (fip) Say "The word that is left—'fip'—isn't a real word. Sometimes, the word won't be a real word.

> **NOTE:** *Give the letter sound, not the letter name. Use pictured items and/or manipulatives if necessary. Use any of the following stimulus words and/or others you select from the story. The correct answers are in parentheses.*

Stimulus items:

"Say 'nest' without /s/." (net)

"Say 'Spain' without /p/." (sane)

"Say 'tree' without /r/." (tee)

"Say 'blow' without /l/." (bow)

"Say 'true' without /r/." (too)

"Say 'floor' without /l/." (for)

"Say 'toast' without /s/." (tote)

"Say 'group' without /r/." (goop)

"Say 'dream' without /r/." (deem)

"Say 'snow' without /n/." (so)

22. Substituting consonants in words having a two-sound cluster.

What to say to the student: "We're going to substitute sounds in words."

> **EXAMPLE** "Say '_____.'" (stimulus word) "Instead of / /" (stimulus sound), "say / /." (stimulus sound) (e.g., "Say 'stop.' Instead of /t/, say /l/.") (slop) Say: "Sometimes, the new word won't be a real word."

> **NOTE:** *Give the letter sound, not the letter name. Use pictured items and/or manipulatives if necessary. Use any of the following stimulus words and/or others you select from the story. The correct answers are in parentheses.*

Stimulus items:

"Say 'blow.' Instead of /l/, say /r/." (bro)

"Say 'snow.' Instead of /n/, say /l/." (slow)

"Say 'gust.' Instead of /t/, say /p/." (gusp)

"Say 'laps.' Instead of /p/, say /k/." (lacks)

"Say 'and.' Instead of /d/, say /t/." (ant)

"Say 'slide.' Instead of /l/, say /p/." (spied)

"Say 'Spain.' Instead of /p/, say /l/." (slain)

"Say 'spout.' Instead of /p/, say /k/." (scout)

"Say 'slippery.' Instead of /l/, say /k/." (skippery)

"Say 'crocodile.' Instead of /r/, say /l/." (clockodile)

23. Phoneme reversing.

What to say to the student: "We're going to say words backward."

> **EXAMPLE** "Say the word '_____'" (stimulus word) "backward." (e.g., "Say 'peep' backward.") (peep)

> **NOTE:** *This is a difficult phoneme-level task and should only be done with older students. Give the letter sound, not the letter name. Use pictured items and/or manipulatives if necessary. Use any of the following stimulus words and/or others you select from the story. The correct answers are in parentheses.*

Stimulus items:

eat (tea)

ice (sigh)

lap (pal)

sell (less)

nice (sign)

more (roam)

Spain (napes)

spill (lips)

roar (roar)

my (I'm)

24. Phoneme switching.

What to say to the student: "We're going to switch the first sounds in two words."

> **EXAMPLE** "Switch the first sounds in '_____' and '_____.'" (stimulus words) (e.g., "Switch the first sounds in 'so' and 'hot.'") (ho sot)

NOTE: *This is a difficult phoneme-level task and should only be done with older students. Give the letter sound, not the letter name. Use pictured items and/or manipulatives if necessary. Use any of the following stimulus words and/or others you select from the story. The correct answers are in parentheses.*

Stimulus items:

so nice (no sice)

be my (me by)

my soup (sy moup)

hot soup (sot hoop)

my nest (ny mest)

soup bowls (boop soles)

will go (gill woe)

soupy Nile (noopy sile)

with rice (rith wice)

chicken soup (sicken choop)

25. Pig Latin.

What to say to the student: "We're going to speak a secret language by using words from the story. In pig Latin, you take off the first sound of a word, put it at the end of the word, and add an 'ay' sound."

EXAMPLE "Say 'dog' in pig Latin." (ogday)

NOTE: *This is a difficult phoneme-level task and should only be done with older students. Use pictured items and/or manipulatives if necessary. Use any of the following stimulus words and/or others you select from the story. The correct answers are in parentheses.*

Stimulus items:

fish (ishfay)

rose (oseray)

rice (iceray)

June (unejay)

take (aketay)

soup (oopsay)

toast (oasttay)

goblin (oblingay)

chicken (ickenchay)

whale (aleway)

From Phonological Awareness into Print

NOTE: *Only five examples per activity are included in this resource due to space. You are encouraged to add many more words into this section that you feel your student(s) is(are) ready to write.*

1. Substituting the initial sound or letter in words.

NOTE: *Use lined paper or copy the sheet of lined paper included in the back of this book.*

Stimulus items:

1.1 to/do

Task a. "Say 'to.' Instead of /t/, say /d/. What's your new word?" (do) "Write/copy 'to' and 'do.'"

Task b. "Circle the **letters** that make the words different." ([t], [d])

Task c. "What **sounds** do these letters make?" (/t/, /d/)

1.2 be/me

Task a. "Say 'be.' Instead of /b/, say /m/. What's your new word?" (me) "Write/copy 'be' and 'me.'"

Task b. "Circle the **letters** that make the words different." ([b], [m])

Task c. "What **sounds** do these letters make?" (/b/, /m/)

1.3 rice/nice

Task a. "Say 'rice.' Instead of /r/, say /n/. What's your new word?" (nice) "Write/copy 'rice' and 'nice.'"

Task b. "Circle the **letters** that make the words different." ([r], [n])

Task c. "What **sounds** do these letters make?" (/r/, /n/)

1.4 gale/tale

Task a. "Say 'gale.' Instead of /g/, say /t/. What's your new word?" (tale) "Write/copy 'gale' and 'tale.'"

Task b. "Circle the **letters** that make the words different." ([g], [t])

Task c. "What **sounds** do these letters make?" (/g/, /t/)

1.5 hot/pot

Task a. "Say 'hot.' Instead of /h/, say /p/. What's your new word?" (pot) "Write/copy 'hot' and 'pot.'"

Task b. "Circle the **letters** that make the words different." ([h], [p])

Task c. "What **sounds** do these letters make?" (/h/, /p/)

2. Substituting the final sound or letter in words.

NOTE: *Use lined paper or copy the sheet of lined paper included in the back of this book.*

Stimulus items:

2.1 me/my
> **Task a.** "Say 'me.' Instead of /long E/, say /long I/. What's your new word?" (my) "Write/copy 'me' and 'my.'"
>
> **Task b.** "Circle the **letters** that make the words different." ([e], [y])
>
> **Task c.** "What **sounds** do these letters make?" (/long E/, /long I/)

2.2 up/us
> **Task a.** "Say 'up.' Instead of /p/, say /s/. What's your new word?" (us) "Write/copy 'up' and 'us.'"
>
> **Task b.** "Circle the **letters** that make the words different." ([p], [s])
>
> **Task c.** "What **sounds** do these letters make?" (/p/, /s/)

2.3 not/nod
> **Task a.** "Say 'not.' Instead of /t/, say /d/. What's your new word?" (nod) "Write/copy 'not' and 'nod.'"
>
> **Task b.** "Circle the **letters** that make the words different." ([t], [d])
>
> **Task c.** "What **sounds** do these letters make?" (/t/, /d/)

2.4 cheep/cheek
> **Task a.** "Say 'cheep.' Instead of /p/, say /k/. What's your new word?" (cheek) "Write/copy 'cheep' and 'cheek.'"
>
> **Task b.** "Circle the **letters** that make the words different." ([p], [k])
>
> **Task c.** "What **sounds** do these letters make?" (/p/, /k/)

2.5 wind/wins
> **Task a.** "Say 'wind.' Instead of /d/, say /z/. What's your new word?" (wins) "Write/copy 'wind' and 'wins.'"
>
> **Task b.** "Circle the **letters** that make the words different." ([d], [s])
>
> **Task c.** "What **sounds** do these letters make?" (/d/, /z/)

3. Substituting the middle sound or letter in words.

NOTE: *Use lined paper or copy the sheet of lined paper included in the back of this book.*

Stimulus items:

3.1 pot/pet
> **Task a.** "Say 'pot.' Instead of /ah/, say /short E/. What's your new word?" (pet) "Write/copy 'pot' and 'pet.'"
>
> **Task b.** "Circle the **letters** that make the words different." ([o], [e])
>
> **Task c.** "What **sounds** do these letters make?" (/ah/, /short E/)

3.2 him/ham

Task a. "Say 'him.' Instead of /short I/, say /short A/. What's your new word?" (ham) "Write/copy 'him' and 'ham.'"

Task b. "Circle the **letters** that make the words different." ([i], [a])

Task c. "What **sounds** do these letters make?" (/short I/, /short A/)

3.3 rose/rise

Task a. "Say 'rose.' Instead of /long O/, say /long I/. What's your new word?" (rise) "Write/copy 'rose' and 'rise.'"

Task b. "Circle the **letters** that make the words different." ([o], [i])

Task c. "What **sounds** do these letters make?" (/long O/, /long I/)

3.4 sip/sap

Task a. "Say 'sip.' Instead of /short I/, say /short A/. What's your new word?" (sap) "Write/copy 'sip' and 'sap.'"

Task b. "Circle the **letters** that make the words different." ([i], [a])

Task c. "What **sounds** do these letters make?" (/short I/, /short A/)

3.5 June/Jane

Task a. "Say 'June.' Instead of /oo/, say /long A/. What's your new word?" (Jane) "Write/copy 'June' and 'Jane.'"

Task b. "Circle the **letters** that make the words different." ([u], [a])

Task c. "What **sounds** do these letters make?" (/oo/, /long A/)

4. Supplying the initial sound or letter in words.

NOTE: *Use lined paper or copy the sheet of lined paper included in the back of this book.*

Stimulus items:

4.1 rice/ice

Task a. "Say 'rice,' say 'ice.' What sound did you hear in 'rice' that is missing in 'ice'?" (/r/) "Now we'll change the **letter.** Write/copy 'rice' and 'ice.'"

Task b. "Circle the beginning **letter** that makes the words different." ([r])

Task c. "What **sound** does this letter make?" (/r/)

4.2 tail/ail

Task a. "Say 'tail,' say 'ail.' What sound did you hear in 'tail' that is missing in 'ail'?" (/t/) "Now we'll change the **letter.** Write/copy 'tail' and 'ail.'"

Task b. "Circle the beginning **letter** that makes the words different." ([t])

Task c. "What **sound** does this letter make?" (/t/)

4.3 more/ore

Task a. "Say 'more,' say 'ore.' What sound did you hear in 'more' that is missing in 'ore'?" (/m/) "Now we'll change the **letter.** Write/copy 'more' and 'ore.'"

Task b. "Circle the beginning **letter** that makes the words different." ([m])

Task c. "What **sound** do these letters make?" (/m/)

4.4 blow/low

Task a. "Say 'blow,' say 'low.' What sound did you hear in 'blow' that is missing in 'low'?" (/b/) "Now we'll change the **letter.** Write/copy 'blow' and 'low.'"

Task b. "Circle the beginning **letter** that makes the words different." ([b])

Task c. "What **sound** does this letter make?" (/b/)

4.5 spill/pill

Task a. "Say 'spill,' say 'pill.' What sound did you hear in 'spill' that is missing in 'pill'?" (/s/) "Now we'll change the **letter.** Write/copy 'spill' and 'pill.'"

Task b. "Circle the beginning **letter** that makes the words different." ([s])

Task c. "What **sound** does this letter make?" (/s/)

5. Supplying the final sound or letter in words.

NOTE: *Use lined paper or copy the sheet of lined paper included in the back of this book.*

Stimulus items:

5.1 laps/lap

Task a. "Say 'laps,' say 'lap.' What sound did you hear in 'laps' that is missing in 'lap'?" (/s/) "Now we'll change the **letter.** Write/copy 'laps' and 'lap.'"

Task b. "Circle the ending/last **letter** that makes the words different." ([s])

Task c. "What **sound** does this letter make?" (/s/)

5.2 its/it

Task a. "Say 'its,' say 'it.' What sound did you hear in 'its' that is missing in 'it'?" (/s/) "Now we'll change the **letter.** Write/copy 'its' and 'it.'"

Task b. "Circle the ending/last **letter** that makes the words different." ([s])

Task c. "What **sound** does this letter make?" (/s/)

5.3 wind/win

Task a. "Say 'wind,' say 'win.' What sound did you hear in 'wind' that is missing in 'win'?" (/d/) "Now we'll change the **letter.** Write/copy 'wind' and 'win.'"

Task b. "Circle the ending/last **letter** that makes the words different." ([d])

Task c. "What **sound** does this letter make?" (/d/)

5.4 bowls/bowl

Task a. "Say 'bowls,' say 'bowl.' What sound did you hear in 'bowls' that is missing in 'bowl'?" (/z/) "Now we'll change the **letter.** Write/copy 'bowls' and 'bowl.'"

Task b. "Circle the ending/last **letter** that makes the word different." ([s])

Task c. "What **sound** does this letter make?" (/z/)

5.5 whoopy/whoop

Task a. "Say 'whoopy,' say 'whoop.' What sound did you hear in 'whoopy' that is missing in 'whoop'?" (/long E/) "Now we'll change the **letter.** Write/copy 'whoopy' and 'whoop.'"

Task b. "Circle the ending/last **letter** that makes the words different." ([y])

Task c. "What **sound** does this letter make?" (/long E/)

6. Switching the first sound and letter in words (ADVANCED).

NOTE: *Use lined paper or copy the sheet of lined paper included in the back of this book.*

Stimulus items:

6.1 so nice

Task a. "Say 'so,' say 'nice.' What sound do you hear at the beginning of 'so'?" (/s/) "What sound do you hear at the beginning of 'nice'?" (/n/) "Switch the first sounds in those words." (no sice) "Now we'll change the **letters.** Write/copy 'so nice' and 'no sice.'"

Task b. "Circle the beginning **letters** that change the words." ([s], [n])

Task c. "What **sounds** do those letters make?" (/s/, /n/)

6.2 be my

Task a. "Say 'be,' say 'my.' What sound do you hear at the beginning of 'be'?" (/b/) "What sound do you hear at the beginning of 'my'?" (/m/) "Switch the first sounds in those words." (me by) "Now we'll change the **letters.** Write/copy 'be my' and 'me by.'"

Task b. "Circle the beginning **letters** that change the words." ([b], [m])

Task c. "What **sounds** do those letters make?" (/b/, /m/)

6.3 my nest

Task a. "Say 'my,' say 'nest.' What sound do you hear at the beginning of 'my'?" (/m/) "What sound do you hear at the beginning of 'nest'?" (/n/) "Switch the first sounds in those words." (ny mest) "Now we'll change the **letters.** Write/copy 'my nest' and 'ny mest.'"

Task b. "Circle the beginning **letters** that change the words." ([m], [n])

Task c. "What **sounds** do those letters make?" (/m/, /n/)

6.4 with rice

Task a. "Say 'with,' say 'rice.' What sound do you hear at the beginning of 'with'?" (/w/) "What sound do you hear at the beginning of 'rice'?" (/r/) "Switch the first sounds in those words." (rith wice) "Now we'll change the **letters.** Write/copy 'with rice' and 'rith wice.'"

Task b. "Circle the beginning **letters** that change the words." ([w], [r])

Task c. "What **sounds** do those letters make?" (/w/, /r/)

6.5 my soup

Task a. "Say 'my,' say 'soup.' What sound do you hear at the beginning of 'my'?" (/m/) "What sound do you hear at the beginning of 'soup'?" (/s/) "Switch the first sounds in those words." (sy moup) "Now we'll change the **letters.** Write/copy 'my soup' and 'sy moup.'"

Task b. "Circle the beginning **letters** that change the words." ([m], [s])

Task c. "What **sounds** do those letters make?" (/m/, /s/)

CHAPTER 6

Phonological Awareness Activities to Use with *Chrysanthemum*

Text version used for selection of stimulus items:

Henkes, K. (1991). *Chrysanthemum*. New York: Scholastic, Inc.

Phonological Awareness Activities at the Word Level

1. Counting words.

What to say to the student: "We're going to count words."

> **EXAMPLE** "How many words do you hear in this sentence (or phrase)? 'her name?'" (2)

Note: *Use pictured items and/or manipulatives if necessary. Use any of the following stimulus phrases or sentences and/or others you select from the story. The correct answers are in parentheses.*

Stimulus items:

bathroom mirror (2)

fat orange (2)

Chrysanthemum wilted (2)

raised her hand (3)

and it was (3)

on the first day (4)

your name is beautiful (4)

now put your head down (5)

lined up to go home (5)

school is no place for me (6)

2. Identifying the missing word from a list.

What to say to the student: "Listen to the words I say. I'll say them again. You tell me which word I leave out."

EXAMPLE "Listen to the words I say: 'dainty, pixie.' I'll say them again. Tell me which one I leave out: 'dainty.'" (pixie)

Note: *Use pictured items and/or manipulatives if necessary. Use any of the following stimulus words and/or others you select from the story. The correct answers are in parentheses.*

Stimulus set #1	Stimulus set #2
tag, flower	flower (tag)
Chrysanthemum, feet	feet (Chrysanthemum)
naptime, favorite, Lily	naptime, Lily (favorite)
fairy, macaroni, outfit	fairy, macaroni (outfit)
baby, sunniest, hooray	sunniest, hooray (baby)
Victoria, ketchup, night	Victoria, night (ketchup)
chocolate, winsome, teacher	chocolate, teacher (winsome)
valley, mistake, fascinating	valley, mistake (fascinating)
crayon, delphinium, butterfly	delphinium, butterfly (crayon)
Parcheesi, loaded, scrawny	Parcheesi, scrawny (loaded)

3. Identifying the missing word in a phrase or sentence.

What to say to the student: "Listen to the sentence I read. Tell me which word is missing the second time I read the sentence."

EXAMPLE "'gets ready for.' Listen again and tell me which word I leave out. 'gets ready _____.'" (for)

Note: *Use pictured items and/or manipulatives if necessary. Use any of the following stimulus sentences and/or others you select from the story. The correct answers are in parentheses.*

Stimulus items:

her name. her _____. (name)

grew and grew. grew and _____. (grew)

loved her name. loved her _____. (name)

on her birthday cake. _____ her birthday cake. (on)

"Hooray," said Chrysanthemum. "Hooray," said _____. (Chrysanthemum)

My name is too long. My _____ is too long. (name)

upon hearing Chrysanthemum's name. upon _____ Chrysanthemum's name. (hearing)

You're named after a flower. You're named _____ a flower. (after)

Now put your head down. Now put _____ head down. (your)

"Welcome home," said her mother. "Welcome _____," said her mother. (home)

4. Supplying the missing word as an adult reads.

What to say to the student: "I want you to help me read the story. You fill in the words I leave out."

> **EXAMPLE** "Mrs. _____." (Chud)

> **Note:** *Use pictured items and/or manipulatives if necessary. Use any of the following stimulus sentences and/or others you select from the story. The correct answers are in parentheses.*

Stimulus items:

She's _____. (perfect)

wore her _____ dress. (sunniest)

absolutely _____. (perfect)

macaroni and cheese and _____. (ketchup)

hugs and _____ and Parcheesi. (kisses)

She even looks like a _____. (flower)

I just cannot _____ your name. (believe)

Now put your head _____. (down)

She sprouted _____ and petals. (leaves)

Chrysanthemum could scarcely believe her _____. (ears)

5. Rearranging words.

What to say to the student: "I'll say some words out of order. You put them in the right order so they make sense."

> **EXAMPLE** " 'bloomed she.' Put those words in the right order." (she bloomed)

> **Note:** *Use pictured items and/or manipulatives if necessary. Use any of the following stimulus words and/or others you select from the story. The correct answers are in parentheses. This word-level activity can be more difficult than some of the syllable- or phoneme-level activities because of the memory load. If your students are only able to deal with two or three words to be rearranged, add more two- and three-word samples from the story and omit the four-word level items.*

Stimulus items:

it she loved (She loved it)

on cake her birthday (on her birthday cake)

she her sunniest dress wore (She wore her sunniest dress)

with her most possessions prized (with her most prized possessions)

it absolutely was dreadful (It was absolutely dreadful)

I'd it Victoria said change (I'd change it, Victoria said)

your is beautiful name (Your name is beautiful)

and I'm after a flower named (And I'm named after a flower)

chosen as the butterfly spiffy princess (chosen as the spiffy butterfly princess)

my name is Valley Lily of the (My name is Lily of the Valley)

Phonological Awareness Activities at the Syllable Level

1. Syllable counting.

What to say to the student: "We're going to count syllables (or parts) of words."

> **EXAMPLE** "How many syllables do you hear in '_____'?" (stimulus word)
> (e.g., "How many syllables do you hear in 'birth'?") (1)

Note: *Use pictured items and/or manipulatives if necessary. Use any of the following stimulus words and/or others you select from the story. Use any group of 10 stimulus items you select per teaching set.*

Stimulus items:

One-syllable words: put, place, pick, born, be, birth, took, tag, day, down, dream, dirt, cake, call, could, class, queen, course, Ken, could, grew, good, girl, gave, Chud, change, cheese, charms, just, Jo, Jane, must, much, most, make, made, Max, my, name, now, night, nick, knew, not, no, school, so, smell, stem, say, Sue, Sam, fat, first, fits, felt, feet, voice, her, hand, half, home, hugs, huge, wrote, ran, roll, rest, long, looks, left, life, led, luck, lines, Les, like, led, woke, wore, wish, worms, worst, went, way, she, thought, thank, think, your, would, I, Eve, each, on, all

Two-syllable words: perfect, pointing, precious, priceless, pleasant, playground, petals, pockets, princess, Pixie, bathroom, birthday, brightest, better, believe, trifle, teacher, Twinkle, dinner, dreadful, during, dirty, dessert, dainty, daisy, ketchup, kisses, cannot, giggled, garden, chosen, chanted, jumper, jealous, jaundiced, mother, mirror, morning, music, mistake, Mrs., naptime, neither, nothing, sounded, started, smile, scarcely, students, slowly, sprouted, scrawny, something, spiffy, speechless, success, father, flower, frosting, fairy, funny, forgot, valley, herself, hooray, hearing, healthy, written, really, Rita, letters, loaded, longest, Lily, Lois, whisper, wilted, welcome, winsome, thirteen, thinking, throughout, informed, after, answer, upon, until, about, outfit

Three-syllable words: Parcheesi, pretended, possessions, possible, beautiful, begrudging, buttercream, butterfly, carnation, completely, grandmother, chocolate, Marigold, humorous, longingly, exactly, introduced, impression, important, alphabet, exactly, extremely, envious, every, another, envelope

Four-syllable words: Delphinium, Chrysanthemum, miserably, macaroni, Victoria, appreciate, absolutely

2. Initial syllable deleting.

What to say to the student: "We're going to leave out syllables (or parts of words)."

> **EXAMPLE**   "Say '_____.'" (stimulus word) "Say it again without '_____.'"
> (stimulus syllable) (e.g., "Say 'dreadful.' Say it again without 'dread.'") (-ful)

> **Note:** *Use pictured items and/or manipulatives if necessary. Use any of the following stimulus words and/or others you select from the story. The correct answers are in parentheses.*

Stimulus items:

"Say 'grandmother' without 'grand.'" (mother)

"Say 'winsome' without 'win.'" (some)

"Say 'throughout' without 'through.'" (out)

Say 'birthday' without 'birth.'" (day)

"Say 'speechless' without 'speech.'" (less)

"Say 'garden' without 'gar.'" (den)

"Say 'Parcheesi' without 'par.'" (cheesy)

"Say 'carnation' without 'car.'" (nation)

"Say 'marigold' without 'mare.'" (-igold)

"Say 'hooray' without 'who.'" (ray)

3. Final syllable deleting.

What to say to the student: "We're going to leave out syllables (or parts of words)."

> **EXAMPLE**   "Say '_____.'" (stimulus word) "Say it again without '_____.'"
> (stimulus syllable) (e.g., "Say 'chanted' without '-ed.'") (chant)

> **Note:** *Use pictured items and/or manipulatives if necessary. Use any of the following stimulus words and/or others you select from the story. The correct answers are in parentheses.*

Stimulus items:

"Say 'birthday' without 'day.'" (birth)

"Say 'fascinating' without '-ing.'" (fascinate)

"Say 'ketchup' without 'up.'" (ketch-)

"Say 'something' without 'thing.'" (some)

"Say 'longingly' without 'lee.'" (longing)

"Say 'alphabet' without 'bet.'" (alpha)

"Say 'sunniest' without '-est.'" (sunny)

"Say 'Beaker' without '-er.'" (beak)

"Say 'carnation' without '-tion.'" (carnay-)

"Say 'Chrysanthemum' without 'mum.'" (Chrysanthe-)

4. Initial syllable adding.

What to say to the student: "Now let's add syllables (or parts) to words."

> `EXAMPLE` "Add '_____'" (stimulus syllable) "to the beginning of '_____.'" (stimulus syllable) (e.g., "Add 'low' to the beginning of 'iss.'") (Lois)

> **Note:** *Use pictured items and/or manipulatives if necessary. Use any of the following stimulus words and/or others you select from the story. The correct answers are in parentheses.*

Stimulus items:

"Add 'ketch' to the beginning of 'up.'" (ketchup)

"Add 'dread' to the beginning of 'full.'" (dreadful)

"Add 'in' to the beginning of 'formed.'" (informed)

"Add 'win' to the beginning of 'some.'" (winsome)

"Add 'out' to the beginning of 'fit.'" (outfit)

"Add 'point' to the beginning of '-ing.'" (pointing)

"Add 'speech' to the beginning of 'less.'" (speechless)

"Add 'ab' to the beginning of 'solutely.'" (absolutely)

"Add 'long' to the beginning of 'ingly.'" (longingly)

"Add 'be' to the beginning of 'grudging.'" (begrudging)

5. Final syllable adding.

What to say to the student: "Now let's add syllables (or parts) to words."

> `EXAMPLE` "Add '_____'" (stimulus syllable) "to the end of '_____.'" (stimulus syllable) (e.g., "Add '-est' to the end of 'long.'") (longest)

> **Note:** *Use pictured items and/or manipulatives if necessary. Use any of the following stimulus words and/or others you select from the story. The correct answers are in parentheses.*

Stimulus items:

"Add 'time' to the end of 'nap.'" (naptime)

"Add 'er' to the end of 'teach.'" (teacher)

"Add 'ing' to the end of 'frost.'" (frosting)

"Add 'ful' to the end of 'dread.'" (dreadful)

"Add 'gold' to the end of 'mari.'" (Marigold)

"Add 'it' to the end of 'favor.'" (favorite)

"Add 'less' to the end of 'speech.'" (speechless)

"Add 'us' to the end of 'gel.'" (jealous)

"Add 'ing' to the end of 'frost.'" (frosting)

"Add 'fly' to the end of 'butter.'" (butterfly)

6. Syllable substituting.

What to say to the student: "Let's make up some new words."

> **EXAMPLE** "Say '_____.'" (stimulus word) "Instead of '_____'" (stimulus syllable), "say '_____.'" (stimulus syllable) (e.g., "Say 'jumper.' Instead of 'jump,' say 'camp.' The new word is 'camper.'")

> **Note:** *Use pictured items and/or manipulatives if necessary. Use of the following stimulus words and/or others you select from the story. The correct answers are in parentheses.*

Stimulus items:

"Say 'herself.' Instead of 'her,' say 'him.'" (himself)

"Say 'pretended.' Instead of 'ed,' say 'ing.'" (pretending)

"Say 'dreadful.' Instead of 'ful,' say 'ing.'" (dreading)

"Say 'sunniest.' Instead of 'sun,' say 'fun'.'" (funniest)

"Say 'pointed.' Instead of 'ed,' say 'ing.'" (pointing)

"Say 'jealous.' Instead of 'gel,' say 'presh.'" (precious)

"Say 'throughout.' Instead of 'through,' say 'with.'" (without)

"Say 'overall.' Instead of 'all,' say 'run.'" (overrun)

"Say 'dreadful.' Instead of 'dread,' say 'hand.'" (handful)

"Say 'bathroom.' Instead of 'room,' say 'tub.'" (bathtub)

Phonological Awareness Activities at the Phoneme Level

1. Counting sounds.

What to say to the student: "We're going to count sounds in words."

> **EXAMPLE** "How many sounds do you hear in this word? 'Pat.'" (3)

> **Note:** *Use pictured items and/or manipulatives if necessary. Use any of the following stimulus words and/or others you select from the story. Be sure to give the letter sound, not the letter name. Use any group of 10 stimulus items you select per teaching set.*

Stimulus words with two sounds: Sue, be, day, Jo, my, so, say, I'm, Eve, each, on, up, out, all, Al, Kay

Stimulus words with three sounds: put, pick, Pat, pish, Bill, took, tag, Tom, dirt, Don, cake, call, Ken, could, grew, good, luck, gave, cheese, Jane, much, make, made, Sam, fat, feet, half, home, huge, ran, roll, wrote, route, life, led, Les, like, with, woke, wish, would, each, old, thought

Stimulus words with four sounds: place, better, baby, beamed, teacher, dinner, dress, dream, dirty, daisy, called, class, queen, change, Chud, just, must, many, most, Max, named, school, smile, smell, stem, seemed, fits, flower, filled, fairy, funny, hugs, rest, raised, roles, Rita, lives, loved, looked, lined, looks, leaves, left, Lily, Lois, worst, went, that's

Stimulus words with five sounds: plucked, prized, believe, blushed, bloomed, trifle, dragged, dessert, dainty, kisses, cannot, jumper, jealous, next, slowly, scales, spiffy, healthy, written, outfit, loaded, another

2. Sound categorization or identifying a rhyme oddity.

What to say to the student: "Guess which word I say doesn't rhyme with the other three words."

> EXAMPLE "Tell me which word does not rhyme with the other three: '_____,' '_____,' '_____,' '_____.'" (stimulus words) (e.g., "'tag,' 'sag,' 'wilted,' 'jag.' Which word doesn't rhyme?") (wilted)

Note: *Use pictured items if necessary. Use any of the following stimulus words and/or others you select from the story. The correct answers are in parentheses.*

Stimulus items:

name, fame, macaroni, same (macaroni)

flower, pockets, rockets, sockets (flower)

fax, Chrysanthemum, jacks, Max (Chrysanthemum)

Lily, silly, frilly, Marigold (Marigold)

hugs, Victoria, slugs, mugs (Victoria)

Chud, mud, sud, mirror (mirror)

cheese, please, chanted, tease (chanted)

birthday, feature, teacher, preacher (birthday)

cake, Delphinium, bake, make (Delphinium)

teacher, preacher, Twinkle, feature (Twinkle)

3. Matching rhyme.

What to say to the student: "We're going to think of rhyming words."

> EXAMPLE "Which word rhymes with '_____'?" (stimulus word) (e.g., "Which word rhymes with 'cake': 'name,' 'charms,' 'bake,' 'crayon'?") (bake)

Note: *Use pictured items if necessary. Use any of the following stimulus words and/or others you select from the story. The correct answers are in parentheses.*

Stimulus items:

jumper: Parcheesi, hooray, bumper, blushed (bumper)

spiffy: jiffy, carnation, beamed, beautiful (jiffy)

name: Chrysanthemum, lame, humorous, dessert (lame)

worms: completely, bathroom, frosting, firms (firms)

dreamed: begrudging, dainty, seemed, longingly (seemed)

chanted: macaroni, speechless, longest, ranted (ranted)

route: possessions, flower, pout, indescribable (pout)

Twinkle: something, Marigold, sprinkle, Delphinium (sprinkle) bloomed: zoomed, buttercream, impression, alphabet (zoomed)

Lily: whispered, miserably, grandmother, silly (silly)

4. Producing rhyme.

What to say to the student: "Now we'll say rhyming words."

> **EXAMPLE** "Tell me a word that rhymes with '_____.'" (stimulus word)
> (e.g., "Tell me a word that rhymes with 'flower.' You can make up a word if you want.") (power)

> **Note:** *Use pictured items if necessary. Use any of the following stimulus words and/or others you select from the story (i.e., you say a word from the list below and the student is to think of a rhyming word). Use any group of 10 stimulus items you select per teaching set.*

Stimulus items:

/p/: parents, perfect, pointing, put, place, precious, priceless, Parcheesi, pleasant, playground, pick, pretended, petals, plucked, pockets, prized, possessions, possible, princess, Pixie, Pat, pish

/b/: born, be, bathroom, birthday, brightest, better, beautiful, believe, begrudging, buttercream, butterfly, baby, blushed, beamed, bloomed, birth, Bill

/t/: took, tag, trifle, teacher, Tom, Twinkle

/d/: day, dinner, dress, dreadful, during, down, diner, Don, dream, dragged, dirty, dreamed, discontented, dessert, dainty, daisy, Delphinium

/k/: Chrysanthemum, called, cake, crayon, call, could, ketchup, kisses, comfortable, cannot, class, queen, considering, carnation, completely, course, Ken, Kay

/g/: grew, giggled, grandmother, garden, good, girl, gave

/ch/: Chud, change, cheese, chocolate, charms, chosen, chanted

/dz/ (as in gem): jumper, just, jealous, jaundiced, Jo, Jane

/m/: mother, must, mirror, many, miserably, much, macaroni, most, morning, music, make, musical, messenger, Marigold, made, mistake, Max, Mrs., my

/n/: name, naptime, now, night, neither, nothing, next, nice, knew, not, no, named

/s/: sounded, started, school, sunniest, smile, so, scarcely, spelled, students, slowly, smell, sprouted, scrawny, stem, seven, stopped, stared, seemed, say, something, scales, spiffy, speechless, success, Sue, Sam, said

/f/: father, fat, first, fits, flower, fascinating, felt, favorite, filled, feet, frosting, fairy, funny, forgot

/v/: voice, valley, Victoria

/h/: her, happiest, herself, hooray, hearing, hand, half, home, hugs, humorous, huge, healthy

/r/: written, wrote, ran, roll, rest, raised, really, route, roles, Rita

/l/: lives, loved, looked, long, letters, lined, looks, leaves, left, life, loaded, longest, led, luck, longingly, Lily, lines, Lois, Les, like

/w/, /wh/: with, what, when, woke, whispered, wore, wilted, wish, welcome, winsome, walked, worms, wouldn't, worst, wonder, went, way, wildly

/sh/: she, sharing

/voiceless th/: thought, thirteen, thank, things, thinking, throughout, think

/voiced th/: that's, there, then, the

/y/ (as in yellow): your

/short A/: absolutely, after, alphabet, answer, Al

/short U/: appreciate, up, upon, another, until, about, assigned

/short E/: everything, everyone, entire, explained, extremely, entered, envious, else, every

/short I/: in, informed, introduced, indescribable, impression, important, it, if

/long E/: enough, ink, evening, ears, eventually, Eve, exactly, each

/long I/: I, I'm, icing

/long O/: old, orange, overall

/ah/: all, on

/ou/: out, outfit

5. Sound matching (initial).

What to say to the student: "Now we'll listen for the first sound in words."

> **EXAMPLE** "Listen to this sound: / /." (stimulus sound). "Guess which word I say begins with that sound: '_____,' '_____,' '_____,' '_____.'" (stimulus words) (e.g., "Listen to this sound: /ch/. Guess which word I say begins with that sound: 'frosting,' 'nothing,' 'cheese,' 'giggled.'") (cheese)

> **Note:** *Give the letter sound, not the letter name. Use pictured items if necessary. Use any of the following stimulus words and/or others you select from the story. The correct answers are in parentheses.*

Stimulus items:

/k/: students, speechless, Chrysanthemum, favorite (Chrysanthemum)

/p/: Marigold, possessions, considering, hooray (possessions)

/w/: extremely, throughout, Delphinium, whispered (whispered)

/b/: sunniest, leaves, butterfly, longingly (butterfly)

/f/: happiest, fascinating, discontented, grandmother (fascinating)

/s/: completely, beautiful, scrawny, humorous (scrawny)

/ch/: chocolate, Parcheesi, happiest, appreciate (chocolate)

/short E/: wouldn't, thirteen, indescribable, envious (envious)

/t/: dreadful, teacher, jaundiced, miserably (teacher)

/m/: frosting, letters, sunniest, macaroni (macaroni)

6. Sound matching (final).

What to say to the student: "Now we'll listen for the last sound in words."

EXAMPLE "Listen to this sound: / /" (stimulus sound). "Guess which word I say ends with that sound: '_____,' '_____,' '_____,' _____.'" (stimulus words) (e.g., "Listen to this sound: /t/. Guess which word I say ends with that sound: 'home,' 'priceless,' 'enough,' 'happiest.'") (happiest)

Note: *Give the letter sound, not the letter name. Use pictured items and/or manipulatives if necessary. Use any of the following stimulus words and/or others you select from the story. The correct answers are in parentheses.*

Stimulus items:

/p/: throughout, music, ketchup, possessions (ketchup)

/s/: Chrysanthemum, jealous, beautiful, mistake (jealous)

/d/: bloomed, Delphinium, chocolate, macaroni (bloomed)

/long E/: comfortable, priceless, Parcheesi, humorous (Parcheesi)

/d/: grandmother, Chud, miserably, huge (Chud)

/t/: begrudging, chosen, outfit, longingly (outfit)

/voiceless th/: envelope, birth, Marigold, brightest (birth)

/n/: enough, considering, buttercream, impression (impression)

/long A/: eventually, birthday, mother, messenger (birthday)

/l/: frosting, butterfly, humorous, beautiful (beautiful)

7. Identifying the initial sound in words.

What to say to the student: "I'll say a word two times. Tell me what sound is missing the second time: '_____,' '_____.'" (stimulus words)

EXAMPLE "What sound do you hear in '_____'" (stimulus word) "that is missing in '_____'?" (stimulus word) (e.g., "What sound do you hear in 'made' that is missing in 'aid'?") (/m/)

Note: *Give the letter sound, not the letter name. Use pictured items and/or manipulatives if necessary. Use any of the following stimulus words and/or others you select from the story. The correct answers are in parentheses.*

Stimulus items:

"cake, ache. What sound do you hear in 'cake' that is missing in 'ache'?" (/k/)

"fairy, airy. What sound do you hear in 'fairy' that is missing in 'airy'?" (/f/)

"charms, arms. What sound do you hear in 'charms' that is missing in 'arms'?" (/ch/)

"name, aim. What sound do you hear in 'name' that is missing in 'aim'?" (/n/)

"school, cool. What sound do you hear in 'school' that is missing in 'cool'?" (/s/)

"hand, and. What sound do you hear in 'hand' that is missing in 'and'?" (/h/)

"cheese, ease. What sound do you hear in 'cheese' that is missing in 'ease'?" (/ch/)

"birth, earth. What sound do you hear in 'birth' that is missing in 'earth'?" (/b/)

"mother, other. What sound do you hear in 'mother' that is missing in 'other'?" (/m/)

"assigned, signed. What sound do you hear in 'assigned' that is missing in 'signed'?" (/uh/)

8. Identifying the final sound in words.

What to say to the student: "I'll say a word two times. Tell me what sound is missing the second time: '_____,' '_____.'" (stimulus words)

> **EXAMPLE** "What sound do you hear in '_____'" (stimulus word) "that is missing in '_____'?" (stimulus word) (e.g., "What sound do you hear in 'things' that is missing in 'thing'?") (/z/)

> **Note:** *Give the letter sound, not the letter name. Use pictured items and/or manipulatives if necessary. Use any of the following stimulus words and/or others you select from the story. The correct answers are in parentheses.*

Stimulus items:

"worms, worm. What sound do you hear in 'worms' that is missing in 'worm'?" (/z/)

"worst, worse. What sound do you hear in 'worst' that is missing in 'worse'?" (/t/)

"born, bore. What sound do you hear in 'born' that is missing in 'bore'?" (/n/)

"woke, woe. What sound do you hear in 'woke' that is missing in 'woe'?" (/k/)

"dirty, dirt. What sound do you hear in 'dirty' that is missing in 'dirt'?" (/long E/)

"stopped, stop. What sound do you hear in 'stopped' that is missing in 'stop'?" (/t/)

"hugs, hug. What sound do you hear in 'hugs' that is missing in 'hug'?" (/z/)

"like, lie. What sound do you hear in 'like' that is missing in 'lie'?" (/k/)

"Lily, Lil. What sound do you hear in 'Lily' that is missing in 'Lil'?" (/long E/)

"Max, Mack. What sound do you hear in 'Max' that is missing in 'Mack'?" (/s/)

9. Segmenting the initial sound in words.

What to say to the student: "Listen to the word I say and tell me the first sound you hear."

> **EXAMPLE** "What's the first sound in '_____'?" (stimulus word) (e.g., "What's the first sound in 'valley'?") (/v/)

> **Note:** *Give the letter sound, not the letter name. Use pictured items and/or manipulatives if necessary. Use any of the following stimulus words and/or others you select from the story. Use any group of 10 stimulus items you select per teaching set.*

Stimulus items:

/p/: parents, perfect, pointing, put, place, precious, priceless, Parcheesi, pleasant, playground, pick, pretended, petals, plucked, pockets, prized, possessions, possible, princess, Pixie, Pat, pish

/b/: born, be, bathroom, birthday, brightest, better, beautiful, believe, begrudging, buttercream, butterfly, baby, blushed, beamed, bloomed, birth, Bill

/t/: took, tag, trifle, teacher, Tom, Twinkle

/d/: day, dinner, dress, dreadful, during, down, diner, Don, dream, dragged, dirty, dreamed, discontented, dessert, dainty, daisy, Delphinium

/k/: Chrysanthemum, called, cake, crayon, call, could, ketchup, kisses, comfortable, cannot, class, queen, considering, carnation, completely, course, Ken, Kay

/g/: grew, giggled, grandmother, garden, good, girl, gave

/ch/: Chud, change, cheese, chocolate, charms, chosen, chanted

/dz/ (as in gem): jumper, just, jealous, jaundiced, Jo, Jane

/m/: mother, must, mirror, many, miserably, much, macaroni, most, morning, music, make, musical, messenger, Marigold, made, mistake, Max, Mrs., my

/n/: name, naptime, now, night, neither, nothing, next, nice, knew, not, no, named

/s/: sounded, started, school, sunniest, smile, so, scarcely, spelled, students, slowly, smell, sprouted, scrawny, stem, seven, stopped, stared, seemed, say, something, scales, spiffy, speechless, success, Sue, Sam, said

/f/: father, fat, first, fits, flower, fascinating, felt, favorite, filled, feet, frosting, fairy, funny, forgot

/v/: voice, valley, Victoria

/h/: her, happiest, herself, hooray, hearing, hand, half, home, hugs, humorous, huge, healthy

/r/: written, wrote, ran, roll, rest, raised, really, route, roles, Rita

/l/: lives, loved, looked, long, letters, lined, looks, leaves, left, life, loaded, longest, led, luck, longingly, Lily, lines, Lois, Les, like

/w/, /wh/: with, what, when, woke, whispered, wore, wilted, wish, welcome, winsome, walked, worms, wouldn't, worst, wonder, went, way, wildly

/sh/: she, sharing

/voiceless th/: thought, thirteen, thank, things, thinking, throughout, think

/voiced th/: that's, there, then, the

/y/ (as in yellow): your

/short A/: absolutely, after, alphabet, answer, Al

/short U/: appreciate, up, upon, another, until, about, assigned

/short E/: everything, everyone, entire, explained, extremely, entered, envious, else, every

/short I/: in, informed, introduced, indescribable, impression, important, it, if

/long E/: enough, ink, evening, ears, eventually, Eve, exactly, each

/long I/: I, I'm, icing

/long O/: old, orange, overall

/ah/: all, on

/ou/: out, outfit

10. Segmenting the final sound in words.

What to say to the student: "Listen to the word I say and tell me the last sound you hear."

EXAMPLE "What's the last sound in the word '_____'?" (stimulus word)
(e.g., "What's the last sound in the word 'half'?") (/f/)

Note: *Give the letter sound, not the letter name. Use pictured items and/or manipulatives if necessary. Use any of the following stimulus words and/or others you select from the story. Use any group of 10 stimulus items you select per teaching set.*

Stimulus items:

/p/: up, ketchup

/t/: happiest, perfect, must, appreciate, looked, wrote, fat, thought, first, sunniest, brightest, rest, alphabet, thought, felt, favorite, night, pleasant, next, most, walked, feet, dirty, just, cannot, wouldn't, dessert, chocolate, picked, left, worst, outfit, longest, route, stopped, introduced, out, about, went, important, blushed, forgot, throughout

/d/: named, old, loved, sounded, called, whispered, started, giggled, wilted, raised, hand, informed, spelled, head, lined, could, filled, dreamed, dragged, entered, playground, pretended, discontented, jaundiced, sprouted, loaded, prized, stared, seemed, good, led, assigned, chanted, beamed, bloomed, Marigold

/k/: woke, cake, took, think, thank, pick, look, luck, music, like, make, mistake

/g/: tag

/m/: Chrysanthemum, name, bathroom, naptime, home, welcome, winsome, dream, buttercream, stem, Delphinium, Tom

/n/: born, when, written, crayon, then, ran, everyone, upon, thirteen, down, even, garden, one, seven, impression, chosen, queen, carnation, Jane

/ng/: everything, icing, hearing, long, during, sharing, morning, frosting, evening, nothing, something, evening, thinking, considering

/s/: parents, dress, fits, place, precious, priceless, looks, place, jealous, envious, pockets, students, voice, else, speechless, class, princess, humorous, success, dance, course, Max, Lois, Les

/z/: lives, letters, yours, cheese, hugs, kisses, worms, things, leaves, petals, possessions, scales, roles, ears, lines, Mrs.

/v/: believe, gave, of

/r/: father, mother, dinner, mirror, wore, after, grandmother, flower, better, entire, dinner, wore, jumper, neither, after, there, nightmare, wore, teacher, wonder, messenger, answer

/l/: school, smile, roll, call, dreadful, beautiful, comfortable, smell, all, trifle, until, possible, indescribable, girl, overall, Bill, Twinkle

/sh/: wish, pish

/voiceless th/: birth, with

/long A/: day, birthday, way, hooray, say, they, Kay

/long E/: absolutely, scarcely, exactly, many, miserably, macaroni, Parcheesi, slowly, extremely, dirty, miserably, scrawny, every, dainty, fairy, spiffy, Pixie, daisy, wildly, funny, baby, longingly, Lily, valley, only, completely, eventually, healthy

/long I/: butterfly, my

/long O/: Jo

/oo/: Sue, grew, you, too, knew

/uh/: Victoria, Rita

11. Generating words from the story beginning with a particular sound.

What to say to the student: "Let's think of words from the story that start with certain sounds."

> **EXAMPLE** "Tell me a word from the story that starts with / /." (stimulus sound) (e.g., the sound /f/) (father)

Note: *Give the letter sound, not the letter name. Use pictured items if necessary. Use any of the following stimulus words and/or others you select from the story. You say the sound (e.g., a voiceless /p/ sound), and the student is to say a word from the story that begins with that sound. Use any group of 10 stimulus items you select per teaching set.*

Stimulus items:

/p/: parents, perfect, pointing, put, place, precious, priceless, Parcheesi, pleasant, playground, pick, pretended, petals, plucked, pockets, prized, possessions, possible, princess, Pixie, Pat, pish

/b/: born, be, bathroom, birthday, brightest, better, beautiful, believe, begrudging, buttercream, butterfly, baby, blushed, beamed, bloomed, birth, Bill

/t/: took, tag, trifle, teacher, Tom, Twinkle

/d/: day, dinner, dress, dreadful, during, down, diner, Don, dream, dragged, dirty, dreamed, discontented, dessert, dainty, daisy, Delphinium

/k/: Chrysanthemum, called, cake, crayon, call, could, ketchup, kisses, comfortable, cannot, class, queen, considering, carnation, completely, course, Ken, Kay

/g/: grew, giggled, grandmother, garden, good, girl, gave

/ch/: Chud, change, cheese, chocolate, charms, chosen, chanted

/dz/ (as in gem): jumper, just, jealous, jaundiced, Jo, Jane

/m/: mother, must, mirror, many, miserably, much, macaroni, most, morning, music, make, musical, messenger, Marigold, made, mistake, Max, Mrs., my

/n/: name, naptime, now, night, neither, nothing, next, nice, knew, not, no, named

/s/: sounded, started, school, sunniest, smile, so, scarcely, spelled, students, slowly, smell, sprouted, scrawny, stem, seven, stopped, stared, seemed, say, something, scales, spiffy, speechless, success, Sue, Sam, said

/f/: father, fat, first, fits, flower, fascinating, felt, favorite, filled, feet, frosting, fairy, funny, forgot

/v/: voice, valley, Victoria

/h/: her, happiest, herself, hooray, hearing, hand, half, home, hugs, humorous, huge, healthy

/r/: written, wrote, ran, roll, rest, raised, really, route, roles, Rita

/l/: lives, loved, looked, long, letters, lined, looks, leaves, left, life, loaded, longest, led, luck, longingly, Lily, lines, Lois, Les, like

/w/, /wh/: with, what, when, woke, whispered, wore, wilted, wish, welcome, winsome, walked, worms, wouldn't, worst, wonder, went, way, wildly

/sh/: she, sharing

/voiceless th/: thought, thirteen, thank, things, thinking, throughout, think

/voiced th/: that's, there, then, the

/y/ (as in yellow): your

/short A/: absolutely, after, alphabet, answer, Al

/short U/: appreciate, up, upon, another, until, about, assigned

/short E/: everything, everyone, entire, explained, extremely, entered, envious, else, every

/short I/: in, informed, introduced, indescribable, impression, important, it, if

/long E/: enough, ink, evening, ears, eventually, Eve, exactly, each

/long I/: I, I'm, icing

/long O/: old, orange, overall

/ah/: all, on

/ou/: out, outfit

12. Blending sounds in monosyllabic words divided into onset–rime beginning with a two-consonant cluster + rime.

What to say to the student: "Now we'll put sounds together to make words."

> **EXAMPLE** "Put these sounds together to make a word: / / + / /." (stimulus sounds)
> "What's the word?" (e.g., "dr + ag: What's the word?") (drag)

> **Note:** *Give the letter sound, not the letter name. Use pictured items and/or manipulatives if necessary. Use any of the following stimulus words and/or others you select from the story. The correct answers are in parentheses.*

Stimulus items:

sk + ool (school)

ch + arms (charms)

kw + een (queen)

gr + oo (grew)

st + art (start)

fr + ost (frost)

st + opt (stopped)

bl + oom (bloom)

pl + ace (place)

bl + ush (blush)

13. Blending sounds in monosyllabic words divided into onset/rime beginning with a single consonant + rime.

What to say to the student: "Let's put sounds together to make words."

> **EXAMPLE** "Put these sounds together to make a word: / / + / /." (stimulus sounds)
> "What's the word?" (e.g., "/b/ + orn: What's the word?") (born)

Note: *Give the letter sound, not the letter name. Use pictured items and/or manipulatives if necessary. Use any of the following stimulus words and/or others you select from the story. The correct answers are in parentheses.*

Stimulus items:

/k/ + ache (cake)

/n/ + ame (name)

/p/ + ick (pick)

/t/ + ag (tag)

/h/ + and (hand)

/h/ + Ed (head)

/w/ + ilt (wilt)

/w/ + erms (worms)

/p/ + ish (pish)

/f/ + elt (felt)

14. Blending sounds to form a monosyllabic word beginning with a continuant sound.

What to say to the student: "We'll put sounds together to make words."

> **EXAMPLE** "Put these sounds together to make a word: / / + / / + / /." (stimulus sounds) (e.g., /m/ /uh/ /s/ /t/) (must)

Note: *Give the letter sound, not the letter name. Use pictured items and/or manipulatives if necessary. Use any of the following stimulus words and/or others you select from the story. The correct answers are in parentheses.*

Stimulus items:

/m/ /long O/ /s/ /t/ (most)

/h/ /long O/ /m/ (home)

/l/ /uh/ /k/ (luck)

/f/ /long E/ /t/ (feet)

/s/ /m/ /short E/ /l/ (smell)

/voiceless th/ /ah/ /t/ (thought)

/w/ /short I/ /sh/ (wish)

/v/ /oy/ /s/ (voice)

/m/ /short A/ /k/ /s/ (Max)

/n/ /short E/ /k/ /s/ /t/ (next)

15. Blending sounds to form a monosyllabic word beginning with a noncontinuant sound.

What to say to the student: "We'll put sounds together to make words."

> **EXAMPLE** "Put these sounds together to make a word: / / + / / + / /." (stimulus sounds) (e.g., /p/ /short I/ /k/) (pick)

Note: *Give the letter sound, not the letter name. Use pictured items and/or manipulatives if necessary. Use any of the following stimulus words and/or others you select from the story. The correct answers are in parentheses.*

Stimulus items:

/ch/ /uh/ /d/ (Chud)

/b/ /l/ /oo/ /m/ (bloom)

/dz/ (as in gem) /uh/ /s/ /t/ (just)

/g/ /long A/ /v/ (gave)

/k/ /w/ /long E/ /n/ (queen)

/p/ /l/ /long A/ /s/ (place)

/t/ /short A/ /g/ (tag)

/d/ /r/ /long E/ /m/ (dream)

/ch/ /long E/ /z/ (cheese)

/p/ /l/ /uh/ /k/ (pluck)

16. Substituting the initial sound in words.

What to say to the student: "We're going to change beginning/first sounds in words."

EXAMPLE "Say '_____.'" (stimulus word) "Instead of / /" (stimulus sound), "say / /." (stimulus sound) (e.g., "Say 'gave.' Instead of /g/, say /s/. What's your new word?") (save)

Note: *Give the letter sound, not the letter name. Use pictured items and/or manipulatives if necessary. Use any of the following stimulus words and/or others you select from the story. The correct answers are in parentheses.*

Stimulus items:

"Say 'name.' Instead of /n/, say /f/." (fame)

"Say 'pish.' Instead of /p/, say /d/." (dish)

"Say 'pick.' Instead of /p/, say /s/." (sick)

"Say 'feet.' Instead of /f/, say /m/." (meet)

"Say 'voice.' Instead of /v/, say /ch/." (choice)

"Say 'fairy.' Instead of /f/, say /h/." (hairy)

"Say 'petals.' Instead of /p/, say /m/." (metals)

"Say 'lily.' Instead of /l/, say /s/." (silly)

"Say 'thank.' Instead of /voiceless th/, say /y/." (yank)

"Say 'sharing.' Instead of /sh/, say /k/." (caring)

17. Substituting the final sound in words.

What to say to the student: "We're going to change ending/last sounds in words."

EXAMPLE   "Say '_____.'" (stimulus word) "Instead of / /" (stimulus sound), "say / /." (stimulus sound) (e.g., "Say 'made.' Instead of /d/, say /k/. What's your new word?") (make)

Note: *Give the letter sound, not the letter name. Use pictured items and/or manipulatives if necessary. Use any of the following stimulus words and/or others you select from the story. The correct answers are in parentheses.*

Stimulus items:

"Say 'life.' Instead of /f/, say /t/." (light)

"Say 'with.' Instead of /voiceless th/, say /t/." (wit)

"Say 'gave.' Instead of /v/, say /t/." (gate)

"Say 'place.' Instead of /s/, say /t/." (plate)

"Say 'name.' Instead of /m/, say /t/." (Nate)

"Say 'birth.' Instead of /voiceless th/, say /d/." (bird)

"Say 'night.' Instead of /t/, say /s/." (nice)

"Say 'Chud.' Instead of /d/, say /m/." (chum)

"Say 'home.' Instead of /m/, say /p/." (hope)

"Say 'stem.' Instead of /m/, say /p/." (step)

18. Segmenting the middle sound in monosyllabic words.

What to say to the student: "Tell me the middle sound in the word I say."

EXAMPLE   "What's the middle sound in the word '_____'?" (stimulus word) (e.g., "What's the middle sound in the word 'class'?") (/short A/)

Note: *Give the letter sound, not the letter name. Use pictured items and/or manipulatives if necessary. Use any of the following stimulus words and/or others you select from the story. The correct answers are in parentheses.*

Stimulus items:

name (/long A/)

pick (/short I/)

gave (/long A/)

dirt (/r/)

made (/long A/)

voice (/oy/)

cheese (/long E/)

fat (/short A/)

cake (/long A/)

beam (/long E/)

19. Substituting the middle sound in words.

What to say to the student: "We're going to change the middle sound in words."

> **EXAMPLE** "Say '_____.'" (stimulus word) "Instead of / /" (stimulus sound), "say / /." (stimulus sound) (e.g., "Say 'most.' Instead of /long O/, say /uh/. What's your new word?") (must)

Note: *Give the letter sound, not the letter name. Use pictured items and/or manipulatives if necessary. Use any of the following stimulus words and/or others you select from the story. The correct answers are in parentheses.*

Stimulus items:

"Say 'pick.' Instead of /short I/, say /short A/." (pack)

"Say 'luck.' Instead of /uh/, say /short I/." (lick)

"Say 'wish.' Instead of /short I/, say /ah/." (wash)

"Say 'cheese.' Instead of /long E/, say /long O/." (chose)

"Say 'gave.' Instead of /long A/, say /short I/." (give)

"Say 'beam.' Instead of /long E/, say /short A/." (bam)

"Say 'tag.' Instead of /short A/, say /uh/." (tug)

"Say 'Jane.' Instead of /long A/, say /short A/." (Jan)

"Say 'ran.' Instead of /short A/, say /uh/." (run)

"Say 'nice.' Instead of /long I/, say /long E/." (niece)

20. Identifying all sounds in monosyllabic words.

What to say to the student: "Now tell me all the sounds you hear in the word I say."

> **EXAMPLE** "What sounds do you hear in the word '_____'?" (stimulus word) (e.g., "What sounds do you hear in the word 'pick'?") (/p/ /short I/ /k/)

Note: *Give the letter sound, not the letter name. Use pictured items and/or manipulatives if necessary. Use any of the following stimulus words and/or others you select from the story. The correct answers are in parentheses.*

Stimulus items:

Chud (/ch/ /uh/ /d/)

ran (/r/ /short A/ /n/)

first (/f/ /r/ /s/ /t/)

birth (/b/ /r/ /voiceless th/)

name (/n/ /long A/ /m/)

luck (/l/ /uh/ /k/)

voice (/v/ /oy/ /s/)

blushed (/b/ /l/ /uh/ /sh/ /t/)

place (/p/ /l/ /long A/ /s/)

nap (/n/ /short A/ /p/)

21. Deleting sounds within words.

What to say to the student: "We're going to leave out sounds in words."

EXAMPLE "Say '_____'" (stimulus word) "without / /." (stimulus sound) (e.g., "Say 'grew' without /r/.") (goo) Say "The word that was left, 'goo,' is a real word. Sometimes the word won't be a real word."

Note: *Give the letter sound, not the letter name. Use pictured items and/or manipulatives if necessary. Use any of the following stimulus words and/or others you select from the story. The correct answers are in parentheses.*

Stimulus items:

"Say 'scales' without /k/." (sales)

"Say 'place' without /l/." (pace)

"Say 'queen' without /w/." (keen)

"Say 'prize' without /r/." (pies)

"Say 'play' without /l/." (pay)

"Say 'bright' without /r/." (bite)

"Say 'spell' without /p/." (sell)

"Say 'bloom' without /l/." (boom)

"Say 'stopped' without /t/." (sopped)

"Say 'slow' without /l/." (so)

22. Substituting consonants in words having a two-sound cluster.

What to say to the student: "We're going to substitute sounds in words."

EXAMPLE "Say '_____.'" (stimulus word) "Instead of / /" (stimulus sound), "say / /." (stimulus sound) (e.g., "Say 'stop.' Instead of /t/, say /l/.") (slop) Say: "Sometimes, the new word will be a made-up word."

Note: *Give the letter sound, not the letter name. Use pictured items and/or manipulatives if necessary. Use any of the following stimulus words and/or others you select from the story. The correct answers are in parentheses.*

Stimulus items:

"Say 'prize.' Instead of /p/, say /f/." (fries)

"Say 'play.' Instead of /l/, say /r/." (pray)

"Say 'bright.' Instead of /r/, say /l/." (blight)

"Say 'bloom.' Instead of /l/, say /r/." (broom)

"Say 'climbs.' Instead of /l/, say /r/." (crimes)

"Say 'grand.' Instead of /r/, say /l/." (gland)

"Say 'blush.' Instead of /l/, say /r/." (brush)

"Say 'pleasant.' Instead of /l/, say /r/." (present)

"Say 'grew.' Instead of /r/, say /l/." (glue)

"Say 'smell.' Instead of /m/, say /p/." (spell)

23. Phoneme reversing.

What to say to the student: "We're going to say words backward."

> **EXAMPLE** "Say the word '_____'" (stimulus word) "backward." (e.g., "Say 'bone' backward.") (nobe)

Note: *This is a difficult phoneme-level task and should only be done with older students. Give the letter sound, not the letter name. Use pictured items and/or manipulatives if necessary. Use any of the following stimulus words and/or others you select from the story. The correct answers are in parentheses.*

Stimulus items:

Sam (mass)

Chud (dutch)

pick (Kip)

fit (Tiff)

pish (ship)

made (dame)

name (main)

cake (cake)

day (aid)

stem (mets)

24. Phoneme switching.

What to say to the student: "We're going to switch the first sounds in two words."

> **EXAMPLE** "Switch the first sounds in '_____' and '_____.'" (stimulus words) (e.g., "Switch the first sounds in 'pedals' and 'bike.'") (bedals pike)

Note: *This is a difficult phoneme-level task and should only be done with older students. Give the letter sound, not the letter name. Use pictured items and/or manipulatives if necessary. Use any of the following stimulus words and/or others you select from the story. The correct answers are in parentheses.*

Stimulus items:

name tag (tame nag)

her voice (ver hoice)

first day (dirst fay)

birthday cake (kirthday bake)

head down (dead hown)

much better (buch metter)

hugs kisses (kugs hisses)

name Jane (jame nane)

daisy wilted (wazy dilted)

so long (lo song)

25. Pig Latin.

What to say to the student: "We're going to speak a secret language by using words from the story. In pig Latin, you take off the first sound of a word, put it at the end of the word, and add an 'ay' sound."

> **EXAMPLE**   "Say 'tag' in pig Latin." (agtay)

> **Note:** *This is a difficult phoneme-level task and should only be done with older students. Use pictured items and/or manipulatives if necessary. Use any of the following stimulus words and/or others you select from the story. The correct answers are in parentheses.*

Stimulus items:

Rita (eetaray)

Jane (anejay)

name (aimnay)

mother (othermay)

baby (aybeebay)

dessert (eezertday)

musical (useicalmay)

father (ahtherfay)

Parcheesi (archeesipay)

Victoria (ictoriavay)

From Phonological Awareness into Print

> **Note:** *Only six examples per activity are included in this resource due to space. You are encouraged to add many more words into this section that you feel your student(s) is(are) ready to write.*

1. Substituting the initial sound or letter in words.

> **Note:** *Use lined paper or copy the sheet of lined paper included in the back of this book.*

Stimulus items:

1.1. day/say

> **Task a.** "Say 'day.' Instead of /d/, say /s/. What's your new word?" (say) "Write/copy 'day' and 'say.'"
>
> **Task b.** "Circle the **letters** that make the words different." ([d], [s])
>
> **Task c.** "What **sounds** do these letters make?" (/d/, /s/)

1.2. born/torn

> **Task a.** "Say 'born.' Instead of /b/, say /t/. What's your new word?" (torn) "Write/copy 'born' and 'torn.'"
>
> **Task b.** "Circle the **letters** that make the words different." ([b], [t])
>
> **Task c.** "What **sounds** do these letters make?" (/b/, /t/)

1.3. name/fame

> **Task a.** "Say 'name.' Instead of /n/, say /f/. What's your new word?" (fame) "Write/copy 'name' and 'fame.'"
>
> **Task b.** "Circle the **letters** that make the words different." ([n], [f])
>
> **Task c.** "What **sounds** do these letters make?" (/n/, /f/)

1.4. hug/bug

> **Task a.** "Say 'hug.' Instead of /h/, say /b/. What's your new word?" (bug) "Write/copy 'hug' and 'bug.'"
>
> **Task b.** "Circle the **letters** that make the words different." ([h], [b])
>
> **Task c.** "What **sounds** do these letters make?" (/h/, /b/)

1.5. jumper/bumper

> **Task a.** "Say 'jumper.' Instead of /dz/, as in say /b/. What's your new word?" (bumper) "Write/copy 'jumper' and 'bumper.'"
>
> **Task b.** "Circle the **letters** that make the words different." ([j, [b])
>
> **Task c.** "What **sounds** do these letters make?" (/dz/ [as in gem], /b/)

2. Substituting the final sound or letter in words.

> **Note:** *Use lined paper or copy the sheet of lined paper included in the back of this book.*

Stimulus items:

2.1. feet/fees

> **Task a.** "Say 'feet.' Instead of /t/, say /z/. What's your new word?" (fees) "Write/copy 'feet' and 'fees.'"
>
> **Task b.** "Circle the **letters** that make the words different." ([t], [s])
>
> **Task c.** "What **sounds** do these letters make?" (/t/, /z/)

2.2. ran/rat

Task a. "Say 'ran.' Instead of /n/, say /t/. What's your new word?" (rat) "Write/copy 'ran' and 'rat.'"

Task b. "Circle the **letters** that make the words different." ([n], [t])

Task c. "What **sounds** do these letters make?" (/n/, /t/)

2.3. she/shy

Task a. "Say 'she.' Instead of /long E/, say /long I/. What's your new word?" (shy) "Write/copy 'she' and 'shy.'"

Task b. "Circle the **letters** that make the words different." ([e], [y])

Task c. "What **sounds** do these letters make?" (/long E/, /long I/)

2.4. stem/step

Task a. "Say 'stem.' Instead of /m/, say /p/. What's your new word?" (step) "Write/copy 'stem' and 'step.'"

Task b. "Circle the **letters** that make the words different." ([m], [p])

Task c. "What **sounds** do these letters make?" (/m/, /p/)

2.5. Chud/chum

Task a. "Say 'chud.' Instead of /d/, say /m/. What's your new word?" (chum) "Write/copy 'chud' and 'chum.'"

Task b. "Circle the **letters** that make the words different." ([d], [m])

Task c. "What **sounds** do these letters make?" (/d/, /m/)

3. **Substituting the middle sound or letter in words.**

Note: *Use lined paper or copy the sheet of lined paper included in the back of this book.*

Stimulus items:

3.1. tag/tug

Task a. "Say 'tag.' Instead of /short A/, say /uh/. What's your new word?" (tug) "Write/copy 'tag' and 'tug.'"

Task b. "Circle the **letters** that make the words different." ([a], [u])

Task c. "What **sounds** do these letters make?" (/short A/, /uh/)

3.2. fat/fit

Task a. "Say 'fat.' Instead of /short A/, say /short I/. What's your new word?" (fit) "Write/copy 'fat' and 'fit.'"

Task b. "Circle the **letters** that make the words different." ([a], [i])

Task c. "What **sounds** do these letters make?" (/short A/, /short I/)

3.3. luck/lock

Task a. "Say 'luck.' Instead of /uh/, say /ah/. What's your new word?" (lock). Write/copy 'luck' and 'lock.'"

Task b. "Circle the **letters** that make the words different." ([u], [o])

Task c. "What **sounds** do these letters make?" (/uh/, /ah/)

3.4. pick/pack

Task a. "Say 'pick.' Instead of /short I/, say /short A/. What's your new word?" (pack) "Write/copy 'pick' and 'pack.'"

Task b. "Circle the **letters** that make the words different." ([i], [a])

Task c. "What **sounds** do these letters make?" (/short I/, /short A/)

3.5. pocket/picket

Task a. "Say 'pocket.' Instead of /ah/, say /short I/. What's your new word?" (picket) "Write/copy 'pocket' and 'picket.'"

Task b. "Circle the **letters** that make the words different." ([o], [i])

Task c. "What **sounds** do these letters make?" (/ah/, /short I/)

4. Supplying the initial sound or letter in words.

Note: *Use lined paper or copy the sheet of lined paper included in the back of this book.*

Stimulus items:

4.1. fit/it

Task a. "Say 'fit,' say 'it.' What sound did you hear in 'fit' that is missing in 'it'?" (/f/) "Now we'll change the **letter**. Write/copy 'fit' and 'it.'"

Task b. "Circle the beginning **letter** that makes the words different." ([f])

Task c. "What **sound** does this letter make?" (/f/)

4.2. many/any

Task a. "Say 'many,' say 'any.' What sound did you hear in 'many' that is missing in 'any'?" (/m/) "Now we'll change the **letter**. Write/copy 'many' and 'any.'"

Task b. "Circle the beginning **letter** that makes the words different." ([m])

Task c. "What **sound** does this letter make?" (/m/)

4.3. nice/ice

Task a. "Say 'nice,' say 'ice.' What sound did you hear in 'nice' that is missing in 'ice'?" (/n/) "Now we'll change the **letter**. Write/copy 'nice' and 'ice.'"

Task b. "Circle the beginning **letter** that makes the words different." ([n])

Task c. "What **sound** do these letters make?" (/n/)

4.4. place/lace

> **Task a.** "Say 'place,' say 'lace.' What sound did you hear in 'place' that is missing in 'lace'?" (/p/) "Now we'll change the **letter**. Write/copy 'place' and 'lace.'"
>
> **Task b.** "Circle the beginning **letter** that makes the words different." ([p])
>
> **Task c.** "What **sound** does this letter make?" (p/)

4.5. trifle/rifle

> **Task a.** "Say 'trifle,' say 'rifle.' What sound did you hear in 'trifle' that is missing in 'rifle'?" (/t/) "Now we'll change the **letter**. Write/copy 'trifle' and 'rifle.'"
>
> **Task b.** "Circle the beginning **letter** that makes the words different." ([t])
>
> **Task c.** "What **sound** do this letter make?" (/t/)

5. Supplying the final sound or letter in words.

> **Note:** *Use lined paper or copy the sheet of lined paper included in the back of this book.*

Stimulus items:

5.1. charms/charm

> **Task a.** "Say 'charms,' say 'charm.' What sound did you hear in 'charms' that is missing in 'charm'?" (/z/) "Now we'll change the **letter**. Write/copy 'charms' and 'charm.'"
>
> **Task b.** "Circle the ending/last **letter** that makes the words different." ([s])
>
> **Task c.** "What **sound** does this letter make?" (/z/)

5.2. prized/prize

> **Task a.** "Say 'prized,' say 'prize.' What sound did you hear in 'prized' that is missing in 'prize'?" (/d/) "Now we'll change the **letter**. Write/copy 'prized' and 'prize.'"
>
> **Task b.** "Circle the ending/last **letter** that makes the words different." ([d])
>
> **Task c.** "What **sound** does this letter make?" (/d/)

5.3. leaves/leave

> **Task a.** "Say 'leaves,' say 'leave.' What sound did you hear in 'leaves' that is missing in 'leave'?" (/z/) "Now we'll change the **letter**. Write/copy 'leaves' and 'leave.'"
>
> **Task b.** "Circle the ending/last **letter** that make the words different." ([s])
>
> **Task c.** "What **sound** does this letter make?" (/z/)

5.4. dirty/dirt

> **Task a.** "Say 'dirty,' say 'dirt.' What sound did you hear in 'dirty' that is missing in 'dirt'?" (/long E/) "Now we'll change the **letter**. Write/copy 'dirty' and 'dirt.'"
>
> **Task b.** "Circle the ending/last **letter** that makes the word different." ([y])
>
> **Task c.** "What **sound** does this letter make?" (/long E/)

5.5. raised/raise

Task a. "Say 'raised,' say 'raise.' What sound did you hear in 'raised' that is missing in 'raise'?" (/d/) "Now we'll change the **letter.** Write/copy 'raised' and 'raise.'"

Task b. "Circle the ending/last **letter** that makes the words different." ([d])

Task c. "What **sound** does this letter make?" (/d/)

6. Switching the first sound and letter in words (ADVANCED).

Note: *Use lined paper or copy the sheet of lined paper included in the back of this book.*

Stimulus items:

6.1. so long

Task a. "Say 'so,' say 'long.' What sound do you hear at the beginning of 'so'?" (/s/) "What sound do you hear at the beginning of 'long'?" (/l/) "Switch the first sounds in those words." (lo song) "Now we'll change the **letters.** Write/copy 'so long' and 'lo song.'"

Task b. "Circle the beginning **letters** that change the words." ([s], [l])

Task c. "What **sounds** do those letters make?" (/s/, /l/)

6.2. head down

Task a. "Say 'head' say 'down.' What sound do you hear at the beginning of 'head'?" (/h/) "What sound do you hear at the beginning of 'down'?" (/d/) "Switch the first sounds in those words." (dead hown) "Now we'll change the **letters.** Write/copy 'head down" and 'dead hown.'"

Task b. "Circle the beginning **letters** that change the words." ([h], [d])

Task c. "What **sounds** do those letters make?" (/h/, /d/)

6.3. name tag

Task a. "Say 'name,' say 'tag.' What sound do you hear at the beginning of 'name'?" (/n/) "What sound do you hear at the beginning of 'tag'?" (/t/) "Switch the first sounds in those words." (tame nag) "Now we'll change the **letters.** Write/copy 'name tag' and 'tame nag.'"

Task b. "Circle the beginning **letters** that change the words." ([n], [t])

Task c. "What **sounds** do those letters make?" (/n/, /t/)

6.4. my name

Task a. "Say 'my,' say 'name.' What sound do you hear at the beginning of 'my'?" (/m/) "What sound do you hear at the beginning of 'name'?" (/n/) "Switch the first sounds in those words." (ny mame) "Now we'll change the **letters.** Write/copy 'my name' and 'ny mame.'"

Task b. "Circle the beginning **letters** that change the words." ([m], [n])

Task c. "What **sounds** do those letters make?" (/m/, /n/)

6.5. favorite dinner

Task a. "Say 'favorite,' say 'dinner.' What sound do you hear at the beginning of 'favorite'?" (/f/) "What sound do you hear at the beginning of 'dinner'?" (/d/) "Switch the first sounds in those words." (davorite finner). "Now we'll change the **letters.** Write/copy 'favorite dinner' and 'davorite finner.'"

Task b. "Circle the beginning **letters** that change the words." (f], [d])

Task c. "What **sounds** do those letters make?" (/f/, /d/)

CHAPTER 7

Phonological Awareness Activities to Use with *From Head to Toe*

Text version used for selection of stimulus items:

Carle, E. (1997). *From Head to Toe*. New York: HarperCollins Publishers.

Phonological Awareness Activities at the Word Level

1. Counting words.

What to say to the student: "We're going to count words."

> **EXAMPLE**   "How many words do you hear in this sentence (or phrase): 'a monkey'?" (2)

> **NOTE:** *Use pictured items and/or manipulatives if necessary. Use any of the following stimulus phrases or sentences and/or others you select from the story. The correct answers are in parentheses.*

Stimulus items:

can you (2)

my neck (2)

turn my head (3)

wriggle my hips (3)

I can do it (4)

Can you do it? (4)

And I wriggle my hips (5)

I can kick my legs (5)

I can wiggle my toe (5)

And I clap my hands (5)

2. Identifying the missing word from a list.

What to say to the student: "Listen to the words I say. I'll say them again. You tell me which word I leave out."

> EXAMPLE   "Listen to the words I say: 'seal,' 'penguin.' I'll say them again. Tell me which one I leave out: 'seal.'" (penguin)

NOTE: *Use pictured items and/or manipulatives if necessary. Use any of the following stimulus words and/or others you select from the story. The correct answers are in parentheses.*

Stimulus set #1	Stimulus set #2
toe, neck	neck (toe)
hands, crocodile	hands (crocodile)
cat, stomp, hips	cat, stomp (hips)
wave, elephant, kick	wave, kick (elephant)
gorilla, shoulders, raise	shoulders, raise (gorilla)
seal, cat, buffalo	seal, buffalo (cat)
arms, monkey, clap, chest	arms, clap, chest (monkey)
giraffe, foot, thump, clap	giraffe, foot, thump (clap)
wriggle, seal, monkey, kick	seal, monkey, kick (wriggle)
knees, wiggle, camel, arch	knees, wiggle, arch (camel)

3. Identifying the missing word in a phrase or sentence.

What to say to the student: "Listen to the sentence I read. Tell me which word is missing the second time I read the sentence."

> EXAMPLE   "'can you do it?.' Listen again and tell me which word I leave out. 'can you do _____.'" (it)

NOTE: *Use pictured items and/or manipulatives if necessary. Use any of the following stimulus sentences and/or others you select from the story. The correct answers are in parentheses.*

Stimulus items:

I can. I _____. (can)

wiggle my nose. wiggle my _____. (nose)

I am a cat. I _____ a cat. (am)

Clap my hands. Clap my _____. (hands)

I am a gorilla. I am _____ gorilla. (a)

I can kick my legs. I can _____ my legs. (kick)

I can turn my head. I can turn my _____. (head)

I'm a camel and can bend my knees. I'm a _____ and can bend my knees. (camel)

A gorilla can thump his chest. A _____ can thump his chest. (gorilla)

An elephant can stomp his foot. An elephant can _____ his foot. (stomp)

4. Supplying the missing word as an adult reads.

What to say to the student: "I want you to help me read the story. You fill in the words I leave out."

> **EXAMPLE**   "stomp my _____." (foot)

> **NOTE:** *Use pictured items and/or manipulatives if necessary. Use any of the following stimulus sentences and/or others you select from the story. The correct answers are in parentheses.*

Stimulus items:

I can do _____. (it)

I can turn my _____. (head)

I can clap my _____. (hands)

Can you _____ it? (do)

I can _____ my legs. (kick)

I am a _____. (penguin, giraffe, elephant, buffalo, or any animal named in the book)

I wriggle my _____. (hips)

I can bend my _____. (neck)

I _____ do it. (can)

I raise my _____. (shoulders)

5. Rearranging words.

What to say to the student: "I'll say some words out of order. You put them in the right order so they make sense."

> **EXAMPLE**   " 'you it do.' Put those words in the right order." (you do it)

> **NOTE:** *Use pictured items and/or manipulatives if necessary. Use any of the following stimulus words and/or others you select from the story. The correct answers are in parentheses. This word-level activity can be more difficult than some of the syllable- or phoneme-level activities because of the memory load. If your students are only able to deal with two or three words to be rearranged, add more two- and three-word samples from the story and omit the four-word level items.*

Stimulus items:

buffalo I am a. (I am a buffalo.)

chest thump my (thump my chest)

kick legs my (kick my legs)

do can I it. (I can do it.)

seal am I a. (I am a seal.)

can you it do? (Can you do it?)

neck bend my (bend my neck)

raise shoulders my I. (I raise my shoulders.)

back my I arch. (I arch my back.)

camel bend can knees his a. (A camel can bend his knees.)

Phonological Awareness Activities at the Syllable Level

1. Syllable counting.

What to say to the student: "We're going to count syllables (or parts) of words."

> **EXAMPLE** "How many syllables do you hear in '_____'?" (stimulus word) (e.g., "How many syllables do you hear in 'can'?") (1)

> **NOTE:** *Use pictured items and/or manipulatives if necessary. Use any of the following stimulus words and/or others you select from the story. Use any group of 10 stimulus items you select per teaching set.*

Stimulus items:

One-syllable words: bend, back, turn, toe, do, can, clap, cat, kick, chest, my, neck, knees, seal, stomp, foot, head, hands, hips, raise, thump, you, am, an, and, I, it, arms, arch

Two-syllable words: penguin, donkey, camel, giraffe, monkey, wriggle, shoulders

Three-syllable words: buffalo, crocodile, elephant

2. Initial syllable deleting.

What to say to the student: "We're going to leave out syllables (or parts of words)."

> **EXAMPLE** "Say '_____.'" (stimulus word) "Say it again without '_____.'" (stimulus syllable) (e.g., "Say 'catching.' Say it again without 'catch.'") (ing)

> **NOTE:** *Use pictured items and/or manipulatives if necessary. Use any of the following stimulus words and/or others you select from the story. The correct answers are in parentheses.*

Stimulus items:

"Say 'penguin' without 'pen.'" (gwen)

"Say 'buffalo' without 'buff.'" (alow)

"Say 'donkey' without 'don.'" (key)

3. Final syllable deleting.

What to say to the student: "We're going to leave out syllables (or parts of words)."

> **EXAMPLE** "Say _____.'" (stimulus word) "Say it again without '_____.'" (stimulus syllable) (e.g., "Say 'baking' without 'ing.'") (bake)

> **NOTE:** *Use pictured items and/or manipulatives if necessary. Use any of the following stimulus words and/or others you select from the story. The correct answers are in parentheses.*

Stimulus items:

"Say 'donkey' without 'key.'" (don)

"Say 'camel' without '-ul.'" (cam)

"Say 'penguin' without 'gwen.'" (pen)

"Say 'giraffe' without '-aff.'" (jur)

"Say 'wriggle' without 'ul.'" (rig)

"Say 'monkey' without 'key.'" (mun)

"Say 'wiggle' without 'ul.'" (wig)

"Say 'shoulder' without 'der.'" (shoal)

"Say 'buffalo' without 'low.'" (buffa)

"Say 'elephant' without 'funt.'" (ella)

4. Initial syllable adding.

What to say to the student: "Now let's add syllables (or parts) to words."

> **EXAMPLE** "Add '_____'" (stimulus syllable) "to the beginning of '_____.'" (stimulus syllable) (e.g., "Add 'bake' to the beginning of 'ing.'") (baking)

NOTE: *Use pictured items and/or manipulatives if necessary. Use any of the following stimulus words and/or others you select from the story. The correct answers are in parentheses.*

Stimulus items:

"Add 'buff' to the beginning of 'alow.'" (buffalo)

"Add 'jur' to the beginning of '-aff.'" (giraffe)

"Add 'shoal' to the beginning of 'ders.'" (shoulders)

"Add 'pen' to the beginning of 'gwen.'" (penguin)

"Add 'rig' to the beginning of '-ul.'" (wriggle)

"Add 'don' to the beginning of 'key.'" (donkey)

"Add 'croc' to the beginning of 'odile.'" (crocodile)

"Add 'cam' to the beginning of '-ul.'" (camel)

"Add 'mun' to the beginning of 'key.'" (monkey)

"Add 'wig' to the beginning of '-ul.'" (wiggle)

5. Final syllable adding.

What to say to the student: "Now let's add syllables (or parts) to words."

> **EXAMPLE** "Add '_____'" (stimulus syllable) "to the end of '_____.'" (stimulus syllable) (e.g., "Add '-ing' to the end of 'cut.'") (cutting)

NOTE: *Use pictured items and/or manipulatives if necessary. Use any of the following stimulus words and/or others you select from the story. The correct answers are in parentheses.*

Stimulus items:

"Add 'der' to the end of 'shoal.'" (shoulder)

"Add '-ul' to the end of 'crocodye.'" (crocodile)

"Add '-ul' to the end of 'wig.'" (wiggle)

"Add '-aff' to the end of 'jur.'" (giraffe)
"Add '-ul' to the end of 'rig.'" (wriggle)
"Add 'low' to the end of 'buffa.'" (buffalo)
"Add 'key' to the end of 'don.'" (donkey)
"Add 'gwen' to the end of 'pen.'" (penguin)
"Add 'key' to the end of 'mun.'" (monkey)
"Add '-ul' to the end of 'cam.'" (camel)

6. Syllable substituting.

What to say to the student: "Let's make up some new words."

> EXAMPLE "Say '_____.'" (stimulus word) "Instead of '_____'" (stimulus syllable), "say '_____.'" (stimulus syllable) (e.g., "Say 'cutting.' Instead of 'cut,' say 'bake.' The new word is 'baking.'") Say: "Sometimes, the new word won't be a real word."

> **NOTE:** *Use pictured items and/or manipulatives if necessary. Use of the following stimulus words and/or others you select from the story. The correct answers are in parentheses.*

Stimulus items:

"Say 'donkey.' Instead of 'don,' say 'mun.'" (monkey)
"Say 'penguin.' Instead of 'pen,' say 'buff.'" (buffgwen)
"Say 'buffalo.' Instead of 'low,' say 'key.'" (buffakey)
"Say 'wiggle.' Instead of 'wig,' say 'rig.'" (wriggle)
"Say 'donkey.' Instead of 'key,' say '-ul.'" (donul)
"Say 'giraffe.' Instead of '-aff,' say 'key.'" (jerky)
"Say 'camel.' Instead of 'cam,' say 'wig.'" (wiggle)
"Say 'shoulder.' Instead of 'er,' say 'ing.'" (shoulding)
"Say 'crocodile.' Instead of 'dile,' say 'low.'" (crocolow)
"Say 'monkey.' Instead of 'mun,' say 'don.'" (donkey)

Phonological Awareness Activities at the Phoneme Level

1. Counting sounds.

What to say to the student: "We're going to count sounds in words."

> EXAMPLE "How many sounds do you hear in this word: 'leg'?" (3)

> **NOTE:** *Use pictured items and/or manipulatives if necessary. Use any of the following stimulus words and/or others you select from the story. Be sure to give the letter sound and not the letter name. Use any group of 10 stimulus items you select per teaching set.*

Stimulus words with two sounds: toe, do, my, am, an, it

Stimulus words with three sounds: back, turn, can, cat, kick, neck, knees, seal, foot, head, raise, wave, and

Stimulus words with four sounds: bend, clap, camel, chest, giraffe, hips, legs, wriggle, wiggle, thump

Stimulus words with five sounds: donkey, monkey, stomp, hands

2. Sound categorization or identifying a rhyme oddity.

What to say to the student: "Guess which word I say does not rhyme with the other three words."

> **EXAMPLE** "Tell me which word doesn't rhyme with the other three words: '_____,' '_____,' '_____,' '_____.'" (stimulus words) (e.g., " 'can,' 'pan,' 'camel,' 'fan.' Which word doesn't rhyme?") (camel)

NOTE: *Use pictured items if necessary. Use any of the following stimulus words and/or others you select from the story. The correct answers are in parentheses.*

Stimulus items:

cat, camel, rat, sat (camel)

stomp, romp, wriggle, pomp (wriggle)

knees, wave, crave, pave (knees)

chest, hands, best, crest (hands)

clap, flap, map, back (back)

raise, wiggle, praise, graze (wiggle)

wiggle, giggle, giraffe, wriggle (giraffe)

crocodile, neck, check, peck (crocodile)

shoulder, buffalo, bolder, folder (buffalo)

thump, stomp, bump, lump (stomp)

3. Matching rhyme.

What to say to the student: "We're going to think of rhyming words."

> **EXAMPLE** "Which word rhymes with '_____'?" (stimulus word) (e.g., "Which word rhymes with 'chest': 'giraffe,' 'seal,' 'legs,' 'best'?") (best)

NOTE: *Use pictured items if necessary. Use any of the following stimulus words and/or others you select from the story. The correct answers are in parentheses.*

Stimulus items:

seal: hands, wriggle, peel, thump (peel)

back: tack, cat, buffalo, toe (tack)

knees: penguin, bees, wave, chest (bees)

arch: crocodile, turn, march, bend (march)

hips: hands, lips, wiggle, shoulders (lips)

monkey: stomp, giraffe, funky, arms (funky)

bend: cat, crocodile, send, donkey (send)

wriggle: knees, thump, elephant, wiggle (wiggle)

wave: wriggle, cave, gorilla, stomp (cave)

wiggle: camel, giggle, buffalo, cat (giggle)

4. Producing rhyme.

What to say to the student: "Now we'll say rhyming words."

> **EXAMPLE** "Tell me a word that rhymes with '_____.'" (stimulus word) (e.g., "Tell me a word that rhymes with 'cat.' You can make up a word if you want.") (rat, sat, bat, hat, mat, etc.)

> **NOTE:** *Use pictured items if necessary. Use any of the following stimulus words and/or others you select from the story (i.e., you say a word from the list below and the student is to think of a rhyming word). Use any group of 10 stimulus items you select per teaching set.*

Stimulus items:

/p/: penguin

/b/: bend, buffalo, back

/t/: turn, toe

/d/: do, donkey

/k/: can, clap, cat, crocodile, camel, kick

/g/: gorilla

/ch/: chest

/dz/ (as in gem): giraffe

/m/: my, monkey

/n/: neck, knees

/s/: seal, stomp

/f/: foot, from

/h/: head, hands, hips

/r/: raise, wriggle

/l/: legs

/w/, /wh/: wave, wiggle

/sh/: shoulders

/voiceless th/: thump

/y/ (as in yellow): you

/short A/: am, an, and

/short U/: a

/short E/: elephant

/ah/: arch, arm

5. Sound matching (initial).

What to say to the student: "Now we'll listen for the first sound in words."

> **EXAMPLE** "Listen to this sound: / /." (stimulus sound). "Guess which word I say begins with that sound: '_____,' '_____,' '_____,' '_____.'" (stimulus words) (e.g., "Listen to this sound: /d/. Guess which word I say begins with that sound: 'donkey,' 'foot,' 'head,' 'thump.'") (donkey)

> **NOTE:** *Give the letter sound, not the letter name. Use pictured items if necessary. Use any of the following stimulus words and/or others you select from the story. The correct answers are in parentheses.*

Stimulus items:

/r/: hands, wriggle, raise, elephant (raise)

/g/: buffalo, neck, thump, gorilla (gorilla)

/f/: fine, good, paper, brother (fine)

/b/: shoulders, back, monkey, seal (back)

/sh/: wriggle, knees, shoulders, cat (shoulders)

/dz/ (as in gem): giraffe, gorilla, seal, thump (giraffe)

/k/: neck, legs, crocodile, buffalo (crocodile)

/h/: donkey, penguin, hands, kick (hands)

/ch/: clap, camel, chest, wiggle (chest)

/t/: crocodile, gorilla, toe, seal (toe)

6. Sound matching (final).

What to say to the student: "Now we'll listen for the last sound in words."

> **EXAMPLE** "Listen to this sound: / /." (stimulus sound) "Guess which word I say ends with that sound: '_____,' '_____,' '_____,' '_____.'" (stimulus words) (e.g., "Listen to this sound: /t/. Guess which word I say ends with that sound: 'camel,' 'cat,' 'bend,' 'wave.'") (cat)

> **NOTE:** *Give the letter sound, not the letter name. Use pictured items and/or manipulatives if necessary. Use any of the following stimulus words and/or others you select from the story. The correct answers are in parentheses.*

Stimulus items:

/l/: arch, wriggle, stomp, monkey (wriggle)

/t/: stomp, elephant, arms, giraffe (elephant)

/n/: penguin, raise, camel, buffalo (penguin)

/z/: foot, wiggle, raise, crocodile (raise)

/k/: wiggle, donkey, back, chest (back)

/long E/: stomp, donkey, knees, thump (donkey)

/s/: giraffe, camel, hips, arch (hips)

/d/: chest, penguin, crocodile, bend (bend)

/m/: from, turn, elephant, camel (from)

/p/: penguin, monkey, thump, kick (thump)

7. Identifying the initial sound in words.

What to say to the student: "I'll say a word two times. Tell me what sound is missing the second time: '_____,' '_____.' " (stimulus words)

> **EXAMPLE** "What sound do you hear in '_____' " (stimulus word) "that is missing in '_____'?" (stimulus word) (e.g., "What sound do you hear in 'his' that's missing in 'is'?") (/h/)

NOTE: *Give the letter sound, not the letter name. Use pictured items and/or manipulatives if necessary. Use any of the following stimulus words and/or others you select from the story. The correct answers are in parentheses.*

Stimulus items:

"can, an. What sound do you hear in 'can' that is missing in 'an'?" (/k/)

"my, I. What sound do you hear in 'my' that is missing in 'I'?" (/m/)

"cat, at. What sound do you hear in 'cat' that is missing in 'at'?" (/k/)

"bend, end. What sound do you hear in 'bend' that is missing in 'end'?" (/b/)

"leg, egg. What sound do you hear in 'leg' that is missing in 'egg'?" (/l/)

"turn, urn. What sound do you hear in 'turn' that is missing in 'urn'?" (/t/)

"seal, eel. What sound do you hear in 'seal' that is missing in 'eel'?" (/s/)

"kick, ick. What sound do you hear in 'kick' that is missing in 'ick'?" (/k/)

"head, Ed. What sound do you hear in 'head' that is missing in 'Ed'?" (/h/)

"clap, lap. What sound do you hear in 'clap' that is missing in 'lap'?" (/k/)

8. Identifying the final sound in words.

What to say to the student: "I'll say a word two times. Tell me what sound is missing the second time: '_____,' '_____.' " (stimulus words)

> **EXAMPLE** "What sound do you hear in '_____' " (stimulus word) "that is missing in '_____'?" (stimulus word) (e.g., "What sound do you hear in 'hips' that is missing in 'hip'?") (/s/)

NOTE: *Give the letter sound, not the letter name. Use pictured items and/or manipulatives if necessary. Use any of the following stimulus words and/or others you select from the story. The correct answers are in parentheses.*

Stimulus items:

"and, an. What sound do you hear in 'and' that is missing in 'an'?" (/d/)

"legs, leg. What sound do you hear in 'legs' that is missing in 'leg'?" (/z/)

"wave, way. What sound do you hear in 'wave' that is missing in 'way'?" (/v/)

"hands, hand. What sound do you hear in 'hands' that is missing in 'hand'?" (/z/)

"seal, sea. What sound do you hear in 'seal' that is missing in 'sea'?" (/l/)

"knees, knee. What sound do you hear in 'knees' that is missing in 'knee'?" (/z/)

"shoulders, shoulder. What sound do you hear in 'shoulders' that is missing in 'shoulder'?" (/z/)

"thump, thumb. What sound do you hear in 'thump' that is missing in 'thumb'?" (/p/)

"chest, chess. What sound do you hear in 'chest' that is missing in 'chess'?" (/t/)

"monkey, monk. What sound do you hear in 'monkey' that is missing in 'monk'?" (/long E/)

9. Segmenting the initial sound in words.

What to say to the student: "Listen to the word I say and tell me the first sound you hear."

> **EXAMPLE** "What's the first sound in '_____'?" (stimulus word) (e.g., "What's the first sound in 'bend'?") (/b/)

NOTE: *Give the letter sound, not the letter name. Use pictured items and/or manipulatives if necessary. Use any of the following stimulus words and/or others you select from the story. Use any group of 10 stimulus items you select per teaching set.*

Stimulus items:

/p/: penguin

/b/: bend, buffalo, back

/t/: turn, toe

/d/: do, donkey

/k/: can, clap, cat, crocodile, camel, kick

/g/: gorilla

/ch/: chest

/dz/ (as in gem): giraffe

/m/: my, monkey

/n/: neck, knees

/s/: seal, stomp

/f/: foot, from

/h/: head, hands, hips

/r/: raise, wriggle

/l/: legs

/w/, /wh/: wave, wiggle

/sh/: shoulders

/voiceless th/: thump

/y/ (as in yellow): you

/short A/: am, an, and

/short U/: a

/short E/: elephant

/ah/: arch, arm

10. Segmenting the final sound in words.

What to say to the student: "Listen to the word I say and tell me the last sound you hear."

> **EXAMPLE**   "What's the last sound in the word '_____'?" (stimulus word)
> (e.g., "What's the last sound in the word 'cat'?") (/t/)

> **NOTE:** *Give the letter sound, not the letter name. Use pictured items and/or manipulatives if necessary. Use any of the following stimulus words and/or others you select from the story. Use any group of 10 stimulus items you select per teaching set.*

Stimulus items:

/p/: clap, thump, stomp

/t/: it, chest, cat, elephant, foot

/d/: and, head, bend

/k/: neck, back, kick

/m/: am, from

/n/: penguin, turn, can

/s/: hips

/z/: raise, shoulders, arms, hands, knees, legs

/f/: giraffe

/v/: wave

/l/: seal, crocodile, wriggle, camel, wiggle

/long E/: monkey, donkey

/long I/: I, my

/long O/: buffalo, toe

/oo/: you, do, to

11. Generating words from the story beginning with a particular sound.

What to say to the student: "Let's think of words from the story that start with certain sounds."

> **EXAMPLE**   "Tell me a word from the story that starts with / /." (stimulus sound)
> (e.g., the sound /p/) (penguin)

> **NOTE:** *Give the letter sound, not the letter name. Use pictured items if necessary. Use any of the following stimulus words and/or others you select from the story. You say the sound (e.g., a voiceless /p/ sound), and the student is to say a word from the story that begins with that sound. Use any group of 10 stimulus items you select per teaching set.*

Stimulus items:

/p/: penguin

/b/: bend, buffalo, back

/t/: turn, toe

/d/: do, donkey

/k/: can, clap, cat, crocodile, camel, kick

/g/: gorilla

/ch/: chest

/dz/ (as in gem): giraffe

/m/: my, monkey

/n/: neck, knees

/s/: seal, stomp

/f/: foot, from

/h/: head, hands, hips

/r/: raise, wriggle

/l/: legs

/w/, /wh/: wave, wiggle

/sh/: shoulders

/voiceless th/: thump

/y/ (as in yellow): you

/short A/: am, an, and

/short U/: a

/short E/: elephant

12. Blending sounds in monosyllabic words divided into onset/rime beginning with a two-consonant cluster + rime.

What to say to the student: "Now we'll put sounds together to make words."

EXAMPLE "Put these sounds together to make a word: / / + / /." (stimulus sounds) "What's the word?" (e.g., "fl + ip: What's the word?") (flip)

NOTE: *Give the letter sound, not the letter name. Use pictured items and/or manipulatives if necessary. Use any of the following stimulus words and/or others you select from the story. The correct answers are in parentheses.*

Stimulus items:

fr + um (from)

cl + ap (clap)

st + omp (stomp)

Sourcebook users are encouraged to add stimulus items into this activity from curriculum materials they may be using with *From Head to Toe*.

13. Blending sounds in monosyllabic words divided into onset/rime beginning with a single consonant + rime.

What to say to the student: "Let's put sounds together to make words."

> **EXAMPLE** "Put these sounds together to make a word (/ / + / /)." (stimulus sounds) "What's the word?" (e.g., "/g/ + ood: What's the word?") (good)

> **NOTE:** *Give the letter sound, not the letter name. Use pictured items and/or manipulatives if necessary. Use any of the following stimulus words and/or others you select from the story. The correct answers are in parentheses.*

Stimulus items:

/h/ + ip (hip)

/l/ + egg or ehg (leg)

/h/ + Ed (head)

/n/ + eck (neck)

/s/ + eel (seal)

/b/ + end (bend)

/k/ + ick (kick)

/t/ + urn (turn)

/m/ + eye (my)

/t/ + owe (toe)

14. Blending sounds to form a monosyllabic word beginning with a continuant sound.

What to say to the student: "We'll put sounds together to make words."

> **EXAMPLE** "Put these sounds together to make a word (/ / + / / + / /)." (stimulus sounds) (e.g., "/m/ /ah/ /m/.") (mom)

> **NOTE:** *Give the letter sound, not the letter name. Use pictured items and/or manipulatives if necessary. Use any of the following stimulus words and/or others you select from the story. The correct answers are in parentheses.*

Stimulus items:

/m/ /long I/ (my)

/s/ /long E/ /l/ (seal)

/n/ /short E/ /k/ (neck)

/l/ /short E/ or /long A/ /g/ (leg)

/w/ /long A/ /v/ (wave)

/f/ /oo/ /t/ (foot)

/s/ /t/ /ah/ /m/ /p/ (stomp)

/n/ /long E/ /z/ (knees)

/f/ /r/ /uh/ /m/ (from)

/y/ (as in yellow) /oo/ (you)

15. Blending sounds to form a monosyllabic word beginning with a noncontinuant sound.

What to say to the student: "We'll put sounds together to make words."

> **EXAMPLE** "Put these sounds together to make a word (/ / + / / + / /)." (stimulus sounds) (e.g., "/d/ /ah/ /g/.") (dog)

> **NOTE:** *Give the letter sound, not the letter name. Use pictured items and/or manipulatives if necessary. Use any of the following stimulus words and/or others you select from the story. The correct answers are in parentheses.*

Stimulus items:

/t/ /oo/ (to)

/b/ /short E/ /n/ /d/ (bend)

/t/ /long O/ (toe)

/d/ /oo/ (do)

/ch/ /short E/ /s/ /t/ (chest)

/t/ /er/ /n/ (turn)

/b/ /short A/ /k/ (back)

/k/ /l/ /short A/ /p/ (clap)

/k/ /short A/ /t/ (cat)

/k/ /short I/ /k/ (kick)

16. Substituting the initial sound in words.

What to say to the student: "We're going to change beginning/first sounds in words."

> **EXAMPLE** "Say '_____.'" (stimulus word) "Instead of / /" (stimulus sound), "say / /." (stimulus sound) (e.g., "Say 'back.' Instead of /b/, say /p/. What's your new word?") (pack)

> **NOTE:** *Give the letter sound, not the letter name. Use pictured items and/or manipulatives if necessary. Use any of the following stimulus words and/or others you select from the story. The correct answers are in parentheses.*

Stimulus items:

"Say 'cat.' Instead of /k/, say /b/." (bat)

"Say 'toe.' Instead of /t/, say /f/." (foe)

"Say 'seal.' Instead of /s/, say /t/." (teal)

"Say 'neck.' Instead of /n/, say /p/." (peck)

"Say 'chest.' Instead of /ch/, say /r/." (rest)

"Say 'bend.' Instead of /b/, say /s/." (send)

"Say 'back.' Instead of /b/, say /t/." (tack)

"Say 'wave.' Instead of /w/, say /k/." (cave)

"Say 'thump. Instead of /voiceless th/, say /b/." (bump)

"Say 'turn.' Instead of /t/, say /b/." (burn)

17. Substituting the final sound in words.

What to say to the student: "We're going to change ending/last sounds in words."

> **EXAMPLE**   "Say '_____.'" (stimulus word) "Instead of / /" (stimulus sound), "say / /." (stimulus sound) (e.g., "Say 'back.' Instead of /k/, say /t/. What's your new word?") (bat)

NOTE: *Give the letter sound, not the letter name. Use pictured items and/or manipulatives if necessary. Use any of the following stimulus words and/or others you select from the story. The correct answers are in parentheses.*

Stimulus items:

"Say 'my.' Instead of /long I/, say /long A/." (may)

"Say 'can.' Instead of /n/, say /t." (cat)

"Say 'hip.' Instead of /p/, say /t/." (hit)

"Say 'neck.' Instead of /k/, say /t/." (net)

"Say 'wave.' Instead of /v/, say /t/." (wait)

"Say 'back.' Instead of /k/, say /t/." (bat)

"Say 'bend.' Instead of /d/, say /t/." (bent)

"Say 'seal.' Instead of /l/, say /t/." (seat)

"Say 'raise.' Instead of /z/, say /t/." (rate)

"Say 'arm.' Instead of /m/, say /ch/." (arch)

18. Segmenting the middle sound in monosyllabic words.

What to say to the student: "Tell me the middle sound in the word I say."

> **EXAMPLE**   "What's the middle sound in the word '_____'?" (stimulus word) (e.g., "What's the middle sound in the word 'back'?") (/short A/)

NOTE: *Give the letter sound, not the letter name. Use pictured items and/or manipulatives if necessary. Use any of the following stimulus words and/or others you select from the story. The correct answers are in parentheses.*

Stimulus items:

can (/short A/)

back (/short A/)

head (/short E/)

wave (/long A/)

kick (/short I/)

turn (/er/)

and (/n/)

raise (long A/)

hip (/short I/)

seal (/long E/)

19. Substituting the middle sound in words.

What to say to the student: "We're going to change the middle sound in words."

> **EXAMPLE**   "Say '_____.'" (stimulus word) "Instead of / /" (stimulus sound),
> "say / /." (stimulus sound) (e.g., "Say 'flop.' Instead of /ah/, say /short I/.
> What's your new word?") (flip)

> **NOTE:** *Give the letter sound, not the letter name. Use pictured items and/or manipulatives if*
> *necessary. Use any of the following stimulus words and/or others you select from the*
> *story. The correct answers are in parentheses.*

Stimulus items:

"Say 'cat.' Instead of /short A/, say /ah/." (cot)

"Say 'head.' Instead of /short E/, say /short I/." (hid)

"Say 'seal.' Instead of /long E/, say /long A/." (sail)

"Say 'wave.' Instead of /long A/, say /long E/." (weave)

"Say 'back.' Instead of /short A/, say /uh/." (buck)

"Say 'neck.' Instead of /short E/, say /short A/." (knack)

"Say 'cat.' Instead of /short A/, say /uh/." (cut)

"Say 'from.' Instead of /uh/, say /long A/." (frame)

"Say 'hip.' Instead of /short I/, say /ah/." (hop)

"Say 'head.' Instead of /short E/, say /short A/." (had)

20. Identifying all sounds in monosyllabic words.

What to say to the student: "Now tell me all the sounds you hear in the word I say."

> **EXAMPLE**   "What sounds do you hear in the word '_____'?" (stimulus word)
> (e.g., "What sounds do you hear in the word 'dog'?") (/d/ /ah/ /g/)

> **NOTE:** *Give the letter sound, not the letter name. Use pictured items and/or manipulatives if*
> *necessary. Use any of the following stimulus words and/or others you select from the*
> *story. The correct answers are in parentheses.*

Stimulus items:

head (/h/ /short E/ /d/)

neck (/n/ /short E/ /k/)

kick (/k/ /short I/ /k/)

wave (/w/ /long A/ /v/)

seal (/s/ /long E/ /l/)

cat (/k/ /short A/ /t/)

chest (/ch/ /short E/ /s/ /t/)

hip (/h/ /short I/ /p/)

stomp (/s/ /t/ /ah/ /m/ /p/)

thump (/voiceless th/ /uh/ /m/ /p/)

21. Deleting sounds within words.

What to say to the student: "We're going to leave out sounds in words."

> EXAMPLE   "Say '_____'" (stimulus word) "without / /." (stimulus sound) (e.g., "Say 'slid' without /l/.") (sid) Say "The word that was left, 'sid,' is a real word. Sometimes, the new word won't be a real word."

NOTE: *Give the letter sound, not the letter name. Use pictured items and/or manipulatives if necessary. Use any of the following stimulus words and/or others you select from the story. The correct answers are in parentheses.*

Stimulus items:

"Say 'clap' without /l/." (cap)

"Say 'chest' without /s/." (Chet)

"Say 'hand' without /n/." (had)

"Say 'stomp' without /m/." (stop)

"Say 'hips' without /p/." (hiss)

"Say 'bend' without /n/." (bed)

Sourcebook users are encouraged to add stimulus items into this activity from curriculum materials they may be using with *From Head to Toe.*

22. Substituting consonants in words having a two-sound cluster.

What to say to the student: "We're going to substitute sounds in words."

> EXAMPLE   "Say '_____.'" (stimulus word) "Instead of / /" (stimulus sound), "say / /." (stimulus sound) (e.g., "Say 'stop.' Instead of /t/, say /l/.") (slop) Say: "Sometimes, the new word will be a made-up word."

NOTE: *Give the letter sound, not the letter name. Use pictured items and/or manipulatives if necessary. Use any of the following stimulus words and/or others you select from the story. The correct answers are in parentheses.*

Stimulus items:

"Say 'bend.' Instead of /d/, say /t/." (bent)

"Say 'clap.' Instead of /k/, say /s/." (slap)

"Say 'turn.' Instead of /n/, say /p/." (turp)

"Say 'hips.' Instead of /p/, say /t/." (hits)

"Say 'and.' Instead of /d/, say /t/." (ant)

"Say 'chest.' Instead of /s/, say /k/." (checked)

Sourcebook users are encouraged to add stimulus items into this activity from curriculum materials they may be using with *From Head to Toe*.

23. Phoneme reversing.

What to say to the student: "We're going to say words backward."

> EXAMPLE   "Say the word '_____'" (stimulus word) "backward." (e.g., "Say 'bone' backward.") (nobe)

NOTE: *This is a difficult phoneme-level task and should only be done with older students. Give the letter sound, not the letter name. Use pictured items and/or manipulatives if necessary. Use any of the following stimulus words and/or others you select from the story. The correct answers are in parentheses.*

Stimulus items:

my (I'm)

kick (kick)

cat (tack)

back (cab)

can (knack)

seal (lease)

neck (Ken)

toe (oat)

do (ood)

to (oot)

24. Phoneme switching.

What to say to the student: "We're going to switch the first sounds in two words."

> EXAMPLE   "Switch the first sounds in '_____' and '_____.'" (stimulus words) (e.g., "Switch the first sounds in 'can' and 'do.'") (dan koo)

NOTE: *This is a difficult phoneme-level task and should only be done with older students. Give the letter sound, not the letter name. Use pictured items and/or manipulatives if necessary. Use any of the following stimulus words and/or others you select from the story. The correct answers are in parentheses.*

Stimulus items:

cat back (bat cack)

head toe (Ted hoe)

wiggle hips (higgle wips)

turn head (hurn Ted)

bend neck (nend beck)

raise my (maize rye)

seal hands (heal sands)

thump chest (chump thest)

kick legs (lick kegs)

wiggle toes (tiggle woes)

25. Pig Latin.

What to say to the student: "We're going to speak a secret language by using words from the story. In pig Latin, you take off the first sound of a word, put it at the end of the word, and add an 'ay' sound."

> **EXAMPLE**   "Say 'dog' in pig Latin." (ogday)

> **NOTE:** *This is a difficult phoneme-level task and should only be done with older students. Use pictured items and/or manipulatives if necessary. Use any of the following stimulus words and/or others you select from the story. The correct answers are in parentheses.*

Stimulus items:

cat (atkay)

neck (ecknay)

bend (endbay)

raise (azeray)

seal (eelsay)

thump (umpthay)

donkey (awnkeyday)

gorilla (orillagay)

buffalo (uffalobay)

camel (amelkay)

From Phonological Awareness into Print

> **NOTE:** *Only five examples per activity are included in this resource due to space. You are encouraged to add many more words into this section that you feel your student(s) are ready to write.*

1. Substituting the initial sound or letter in words.

> **NOTE:** *Use lined paper or copy the sheet of lined paper included in the back of this book.*

Stimulus items:

1.1 cat/hat

> **Task a.** "Say 'cat.' Instead of /k/, say /h/. What's your new word?" (hat) "Write/copy 'cat' and 'hat.'"
>
> **Task b.** "Circle the **letters** that make the words different." ([c], [h])
>
> **Task c.** "What **sounds** do these letters make?" (/k/, /h/)

1.2 bend/send

> **Task a.** "Say 'bend.' Instead of /b/, say /s/. What's your new word?" (send) "Write/copy 'bend' and 'send.'"
>
> **Task b.** "Circle the **letters** that make the words different." ([b], [s])
>
> **Task c.** "What **sounds** do these letters make?" (/b/, /s/)

1.3 toe/hoe

> **Task a.** "Say 'toe.' Instead of /t/, say /h/. What's your new word?" (hoe) "Write/copy 'toe' and 'hoe.'"
>
> **Task b.** "Circle the **letters** that make the words different." ([t], [h])
>
> **Task c.** "What **sounds** do these letters make?" (/t/, /h/)

1.4 hands/lands

> **Task a.** "Say 'hands.' Instead of /h/, say /l/. What's your new word?" (lands) "Write/copy 'hands' and 'lands.'"
>
> **Task b.** "Circle the **letters** that make the words different." ([h], [l])
>
> **Task c.** "What **sounds** do these letters make?" (/h/, /l/)

1.5 wiggle/giggle

> **Task a.** "Say 'wiggle.' Instead of /w/, say /g/. What's your new word?" (giggle) "Write/copy 'wiggle' and 'giggle.'"
>
> **Task b.** "Circle the **letters** that make the words different." ([w], [g])
>
> **Task c.** "What **sounds** do these letters make?" (/w/, /g/)

2. Substituting the final sound or letter in words.

> **NOTE:** *Use lined paper or copy the sheet of lined paper included in the back of this book.*

Stimulus items:

2.1 cat/cap

> **Task a.** "Say 'cat.' Instead of /t/, say /p/. What's your new word?" (cap) "Write/copy 'cat' and 'cap.'"
>
> **Task b.** "Circle the **letters** that make the words different." ([t], [p])
>
> **Task c.** "What **sounds** do these letters make?" (/t/, /p/)

2.2 bend/bent

> **Task a.** "Say 'bend.' Instead of /d/, say /t/. What's your new word?" (bent) "Write/copy 'bend' and 'bent.'"

Task b. "Circle the **letters** that make the words different." ([d], [t])

Task c. "What **sounds** do these letters make?" (/d/, /t/)

2.3 am/an

Task a. "Say 'am.' Instead of /m/, say /n/. What's your new word?" (an) "Write/copy 'am' and 'an.'"

Task b. "Circle the **letters** that make the words different." ([m], [n])

Task c. "What **sounds** do these letters make?" (/m/, /n/)

2.4 can/cat

Task a. "Say 'can.' Instead of /n/, say /t/. What's your new word?" (cat) "Write/copy 'can' and 'cat.'"

Task b. "Circle the **letters** that make the words different." ([n], [t])

Task c. "What **sounds** do these letters make?" (/n/, /t/)

2.5 hip/hit

Task a. "Say 'hip.' Instead of /p/, say /t/. What's your new word?" (hit) "Write/copy 'hip' and 'hit.'"

Task b. "Circle the **letters** that make the words different." ([p], [t])

Task c. "What **sounds** do these letters make?" (/p/, /t/)

3. Substituting the middle sound or letter in words.

NOTE: *Use lined paper or copy the sheet of lined paper included in the back of this book.*

Stimulus items:

3.1 cat/cut

Task a. "Say 'cat.' Instead of /short A/, say /short U/. What's your new word?" (cut) "Write/copy 'cat' and 'cut.'"

Task b. "Circle the **letters** that make the words different." ([a], [u])

Task c. "What **sounds** do these letters make?" (/short A/, /short U/)

3.2 hip/hop

Task a. "Say 'hip.' Instead of /short I/, say /ah/. What's your new word?" (hop) "Write/copy 'hip' and 'hop.'"

Task b. "Circle the **letters** that make the words different." ([i], [o])

Task c. "What **sounds** do these letters make?" (/short I/, /ah/)

3.3 clap/clip

Task a. "Say 'clap.' Instead of /short A/, say /short I/. What's your new word?" (clip) "Write/copy 'clap' and 'clip.'"

Task b. "Circle the **letters** that make the words different." ([a], [i])

Task c. "What **sounds** do these letters make?" (/short A/, /short I/)

3.4 can/con

    Task a. "Say 'can.' Instead of /short A/, say /ah/. What's your new word?" (con) "Write/copy 'can' and 'con.'"

    Task b. "Circle the **letters** that make the words different." ([a], [o])

    Task c. "What **sounds** do these letters make?" (/short A/, /ah/)

3.5 bend/bond

    Task a. "Say 'bend.' Instead of /short E/, say /ah/. What's your new word?" (bond) "Write/copy 'bend' and 'bond.'"

    Task b. "Circle the **letters** that make the words different." ([e], [o])

    Task c. "What **sounds** do these letters make?" (/short E/, /ah/)

4. Supplying the initial sound or letter in words.

    NOTE: *Use lined paper or copy the sheet of lined paper included in the back of this book.*

Stimulus items:

4.1 can/an

    Task a. "Say 'can,' say 'an.' What sound did you hear in 'can' that is missing in 'an'?" (/k/) "Now we'll change the **letter**. Write/copy 'can' and 'an.'"

    Task b. "Circle the beginning **letter** that makes the words different." ([c])

    Task c. "What **sound** does this letter make?" (/k/)

4.2 bend/end

    Task a. "Say 'bend,' say 'end.' What sound did you hear in 'bend' that's missing in 'end'?" (/b/) "Now we'll change the **letter**. Write/copy 'bend' and 'end.'"

    Task b. "Circle the beginning **letter** that makes the words different." ([b])

    Task c. "What **sound** does this letter make?" (/b/)

4.3 hand/and

    Task a. "Say 'hand,' say 'and.' What sound did you hear in 'hand' that's missing in 'and'?" (/h/) "Now we'll change the **letter**. Write/copy 'hand' and 'and.'"

    Task b. "Circle the beginning **letter** that makes the words different." ([h])

    Task c. "What **sound** do these letters make?" (/h/)

4.4 turn/urn

    Task a. "Say 'turn,' say 'urn.' What sound did you hear in 'turn' that's missing in 'urn'?" (/t/) "Now we'll change the **letter**. Write/copy 'turn' and 'urn.'"

    Task b. "Circle the beginning **letter** that makes the words different." ([t])

    Task c. "What **sound** does this letter make?" (/t/)

4.5 clap/lap

    Task a. "Say 'clap,' say 'lap.' What sound did you hear in 'clap' that's missing in 'lap'?" (/k/) "Now we'll change the **letter**. Write/copy 'clap' and 'lap.'"

    Task b. "Circle the beginning **letter** that makes the words different." ([c])

    Task c. "What **sound** does this letter make?" (/k/)

5. Supplying the final sound or letter in words.

NOTE: *Use lined paper or copy the sheet of lined paper included in the back of this book.*

Stimulus items:

5.1 and/an

Task a. "Say 'and,' say 'an.' What sound did you hear in 'and' that's missing in 'an'?" (/d/) "Now we'll change the **letter**. Write/copy 'and' and 'an.'"

Task b. "Circle the ending/last **letter** that makes the words different." ([d])

Task c. "What **sound** does this letter make?" (/d/)

5.2 hands/hand

Task a. "Say 'hands,' say 'hand.' What sound did you hear in 'hands' that's missing in 'hand'?" (/z/) "Now we'll change the **letter**. Write/copy 'hands' and 'hand.'"

Task b. "Circle the ending/last **letter** that makes the words different." ([s])

Task c. "What **sound** does this letter make?" (/z/)

5.3 knees/knee

Task a. "Say 'knees,' say 'knee.' What sound did you hear in 'knees' that's missing in 'knee'?" (/z/) "Now we'll change the **letter**. Write/copy 'knees' and 'knee.'"

Task b. "Circle the ending/last **letter** that makes the words different." ([s])

Task c. "What **sound** does this letter make?" (/z/)

5.4 bend/ben

Task a. "Say 'bend,' say 'ben.' What sound did you hear in 'bend' that's missing in 'ben'?" (/d/) "Now we'll change the **letter**. Write/copy 'bend' and 'ben' or 'Ben.'"

Task b. "Circle the ending/last **letter** that makes the word different." ([d])

Task c. "What **sound** does this letter make?" (/d/)

5.5 hips/hip

Task a. "Say 'hips,' say 'hip.' What sound did you hear in 'hips' that's missing in 'hip'?" (/s/) "Now we'll change the **letter**. Write/copy 'hips' and 'hip.'"

Task b. "Circle the ending/last **letter** that makes the words different." ([s])

Task c. "What **sound** does this letter make?" (/s/)

6. Switching the first sound and letter in words (ADVANCED).

NOTE: *Use lined paper or copy the sheet of lined paper included in the back of this book.*

Stimulus items:

6.1 cat back

Task a. "Say 'cat,' say 'back.' What sound do you hear at the beginning of 'cat'?" (/k/) "What sound do you hear at the beginning of 'back'?" (/b/) "Switch the first sounds in those words." (bat cack) "Now we'll change the **letters**. Write/copy 'cat back' and 'bat cack.'"

Task b. "Circle the beginning **letters** that change the words." ([c], [b])

Task c. "What **sounds** do those letters make?" (/k/, /b/)

6.2 kick legs

Task a. "Say 'kick,' say 'legs.' What sound do you hear at the beginning of 'kick'?" (/k/) "What sound do you hear at the beginning of 'legs'?" (/l/) "Switch the first sounds in those words." (lick kegs) "Now we'll change the **letters**. Write/copy 'kick legs' and 'lick kegs.'"

Task b. "Circle the beginning **letters** that change the words." ([k], [l])

Task c. "What **sounds** do those letters make?" (/k/, /l/)

6.3 bend neck

Task a. "Say 'bend,' say 'neck.' What sound do you hear at the beginning of 'bend'?" (/b/) "What sound do you hear at the beginning of 'neck'?" (/n/) "Switch the first sounds in those words." (nend beck) "Now we'll change the **letters**. Write/copy 'bend neck' and 'nend beck.'"

Task b. "Circle the beginning **letters** that change the words." ([b], [n])

Task c. "What **sounds** do those letters make?" (/b/, /n/)

6.4 seal hands

Task a. "Say 'seal,' say 'hands.' What sound do you hear at the beginning of 'seal'?" (/s/) "What sound do you hear at the beginning of 'hands'?" (/h/) "Switch the first sounds in those words." (heal sands) "Now we'll change the **letters**. Write/copy 'seal hands' and 'heal sands.'"

Task b. "Circle the beginning **letters** that change the words." ([s], [h])

Task c. "What **sounds** do those letters make?" (/s/, /h/)

6.5 wiggle toes

Task a. "Say 'wiggle,' say 'toes.' What sound do you hear at the beginning of 'wiggle'?" (/w/) "What sound do you hear at the beginning of 'toes'?" (/t/) "Switch the first sounds in those words." (tiggle woes) "Now we'll change the **letters**. Write/copy 'wiggle toes' and 'tiggle woes.'"

Task b. "Circle the beginning **letters** that change the words." ([t], [w])

Task c. "What **sounds** do those letters make?" (/t/, /w/)

Phonological Awareness Activities to Use with *Home for a Bunny*

Text version used for selection of stimulus items:

Wise Brown, M., and Williams, G. (Illustrator). (1956, 1984). Golden Books Publishing Company.

Phonological Awareness Activities at the Word Level

1. Counting words.

What to say to the student: "We're going to count words."

> **EXAMPLE** "How many words do you hear in this sentence (or phrase): It was spring'?" (3)

> **NOTE:** *Use pictured items and/or manipulatives if necessary. Use any of the following stimulus phrases or sentences and/or others you select from the story. The correct answers are in parentheses.*

Stimulus items:

burst out (2)

a home (2)

under a rock (3)

down the road (3)

under a log (3)

so he went on (4)

looking for a home (4)

fall out of the nest (5)

I would fall on the ground. (6)

"Not for me," said the bunny. (6)

2. Identifying the missing word from a list.

What to say to the student: "Listen to the words I say. I'll say them again. You tell me which word I leave out."

> **EXAMPLE**   "Listen to the words I say: 'bunny,' 'home,' 'nest.' I'll say them again. Tell me which one I leave out: 'bunny,' 'home.'" (nest)

> **NOTE:** *Use pictured items and/or manipulatives if necessary. Use any of the following stimulus words and/or others you select from the story. The correct answers are in parentheses.*

Stimulus set #1	Stimulus set #2
burst, sang	burst (sang)
Spring, leaves	leaves (Spring)
going, groundhog, log	going, log (groundhog)
nest, flowers, under	flowers, under (nest)
robin, their, can't	robin, their (can't)
ground, sang, met	ground, met (sang)
under, little, leaves, looking	under, little, leaves (looking)
robins, live, road, asked	robins, road, asked (live)
home, stone, not, no	stone, not, no (home)
drown, bog, water, frog	drown, bog, frog (water)

3. Identifying the missing word in a phrase or sentence.

What to say to the student: "Listen to the sentence I read. Tell me which word is missing the second time I read the sentence."

> **EXAMPLE**   "'It was Spring.' Listen again and tell me which word I leave out: 'It was
> _____.'" (Spring)

> **NOTE:** *Use pictured items and/or manipulatives if necessary. Use any of the following stimulus sentences and/or others you select from the story. The correct answers are in parentheses.*

Stimulus items:

My home. My _____. (home)

Under a stone. _____ a stone. (Under)

Under the ground. Under _____ ground. (the)

Home for a bunny. Home _____ a bunny. (for)

The leaves burst out. The leaves _____ out. (burst)

The flowers burst out. The _____ burst out. (flowers)

Down the road he went. Down the road _____ went. (he)

Can I come in? Can _____ come in? (I)

And that was his home. _____ that was his home. (And)

Where would a bunny find a home? Where _____ a bunny find a home? (would)

4. Supplying the missing word as an adult reads.

What to say to the student: "I want you to help me read the story. You fill in the words I leave out."

EXAMPLE   "It was _____." (Spring)

NOTE: *Use pictured items and/or manipulatives if necessary. Use any of the following stimulus sentences and/or others you select from the story. The correct answers are in parentheses.*

Stimulus items:

Under a _____. (rock, log, stone)

Spring, _____, Spring! (Spring)

The _____ burst out. (leaves, flowers)

A _____ of his own. (home)

A bunny came _____ the road. (down)

A home for a _____. (bunny)

I would _____ out of a nest. (fall)

"Not for me," said the _____. (bunny)

"Here, here, _____," sang the robin. (here)

Here in this nest is _____ home. (my)

5. Rearranging words.

What to say to the student: "I'll say some words out of order. You put them in the right order so they make sense."

EXAMPLE   " 'Spring was it.' Put those words in the right order." (It was Spring.)

NOTE: *Use pictured items and/or manipulatives if necessary. Use any of the following stimulus words and/or others you select from the story. The correct answers are in parentheses. This word-level activity can be more difficult than some of the syllable- or phoneme-level activities because of the memory load. If your students are only able to deal with two or three words to be rearranged, add more two- and three-word samples from the story and omit the four-word level items.*

Stimulus items:

for me not (not for me)

water the under (under the water)

down road the (down the road)

come can in I (can I come in?)

his of own home a (a home of his own)

home where your is (where is your home?)

drown would bog I a in (I would drown in a bog)

on ground the would I fall (I would fall on the ground)

 so road bunny down the went the (so the bunny went down the road)

looking he went on home for a (he went on looking for a home)

Phonological Awareness Activities at the Syllable Level

1. Syllable counting.

What to say to the student: "We're going to count syllables (or parts) of words."

> **EXAMPLE** "How many syllables do you hear in '_____'?" (stimulus word)
> (e.g., "How many syllables do you hear in 'bog'?") (1)

> **NOTE:** *Use pictured items and/or manipulatives if necessary. Use any of the following stimulus words and/or others you select from the story. Use any group of 10 stimulus items you select per teaching set.*

Stimulus items:

> *One-syllable words:* burst, bog, to, down, drown, do, did, came, can, come, can't, ground, my, me, met, nest, not, no, Spring, sang, said, stone, so, road, rock, frog, find, for, fall, he, home, his, here, leaves, log, live, was, where, would, who, were, went, wog, the, their, this, that, your, you, yes, it, out, and, of, eggs, in, is, asked, our, I, on, or

> *Two-syllable words:* bunny, groundhog, going, robin, robins, flowers, little, looking, water, under, about, until

2. Initial syllable deleting.

What to say to the student: "We're going to leave out syllables (or parts of words)."

> **EXAMPLE** "Say '_____.'" (stimulus word) "Say it again without '_____.'"
> (stimulus syllable) (e.g., "Say 'bunny.' Say it again without 'bun.'") (ee)

> **NOTE:** *Use pictured items and/or manipulatives if necessary. Use any of the following stimulus words and/or others you select from the story. The correct answers are in parentheses.*

Stimulus items:

"Say 'groundhog' without 'ground.'" (hog)

"Say 'going' without 'go.'" (ing)

"Say 'robin' without 'rob.'" (in)

"Say 'little' without 'lit.'" (ul)

"Say 'robins' without 'rob.'" (ins)

"Say 'flowers' without 'flau.'" (ers)

"Say 'looking' without 'look.'" (ing)

"Say 'under' without 'un.'" (der)

"Say 'about' without 'uh.'" (bout)

"Say 'until' without 'un.'" (til)

3. Final syllable deleting.

What to say to the student: "We're going to leave out syllables (or parts of words)."

EXAMPLE   "Say '_____.'" (stimulus word) "Say it again without '_____.'" (stimulus syllable) (e.g., "Say 'bunny' without 'ee.'") (bun)

NOTE: *Use pictured items and/or manipulatives if necessary. Use any of the following stimulus words and/or others you select from the story. The correct answers are in parentheses.*

Stimulus items:

"Say 'groundhog' without 'hog.'" (ground)

"Say 'going' without 'ing.'" (go)

"Say 'flowers' without 'ers.'" (flau)

"Say 'until' without 'til.'" (un)

"Say 'about' without 'bout.'" (uh)

"Say 'looking' without 'ing.'" (look)

"Say 'little' without 'ul.'" (lit)

"Say 'robins' without 'ins.'" (rob)

"Say 'under' without 'der.'" (un)

"Say 'robin' without 'in.'" (rob)

4. Initial syllable adding.

What to say to the student: "Now let's add syllables (or parts) to words."

EXAMPLE   "Add '_____'" (stimulus syllable) "to the beginning of '_____.'" (stimulus syllable) (e.g., "'bun' to the beginning of 'ee.'") (bunny)

NOTE: *Use pictured items and/or manipulatives if necessary. Use any of the following stimulus words and/or others you select from the story. The correct answers are in parentheses.*

Stimulus items:

"Add 'ground' to the beginning of 'hog.'" (groundhog)

"Add 'uh' to the beginning of 'bout.'" (about)

"Add 'rob' to the beginning of 'in.'" (robin)

"Add 'un' to the beginning of 'der.'" (under)

"Add 'look' to the beginning of 'ing.'" (looking)

"Add 'flau' to the beginning of 'ers.'" (flowers)

"Add 'lit' to the beginning of 'ul.'" (little)

"Add 'go' to the beginning of 'ing.'" (going)

"Add 'un' to the beginning of 'til.'" (until)

"Add 'rob' to the beginning of 'ins.'" (robins)

5. Final syllable adding.

What to say to the student: "Now let's add syllables (or parts) to words."

> **EXAMPLE** "Add '_____'" (stimulus syllable) "to the end of '_____.'" (stimulus syllable) (e.g., "Add 'ee' to the end of 'bun.'") (bunny)

> **NOTE:** *Use pictured items and/or manipulatives if necessary. Use any of the following stimulus words and/or others you select from the story. The correct answers are in parentheses.*

Stimulus items:

"Add 'hog' to the end of 'ground.'" (groundhog)

"Add 'ins' to the end of 'rob.'" (robins)

"Add 'ers' to the end of 'flau.'" (flowers)

"Add 'bout' to the end of 'uh.'" (about)

"Add 'der' to the end of 'un.'" (under)

"Add 'ing' to the end of 'look.'" (looking)

"Add 'til' to the end of 'un.'" (until)

"Add 'ing' to the end of 'go.'" (going)

"Add 'ul' to the end of 'lit.'" (little)

"Add 'in' to the end of 'rob.'" (robin)

6. Syllable substituting.

What to say to the student: "Let's make up some new words."

> **EXAMPLE** "Say '_____.'" (stimulus word) "Instead of '_____'" (stimulus syllable), "say '_____.'" (stimulus syllable) (e.g., "Say 'bunny.' Instead of 'bun,' say 'fun.' The new word is 'funny.'")

> **NOTE:** *Use pictured items and/or manipulatives if necessary. Use of the following stimulus words and/or others you select from the story. The correct answers are in parentheses.*

Stimulus items:

"Say 'groundhog.' Instead of 'ground,' say 'hedge.'" (hedgehog)

"Say 'little.' Instead of 'ul,' say 'er.'" (litter)

"Say 'going.' Instead of 'go,' say 'show.'" (showing)

"Say 'flowers.' Instead of 'flau,' say 'pow.'" (powers)

"Say 'robins.' Instead of 'ins,' say 'ers.'" (robbers)

"Say 'under.' Instead of 'der,' say 'til.'" (until)

"Say 'looking.' Instead of 'look,' say 'cook.'" (cooking)

"Say 'about.' Instead of 'bout,' say 'frayed.'" (afraid)

"Say 'until.' Instead of 'til,' say 'wind.'" (unwind)

"Say 'robin.' Instead of 'rob,' say 'cab.'" (cabin)

Phonological Awareness Activities at the Phoneme Level

1. Counting sounds.

What to say to the student: "We're going to count sounds in words."

> **EXAMPLE**   "How many sounds do you hear in this word? 'nest.'" (4)

> **NOTE:** *Use pictured items and/or manipulatives if necessary. Use any of the following stimulus words and/or others you select from the story. Be sure to give the letter sound and not the letter name. Use any group of 10 stimulus items you select per teaching set.*

Stimulus words with one sound: a, I

Stimulus words with two sounds: to, do, my, me, no, so, he, who, the, you, it, of, in, own, is, on

Stimulus words with three sounds: bog, did, met, came, can, come, not, said, road, rock, fall, home, his, log, live, was, wog, this, that, yes, and, eggs

Stimulus words with four sounds: burst, bunny, can't, nest, going, stone, frog, find, leaves, little, went, water, under, asked

Stimulus words with five sounds: Spring, robin, until

Stimulus words with six sounds: robins

2. Sound categorization or identifying a rhyme oddity.

What to say to the student: "Guess which word I say does not rhyme with the other three words."

> **EXAMPLE**   "Tell me which word does not rhyme with the other three words: '_____,' '_____,' '_____,' '_____.'" (stimulus words) (e.g., "'came,' 'same,' 'tame,' 'ground.' Which word doesn't rhyme?") (ground)

> **NOTE:** *Use pictured items if necessary. Use any of the following stimulus words and/or others you select from the story. The correct answers are in parentheses.*

Stimulus items:

Spring, ring, sing, sang (sang)

frog, home, log, bog (home)

flowers, stone, powers, showers (stone)

looking, cooking, wog, booking (wog)

water, nest, best, pressed (water)

rock, sock, lock, under (under)

stone, robins, phone, loan (robins)

going, rowing, groundhog, showing (groundhog)

sang, burst, first, thirst (sang)

ground, round, poems, found (poems)

3. Matching rhyme.

What to say to the student: "We're going to think of rhyming words."

> **EXAMPLE** "Which word rhymes with '_____'?" (stimulus word) (e.g., "Which word rhymes with 'Spring': 'nest,' 'can't,' 'sang,' 'ring'?") (ring)

NOTE: *Use pictured items if necessary. Use any of the following stimulus words and/or others you select from the story. The correct answers are in parentheses.*

Stimulus items:

sang: rang, frog, road, down (rang)

looking: cooking, robins, stone, nest (cooking)

wog: flowers, robin, bog, leaves (bog)

frog: asked, log, where, find (log)

stone: bone, sang, road, fall (bone)

home: little, gnome, until, where (gnome)

going: eggs, your, under, rowing (rowing)

bunny: water, where, leaves, money (money)

frog: log, read, alone, right (log)

flowers: under, powers, eggs, asked (powers)

4. Producing rhyme.

What to say to the student: "Now we'll say rhyming words."

> **EXAMPLE** "Tell me a word that rhymes with '_____.'" (stimulus word) (e.g., "Tell me a word that rhymes with 'frog.' You can make up a word if you want.") (dog, bog, wog)

NOTE: *Use pictured items if necessary. Use any of the following stimulus words and/or others you select from the story (i.e., you say a word from the list below and the student is to think of a rhyming word). Use any group of 10 stimulus items you select per teaching set.*

Stimulus items:

/b/: burst, bunny, bog

/t/: to

/d/: down, drown, do, did

/k/: came, can, come, can't

/g/: going, ground

/m/: my, me, met

/n/: nest, not, no

/s/: Spring, sang, said, stone, so

/f/: frog, flowers, find, for, fall

/h/: he, home, his, here

/r/: robin, robins, road, rock

/l/: leaves, log, little, looking, live

/w/, /wh/: was, where, would, were, went, wog, water

/voiced th/: the, their, this, that

/y/ (as in yellow): you, your, yes

vowels: it, out, and, of, eggs, in, own, is, asked, our, on, or

5. Sound matching (initial).

What to say to the student: "Now we'll listen for the first sound in words."

> **EXAMPLE** "Listen to this sound: / /." (stimulus sound). "Guess which word I say begins with that sound: '_____,' '_____,' '_____,' '_____.'" (stimulus words) (e.g., "Listen to this sound: /b/. Guess which word I say begins with that sound: 'frog,' 'bog,' 'sang,' 'nest.'") (bog)

> **NOTE:** *Give the letter sound, not the letter name. Use pictured items if necessary. Use any of the following stimulus words and/or others you select from the story. The correct answers are in parentheses.*

Stimulus items:

/m/: nest, sang, frog, met (met)

/d/: drown, rock, leaves, about (drown)

/f/: home, find, live, here (find)

/h/: log, stone, home, fall (home)

/w/: here, looking, groundhog, water (water)

/l/: leaves, met, rock, find (leaves)

/k/: stone, robins, can't, flowers (can't)

/s/: their, said, not, find (said)

/voiced th/: that, home, stone, rock (that)

/r/: home, about, live, road (road)

6. Sound matching (final).

What to say to the student: "Now we'll listen for the last sound in words."

> **EXAMPLE** "Listen to this sound: / /." (stimulus sound) "Guess which word I say ends with that sound: '_____,' '_____,' '_____,' '_____.'" (stimulus words) (e.g., "Listen to this sound: /g/. Guess which word I say ends with that sound: 'frog,' 'he,' 'the,' 'road.'") (frog)

NOTE: *Give the letter sound, not the letter name. Use pictured items and/or manipulatives if necessary. Use any of the following stimulus words and/or others you select from the story. The correct answers are in parentheses.*

Stimulus items:

/k/: rock, home, log, robin (rock)

/n/: home, robin, yes, said (robin)

/z/: came, this, rock, is (is)

/ng/: Spring, burst, frog, robin (Spring)

/r/: until, frog, come, water (water)

/long O/: fall, so, were, my (so)

/s/: this, going, was, until (this)

/oo/: came, sang, do, here (do)

/r/: under, burst, bunny, the (under)

/l/: and, robin, little, came (little)

7. Identifying the initial sound in words.

What to say to the student: "I'll say a word two times. Tell me what sound is missing the second time: '_____,' '_____.'" (stimulus words)

> EXAMPLE   "What sound do you hear in '_____'" (stimulus word) "that is missing in '_____'?" (stimulus word) (e.g., "What sound do you hear in 'fall' that is missing in 'all'?") (/f/)

NOTE: *Give the letter sound, not the letter name. Use pictured items and/or manipulatives if necessary. Use any of the following stimulus words and/or others you select from the story. The correct answers are in parentheses.*

Stimulus items:

"ground, round. What sound do you hear in 'ground' that's missing in 'round'?" (/g/)

"stone, tone. What sound do you hear in 'stone' that's missing in 'tone'?" (/s/)

"road, owed. What sound do you hear in 'road' that's missing in 'owed'?" (/r/)

"came, aim. What sound do you hear in 'came' that's missing in 'aim'?" (/k/)

"about, bout. What sound do you hear in 'about' that's missing in 'bout'?" (/short U/)

"leaves, eaves. What sound do you hear in 'leaves' that's missing in 'eaves'?" (/l/)

"fall, all. What sound do you hear in 'fall' that's missing in 'all'?" (/f/)

"no, owe. What sound do you hear in 'no' that's missing in 'owe'?" (/n/)

"that, at. What sound do you hear in 'that' that's missing in 'at'?" (/voiced th/)

"his, is. What sound do you hear in 'his' that's missing in 'is'?" (/h/)

8. Identifying the final sound in words.

What to say to the student: "I'll say a word two times. Tell me what sound is missing the second time: '_____,' '_____.' " (stimulus words)

> **EXAMPLE** "What sound do you hear in '_____' " (stimulus word) "that is missing in '_____'?" (stimulus word) (e.g., "What sound do you hear in 'flowers' that is missing in 'flower'?") (/z/)

> **NOTE:** *Give the letter sound, not the letter name. Use pictured items and/or manipulatives if necessary. Use any of the following stimulus words and/or others you select from the story. The correct answers are in parentheses.*

Stimulus items:

"asked, ask. What sound do you hear in 'asked' that's missing in 'ask'?" (/t/)

"bunny, bun. What sound do you hear in 'bunny' that's missing in 'bun'?" (/long E/)

"robins, robin. What sound do you hear in 'robins' that's missing in 'robin'?" (/z/)

"stone, stowe. What sound do you hear in 'stone' that's missing in 'stowe'?" (/n/)

"can't, can. What sound do you hear in 'can't' that's missing in 'can'?" (/t/)

"eggs, egg. What sound do you hear in 'eggs' that's missing in 'egg'?" (/z/)

"find, fine. What sound do you hear in 'find' that's missing in 'fine'?" (/d/)

"own, owe. What sound do you hear in 'own' that's missing in 'owe'?" (/n/)

"home, hoe. What sound do you hear in 'home' that's missing in 'hoe'?" (/m/)

"flowers, flower. What sound do you hear in 'flowers' that's missing in 'flower'?" (/z/)

9. Segmenting the initial sound in words.

What to say to the student: "Listen to the word I say and tell me the first sound you hear."

> **EXAMPLE** "What's the first sound in '_____'?" (stimulus word) (e.g., "What's the first sound in 'bog'?") (/b/)

> **NOTE:** *Give the letter sound, not the letter name. Use pictured items and/or manipulatives if necessary. Use any of the following stimulus words and/or others you select from the story. Use any group of 10 stimulus items you select per teaching set.*

Stimulus items:

/b/: burst, bunny, bog

/t/: to

/d/: down, drown, do, did

/k/: came, can, come, can't

/g/: groundhog, going, ground

/m/: my, me, met

/n/: nest, not, no

/s/: Spring, sang, said, stone, so

/f/: frog, flowers, find, for, fall

/h/: he, home, his, here, who

/r/: robin, robins, road, rock

/l/: leaves, log, little, looking, live

/w/, /wh/: was, where, would, were, went, wog, water

/voiced th/: the, their, this, that

/y/ (as in yellow): your, you, yes

vowels: it, and, of, eggs, in, own, under, is, asked, about, on, until

10. Segmenting the final sound in words.

What to say to the student: "Listen to the word I say and tell me the last sound you hear."

EXAMPLE "What's the last sound in the word '_____'?" (stimulus word) (e.g., "What's the last sound in the word 'bog'?") (/g/)

NOTE: *Give the letter sound, not the letter name. Use pictured items and/or manipulatives if necessary. Use any of the following stimulus words and/or others you select from the story. Use any group of 10 stimulus items you select per teaching set.*

Stimulus items:

/t/: it, burst, out, asked, nest, about, not, went, can't, met, that

/d/: said, and, road, find, ground, would, did

/k/: rock

/g/: frog, groundhog, log, wog, bog

/m/: came, home, come

/n/: robin, in, down, own, stone, on, drown, can

/ng/: Spring, looking, sang, going

/s/: this, yes

/z/: was, leaves, flowers, robins, eggs, his, is

/v/: of

/r/: their, for, under, or, where, your, here, were, our, water

/l/: little, fall, until

/long E/: bunny, he, me

/long I/: my

/long O/: so, no

/short U/: the

/oo/: do, you

11. Generating words from the story beginning with a particular sound.

What to say to the student: "Let's think of words from the story that start with certain sounds."

> **EXAMPLE** "Tell me a word from the story that starts with / /." (stimulus sound)
> (e.g., the sound /b/) (bog)

> **NOTE:** *Give the letter sound, not the letter name. Use pictured items if necessary. Use any of the following stimulus words and/or others you select from the story. You say the sound (e.g., a voiceless /p/ sound), and the student is to say a word from the story that begins with that sound. Use any group of 10 stimulus items you select per teaching set.*

Stimulus items:

/b/: burst, bunny, bog

/t/: to

/d/: down, drown, do, did

/k/: came, can, come, can't

/g/: groundhog, going, ground

/m/: my, me, met

/n/: nest, not, no

/s/: Spring, sang, said, stone, so

/f/: frog, flowers, find, for, fall

/h/: he, home, his, here, who

/r/: robin, robins, road, rock

/l/: leaves, log, little, looking, live

/w/, /wh/: was, where, would, were, went, wog, water

/voiced th/: the, their, this, that

/y/ (as in yellow): your, you, yes

vowels: it, and, of, eggs, in, own, under, is, asked, about, on, until

12. Blending sounds in monosyllabic words divided into onset/rime beginning with a two-consonant cluster + rime.

What to say to the student: "Now we'll put sounds together to make words."

> **EXAMPLE** "Put these sounds together to make a word (/ / + / /)." (stimulus sounds)
> "What's the word?" (e.g., "st + ick: What's the word?") (stick)

> **NOTE:** *Give the letter sound, not the letter name. Use pictured items and/or manipulatives if necessary. Use any of the following stimulus words and/or others you select from the story. The correct answers are in parentheses.*

Stimulus items:

    st + one (stone)

    dr + own (drown)

    fr + og (frog)

    gr + ound (ground)

Sourcebook users are encouraged to add stimulus items into this activity from curriculum materials they may be using with *Home for a Bunny*.

13. Blending sounds in monosyllabic words divided into onset/rime beginning with a single consonant + rime.

What to say to the student: "Let's put sounds together to make words."

> **EXAMPLE** "Put these sounds together to make a word (/ / + / /)." (stimulus sounds) "What's the word?" (e.g., "/b/ + og: What's the word?") (bog)

> **NOTE:** *Give the letter sound, not the letter name. Use pictured items and/or manipulatives if necessary. Use any of the following stimulus words and/or others you select from the story. The correct answers are in parentheses.*

Stimulus items:

    /d/ + own (down)

    /k/ + ame (came)

    /n/ + est (nest)

    /s/ + ang (sang)

    /h/ + ome (home)

    /voiced th/ + is (this)

    /m/ + et (met)

    /l/ + eaves (leaves)

    /w/ + ent (went)

    /voiced th/ + at (that)

14. Blending sounds to form a monosyllabic word beginning with a continuant sound.

What to say to the student: "We'll put sounds together to make words."

> **EXAMPLE** "Put these sounds together to make a word: / / + / / + / /." (stimulus sounds) (e.g., /n/ /ah/ /t/) (not)

> **NOTE:** *Give the letter sound, not the letter name. Use pictured items and/or manipulatives if necessary. Use any of the following stimulus words and/or others you select from the story. The correct answers are in parentheses.*

Stimulus items:

/l/ /long E/ /v/ /z/ (leaves)

/s/ /short E/ /d/ (said)

/r/ /long O/ /d/ (road)

/h/ /long O/ /m/ (home)

/w/ /short E/ /n/ /t/ (went)

/y/ (as in yellow) /oo/ (you)

/h/ /short I/ /z/ (his)

/f/ /long I/ /n/ /d/ (find)

/voiced th/ /short I/ /s/ (this)

/r/ /ah/ /k/ (rock)

15. Blending sounds to form a monosyllabic word beginning with a noncontinuant sound.

What to say to the student: "We'll put sounds together to make words."

> **EXAMPLE** "Put these sounds together to make a word (/ / + / / + / /)." (stimulus sounds) (e.g., /t/ /oo/) (to)

> **NOTE:** *Give the letter sound, not the letter name. Use pictured items and/or manipulatives if necessary. Use any of the following stimulus words and/or others you select from the story. The correct answers are in parentheses.*

Stimulus items:

/b/ /ah/ /g/ (bog)

/d/ /short I/ /d/ (did)

/k/ /short A/ /n/ (can)

/b/ /r/ /s/ /t/ (burst)

/k/ /long A/ /m/ (came)

/d/ /oo/ (do)

/k/ /short U/ /m/ (come)

/k/ /short A/ /n/ /t/ (can't)

/g/ /long O/ (go)

/k/ /short A/ /n/ (can)

16. Substituting the initial sound in words.

What to say to the student: "We're going to change beginning/first sounds in words."

> **EXAMPLE** "Say '_____.'" (stimulus word) "Instead of / /" (stimulus sound), "say / /." (stimulus sound) (e.g., "Say 'bog.' Instead of /b/. say /l/. What's your new word?") (log)

> **NOTE:** *Give the letter sound, not the letter name. Use pictured items and/or manipulatives if necessary. Use any of the following stimulus words and/or others you select from the story. The correct answers are in parentheses.*

Stimulus items:

"Say 'to.' Instead of /t/, say /d/." (do)

"Say 'came.' Instead of /k/, say /f/." (fame)

"Say 'ground.' Instead of /g/, say /b/." (browned)

"Say 'sang.' Instead of /s/, say /f/." (fang)

"Say 'met.' Instead of /m/, say /p/." (pet)

"Say 'home.' Instead of /h/, say /d/." (dome)

"Say 'that.' Instead of /voiced th/, say /r/." (rat)

"Say 'looking.' Instead of /l/, say /k/." (cooking)

"Say 'drown.' Instead of /d/, say /f/." (frown)

"Say 'nest.' Instead of /n/, say /b/." (best)

17. Substituting the final sound in words.

What to say to the student: "We're going to change ending/last sounds in words."

> **EXAMPLE**   "Say '_____.'" (stimulus word) "Instead of / /" (stimulus sound), "say / /." (stimulus sound) (e.g., "Say 'can.' Instead of /n/, say /t/. What's your new word?") (cat)

NOTE: *Give the letter sound, not the letter name. Use pictured items and/or manipulatives if necessary. Use any of the following stimulus words and/or others you select from the story. The correct answers are in parentheses.*

Stimulus items:

"Say 'my.' Instead of /long I/, say /long E/." (me)

"Say 'can't.' Instead of /t/, say /z/." (cans)

"Say 'stone.' Instead of /n/, say /v/." (stove)

"Say 'road.' Instead of /d/, say /z/." (rose)

"Say 'home.' Instead of /m/, say /p/." (hope)

"Say 'came.' Instead of /m/, say /n/." (cane)

"Say 'me.' Instead of /long E/, say /oo/." (moo)

"Say 'so.' Instead of /long O/, say /long E/." (see)

"Say 'flowers.' Instead of /z/, say /d/." (flowered)

"Say 'yes.' Instead of /s/, say /t/." (yet)

18. Segmenting the middle sound in monosyllabic words.

What to say to the student: "Tell me the middle sound in the word I say."

> **EXAMPLE**   "What's the middle sound in the word '_____'?" (stimulus word) (e.g., "What's the middle sound in the word 'bog'?") (/ah/)

NOTE: *Give the letter sound, not the letter name. Use pictured items and/or manipulatives if necessary. Use any of the following stimulus words and/or others you select from the story. The correct answers are in parentheses.*

Stimulus items:

did (/short I/)

came (/long A/)

come (/short U/)

not (/ah/)

can (/short A/)

met (/short E/)

said (/short E/)

home (/long O/)

live (/short I/)

rock (/ah/)

19. Substituting the middle sound in words.

What to say to the student: "We're going to change the middle sound in words."

> **EXAMPLE**   "Say '_____.'" (stimulus word) "Instead of / /" (stimulus sound), "say / /." (stimulus sound) (e.g., "Say 'bog.' Instead of /ah/, say /short I/. What's your new word?") (big)

NOTE: *Give the letter sound, not the letter name. Use pictured items and/or manipulatives if necessary. Use any of the following stimulus words and/or others you select from the story. The correct answers are in parentheses.*

Stimulus items:

"Say 'did.' Instead of /short I/, say /short A/." (dad)

"Say 'come.' Instead of /short U/, say /long A/." (came)

"Say 'not.' Instead of /ah/, say /short I/." (knit)

"Say 'fall.' Instead of /ah/, say /short I/." (fill)

"Say 'home.' Instead of /long O/, say /short I/." (him)

"Say 'this.' Instead of /short I/, say /short U/." (thus)

"Say 'log.' Instead of /ah/, say /short A/." (lag)

"Say 'live.' Instead of /short I/, say /short U/." (love)

"Say 'can' Instead of /short A/, say /long A/." (cane)

"Say 'his.' Instead of /short I/, say /short A/." (has)

20. Identifying all sounds in monosyllabic words.

What to say to the student: "Now tell me all the sounds you hear in the word I say."

EXAMPLE "What sounds do you hear in the word '_____'?" (stimulus word)
(e.g., "What sounds do you hear in the word 'bog'?") (/b/ /ah/ /g/)

NOTE: *Give the letter sound, not the letter name. Use pictured items and/or manipulatives if necessary. Use any of the following stimulus words and/or others you select from the story. The correct answers are in parentheses.*

Stimulus items:

did (/d/ /short I/ /d/)

to (/t/ /oo/)

nest (/n/ /short E/ /s/ /t/)

came (/k/ /long A/ /m/)

come (/k/ /short U/ /m/)

stone (/s/ /t/ /long O/ /n/)

frog (/f/ /r/ /ah/ /g/)

eggs (/long A/ /g/ /z/)

that (/voiced th/ /short A/ /t/)

burst (/b/ /r/ /s/ /t/)

21. Deleting sounds within words.

What to say to the student: "We're going to leave out sounds in words."

EXAMPLE "Say '_____'" (stimulus word) "without / /." (stimulus sound)
(e.g., "Say 'frog' without /r /.") (fog) Say: "The word that's left—'fog'—is a real word. Sometimes, the new word won't be a real word."

NOTE: *Give the letter sound, not the letter name. Use pictured items and/or manipulatives if necessary. Use any of the following stimulus words and/or others you select from the story. The correct answers are in parentheses.*

Stimulus items:

"Say 'stone' without /t/." (sewn)

"Say 'nest' without /s/." (net)

"Say 'went' without /n/." (wet)

"Say 'ground' without /r/." (gowned)

"Say 'burst' without /s/." (Bert)

"Say 'drown' without /r/." (down)

"Say 'Spring' without /r/." (sping)

"Say 'under' without /n/." (udder)

"Say 'flowers' without /l/." (fowers)

"Say 'can't' without /n/." (cat)

22. Substituting consonants in words having a two-sound cluster.

What to say to the student: "We're going to substitute sounds in words."

> **EXAMPLE** "Say '_____.'" (stimulus word) "Instead of / /" (stimulus sound), "say / /." (stimulus sound) (e.g., "Say 'stone.' Instead of /t/, say /k/.") (scone) Say: "Sometimes, the new word will be a made-up word."

> **NOTE:** *Give the letter sound, not the letter name. Use pictured items and/or manipulatives if necessary. Use any of the following stimulus words and/or others you select from the story. The correct answers are in parentheses.*

Stimulus items:

"Say 'drown.' Instead of /d/, say /b/." (brown)

"Say 'flowers.' Instead of /f/, say /p/." (plowers)

"Say 'can't.' Instead of /n/, say /s/." (cast)

"Say 'burst.' Instead of /s/, say /p/." (burped)

"Say 'ground.' Instead of /g/, say /b/." (browned)

"Say 'went.' Instead of /n/, say /s/." (west)

"Say 'asked.' Instead of /t/, say /s/." (asks)

"Say 'leaves.' Instead of /v/, say /n/." (leans)

"Say 'find.' Instead of /d/, say /z/." (fines)

"Say 'leaves.' Instead of /v/, say /d/." (leads)

23. Phoneme reversing.

What to say to the student: "We're going to say words backward."

> **EXAMPLE** "Say the word '_____'" (stimulus word) "backward." (e.g., "Say 'bog' backward.") (gob)

> **NOTE:** *This is a difficult phoneme-level task and should only be done with older students. Give the letter sound, not the letter name. Use pictured items and/or manipulatives if necessary. Use any of the following stimulus words and/or others you select from the story. The correct answers are in parentheses.*

Stimulus items:

came (make)

did (did)

can (knack)

stone (notes)

said (dess)

met (tem)

not (tahn)

come (muck)

no (own)

my (I'm)

24. Phoneme switching.

What to say to the student: "We're going to switch the first sounds in two words."

EXAMPLE "Switch the first sounds in '_____' and '_____.'" (stimulus words) (e.g., "Switch the first sounds in 'he' and 'went.'") (we hent)

NOTE: *This is a difficult phoneme-level task and should only be done with older students. Give the letter sound, not the letter name. Use pictured items and/or manipulatives if necessary. Use any of the following stimulus words and/or others you select from the story. The correct answers are in parentheses.*

Stimulus items:

bunny find (funny bind)

the road (ruh thoad)

you live (lou yive)

my log (lie mog)

my home (hy mome)

leaves burst (beaves lurst)

flowers burst (blauers first)

not for (fought nor)

the bog (buh thog)

bunny went (wunny bent)

25. Pig Latin.

What to say to the student: "We're going to speak a secret language by using words from the story. In pig Latin, you take off the first sound of a word, put it at the end of the word, and add an 'ay' sound."

EXAMPLE "Say 'bog' in pig Latin." (ogbay)

NOTE: *This is a difficult phoneme-level task and should only be done with older students. Use pictured items and/or manipulatives if necessary. Use any of the following stimulus words and/or others you select from the story. The correct answers are in parentheses.*

Stimulus items:

live (ivelay)

log (oglay)

spring (pringsay)

robins (obinsray)

frog (rogfay)

leaves (eaveslay)

little (ittlelay)

home (omehay)

groundhog (roundhoggay)

bunny (unnybay)

From Phonological Awareness into Print

NOTE: *Only five examples per activity are included in this resource due to space. You are encouraged to add many more words into this section that you feel your student(s) is(are) ready to write.*

1. Substituting the initial sound or letter in words.

NOTE: *Use lined paper or copy the sheet of lined paper included in the back of this book.*

Stimulus items:

1.1 do/to

Task a. "Say 'do.' Instead of /d/, say /t/. What's your new word?" (to) "Write/copy 'do' and 'to.'"

Task b. "Circle the **letters** that make the words different." ([d], [t])

Task c. "What **sounds** do these letters make?" (/d/, /t/)

1.2 live/give

Task a. "Say 'live.' Instead of /l/, say /g/. What's your new word?" (give) "Write/copy 'live' and 'give.'"

Task b. "Circle the **letters** that make the words different." ([l], [g])

Task c. "What **sounds** do these letters make?" (/l/, /g/)

1.3 sang/rang

Task a. "Say 'sang.' Instead of /s/, say /r/. What's your new word?" (rang) "Write/copy 'sang' and 'rang.'"

Task b. "Circle the **letters** that make the words different." ([s], [r])

Task c. "What **sounds** do these letters make?" (/s/, /r/)

1.4 drown/brown

Task a. "Say 'drown.' Instead of /d/, say /b/. What's your new word?" (brown) "Write/copy 'drown' and 'brown.'"

Task b. "Circle the **letters** that make the words different." ([d], [b])

Task c. "What **sounds** do these letters make?" (/d/, /b/)

1.5 looking/cooking

Task a. "Say 'looking.' Instead of /l/, say /k/. What's your new word?" (cooking) "Write/copy 'looking' and 'cooking.'"

Task b. "Circle the **letters** that make the words different." ([l], [c])

Task c. "What **sounds** do these letters make?" (/l/, /k/)

2. Substituting the final sound or letter in words.

NOTE: *Use lined paper or copy the sheet of lined paper included in the back of this book.*

Stimulus items:

2.1 not/nod

Task a. "Say 'not.' Instead of /t/, say /d/. What's your new word?" (nod) "Write/copy 'not' and 'nod.'"

Task b. "Circle the **letters** that make the words different." ([t], [d])

Task c. "What **sounds** do these letters make?" (/t/, /d/)

2.2 home/hope

Task a. "Say 'home.' Instead of /m/, say /p /. What's your new word?" (hope) "Write/copy 'home' and 'hope.'"

Task b. "Circle the **letters** that make the words different." ([m], [p])

Task c. "What **sounds** do these letters make?" (/m/, /p/)

2.3 flowers/flowered

Task a. "Say 'flowers.' Instead of /z/, say /d/. What's your new word?" (flowered) "Write/copy 'flowers' and 'flowered.'"

Task b. "Circle the **letters** that make the words different." ([s], [e], [d])

Task c. "What **sounds** do these letters make?" (/z/, /d/)

2.4 so/see

Task a. "Say 'so.' Instead of /long O/, say /long E/. What's your new word?" (see) "Write/copy 'so' and 'see.'"

Task b. "Circle the **letters** that make the words different." ([o], [e], [e])

Task c. "What **sounds** do these letters make?" (/long O/, /long E/)

2.5 rock/rot

Task a. "Say 'rock.' Instead of /k/, say /t/. What's your new word?" (rot) "Write/copy 'rock' and 'rot.'"

Task b. "Circle the **letters** that make the words different." ([c], [k], [t])

Task c. "What **sounds** do these letters make?" (/k/, /t/)

3. Substituting the middle sound or letter in words.

NOTE: *Use lined paper or copy the sheet of lined paper included in the back of this book.*

Stimulus items:

3.1 not/net

Task a. "Say 'not.' Instead of /ah/, say /short E/. What's your new word?" (net) "Write/copy 'not' and 'net.'"

Task b. "Circle the **letters** that make the words different." ([o], [e])

Task c. "What **sounds** do these letters make?" (/ah/, /e/)

3.2 stone/stain

Task a. "Say 'stone.' Instead of /long O/, say /long A/. What's your new word?" (stain) "Write/copy 'stone' and 'stain.'"

Task b. "Circle the **letters** that make the words different." ([o], [e], [a], [i])

Task c. "What **sounds** do these letters make?" (/long O/, /long A/)

3.3 met/might

Task a. "Say 'met.' Instead of /short E/, say /long I/. What's your new word?" (might) "Write/copy 'met' and 'might.'"

Task b. "Circle the **letters** that make the words different." ([e], [i], [g], [h])

Task c. "What **sounds** do these letters make?" (/short E/, /long I/)

3.4 his/has

Task a. "Say 'his.' Instead of /short I/, say /short A/. What's your new word?" (has) "Write/copy 'his' and 'has.'"

Task b. "Circle the **letters** that make the words different." ([i], [a])

Task c. "What **sounds** do these letters make?" (/short I/, /short A/)

3.5 fall/feel

Task a. "Say 'fall.' Instead of /ah/, say /long E/. What's your new word?" (feel) "Write/copy 'fall' and 'feel.'"

Task b. "Circle the **letters** that make the words different." ([a], [e], [e])

Task c. "What **sounds** do these letters make?" (/ah/, /long E/)

4. Supplying the initial sound or letter in words.

NOTE: *Use lined paper or copy the sheet of lined paper included in the back of this book.*

Stimulus items:

4.1 can't/ant

Task a. "Say 'can't,' say 'ant.' What sound did you hear in 'can't' that's missing in 'ant'?" (/k/) "Now we'll change the **letter.** Write/copy 'can't' and 'ant.'"

Task b. "Circle the beginning **letter** that makes the words different." ([c])

Task c. "What **sound** does this letter make?" (/k/)

4.2 about/bout

Task a. "Say 'about,' say 'bout.' What sound did you hear in 'about' that's missing in 'bout'?" (/short U/) "Now we'll change the **letter.** Write/copy 'about' and 'bout.'"

Task b. "Circle the beginning **letter** that makes the words different." ([a])

Task c. "What **sound** does this letter make?" (/short U/)

4.3 stone/tone

Task a. "Say 'stone,' say 'tone.' What sound did you hear in 'stone' that's missing in 'tone'?" (/s/) "Now we'll change the **letter.** Write/copy 'stone' and 'tone.'"

Task b. "Circle the beginning **letter** that makes the words different." ([s])

Task c. "What **sound** does this letter make?" (/s/)

4.4 ground/round
Task a. "Say 'ground,' say 'round.' What sound did you hear in 'ground' that's missing in 'round'?" (/g/) "Now we'll change the **letter.** Write/copy 'ground' and 'round.'"

Task b. "Circle the beginning **letter** that makes the words different." ([g])

Task c. "What **sound** does this letter make?" (/g/)

4.5 leaves/eaves
Task a. "Say 'leaves,' say 'eaves.' What sound did you hear in 'leaves' that's missing in 'eaves'?" (/l/) "Now we'll change the **letter.** Write/copy 'leaves' and 'eaves.'"

Task b. "Circle the beginning **letter** that makes the words different." ([l])

Task c. "What **sound** does this letter make?" (/l/)

5. Supplying the final sound or letter in words.
NOTE: *Use lined paper or copy the sheet of lined paper included in the back of this book.*

Stimulus items:

5.1 leaves/leave
Task a. "Say 'leaves,' say 'leave.' What sound did you hear in 'leaves' that's missing in 'leave'?" (/z/) "Now we'll change the **letter.** Write/copy 'leaves' and 'leave.'"

Task b. "Circle the ending/last **letter** that makes the words different." ([s])

Task c. "What **sound** does this letter make?" (/z/)

5.2 asked/ask
Task a. "Say 'asked,' say 'ask.' What sound did you hear in 'asked' that's missing in 'ask'?" (/t/) "Now we'll change the **letters.** Write/copy 'asked' and 'ask.'"

Task b. "Circle the ending/last **letters** that make the words different." ([e], [d])

Task c. "What **sound** do these letters make?" (/t/)

5.3 and/an
Task a. "Say 'and,' say 'an.' What sound did you hear in 'and' that's missing in 'an'?" (/d/) "Now we'll change the **letter.** Write/copy 'and' and 'an.'"

Task b. "Circle the ending/last **letter** that makes the words different." ([d])

Task c. "What **sound** does this letter make?" (/d/)

5.4 eggs/egg
Task a. "Say 'eggs,' say 'egg.' What sound did you hear in 'eggs' that's missing in 'egg'?" (/z/) "Now we'll change the **letter.** Write/copy 'eggs' and 'egg.'"

Task b. "Circle the ending/last **letter** that makes the word different." ([s])

Task c. "What **sound** does this letter make?" (/z/)

5.5 can't/can

Task a. "Say 'can't,' say 'can.' What sound did you hear in 'can't' that's missing in 'can'?" (/t/) "Now we'll change the **letter**. Write/copy 'can't' and 'can.'"

Task b. "Circle the ending/last **letter** that makes the words different." ([t])

Task c. "What **sound** does this letter make?" (/t/)

6. Switching the first sound and letter in words (ADVANCED).

NOTE: *Use lined paper or copy the sheet of lined paper included in the back of this book.*

Stimulus items:

6.1 he met

Task a. "Say 'he,' say 'met.' What sound do you hear at the beginning of 'he'?" (/h/) "What sound do you hear at the beginning of 'met'?" (/m/) "Switch the first sounds in those words." (me het) "Now we'll change the **letters**. Write/copy 'he met' and 'me het.'"

Task b. "Circle the beginning **letters** that change the words." ([h], [m])

Task c. "What **sounds** do those letters make?" (/h/, /m/)

6.2 bunny find

Task a. "Say 'bunny,' say 'find.' What sound do you hear at the beginning of 'bunny'?" (/b/) "What sound do you hear at the beginning of 'find'?" (/f/) "Switch the first sounds in those words." (funny bind) "Now we'll change the **letters**. Write/copy 'bunny find' and 'funny bind.'"

Task b. "Circle the beginning **letters** that change the words." ([b], [f])

Task c. "What **sounds** do those letters make?" (/b/, /f/)

6.3 he went

Task a. "Say 'he,' say 'went.' What sound do you hear at the beginning of 'he'?" (/h/) "What sound do you hear at the beginning of 'went'?" (/w/) "Switch the first sounds in those words." (we hent) "Now we'll change the **letters**. Write/copy 'he went' and 'we hent.'"

Task b. "Circle the beginning **letters** that change the words." ([h], [w])

Task c. "What **sounds** do those letters make?" (/h/, /w/)

6.4 leaves burst

Task a. "Say 'leaves,' say 'burst.' What sound do you hear at the beginning of 'leaves'?" (/l/) "What sound do you hear at the beginning of 'burst'?" (/b/) "Switch the first sounds in those words." (beaves lurst) "Now we'll change the **letters**. Write/copy 'leaves burst' and 'beaves lurst.'"

Task b. "Circle the beginning letters that change the words." ([l], [b])

Task c. "What **sounds** do those letters make?" (/l/, /b/)

6.5 would fall

Task a. "Say 'would,' say 'fall.' What sound do you hear at the beginning of 'would'?" (/w/) "What sound do you hear at the beginning of 'fall'?" (/f/) "Switch the first sounds in those words." (fould wall) "Now we'll change the **letters.** Write/copy 'would fall' and 'fould wall.'"

Task b. "Circle the beginning **letters** that change the words." ([w], [f])

Task c. "What **sounds** do those letters make?" (/w/, /f/)

CHAPTER

9

Phonological Awareness Activities to Use with *Liang and the Magic Paintbrush*

Text version used for selection of stimulus items:
Demi. (1980). *Liang and the Magic Paintbrush*. New York: Henry Holt and Company.

Phonological Awareness Activities at the Word Level

1. Counting words.

What to say to the student: "We're going to count words."

> **EXAMPLE** "How many words do you hear in this sentence (or phrase)? 'long ago in China'" (4)

> **NOTE:** *Use pictured items and/or manipulatives if necessary. Use any of the following stimulus phrases or sentences and/or others you select from the story. The correct answers are in parentheses.*

Stimulus items:
  nobody knows (2)
  he painted deer (3)
  far and wide (3)
  use it carefully (3)
  an old man appeared (4)
  Liang jumped for joy. (4)
  Liang began to paint. (4)
  The deer came to life. (5)
  What do you think happened? (5)
  It really was a magic paintbrush. (6)

2. Identifying the missing word from a list.

What to say to the student: "Listen to the words I say. I'll say them again. You tell me which word I leave out."

> **EXAMPLE** "Listen to the words I say: 'rock,' 'reeds,' 'wish.' I'll say them again. Tell me which one I leave out: 'rock,' 'reeds.'" (wish)

NOTE: *Use pictured items and/or manipulatives if necessary. Use any of the following stimulus words and/or others you select from the story. The correct answers are in parentheses.*

Stimulus set #1	Stimulus set #2
teach, paint	teach (paint)
royal, life	life (royal)
China, paint, lanterns	China, paint (lanterns)
wish, emperor, life	emperor, life (wish)
word, village, paintbrush	word, paintbrush (village)
magic, enormous, enough	magic, enormous (enough)
rooster, house, phoenix, night	rooster, house, phoenix (night)
soldiers, accident, mountains, joy	soldiers, mountains, joy (accident)
roamed, knew, gold, crashing	knew, gold, crashing (roamed)
school, Liang, imprisoned, wished	school, Liang, wished (imprisoned)

3. Identifying the missing word in a phrase or sentence.

What to say to the student: "Listen to the sentence I read. Tell me which word is missing the second time I read the sentence."

> **EXAMPLE** " 'The emperor.' Listen again and tell me which word I leave out: 'The _____.' " (emperor)

NOTE: *Use pictured items and/or manipulatives if necessary. Use any of the following stimulus sentences and/or others you select from the story. The correct answers are in parentheses.*

Stimulus items:

Nobody knows. Nobody _____. (knows)

More wind! _____ wind! (more)

The royal family. The _____ family. (royal)

The emperor asked. _____ emperor asked. (The)

Paint me the sea. Paint _____ the sea. (me)

Where are the fish? Where are the _____ ? (fish)

A sea full of fish. A _____ full of fish. (sea)

Liang drew and drew. Liang _____ and drew. (drew)

Bobbling about on the water. _____ about on the water. (Bobbling)

The boat began to rock. The boat _____ to rock. (began)

4. Supplying the missing word as an adult reads.

What to say to the student: "I want you to help me read the story. You fill in the words I leave out."

EXAMPLE   "The magic _____." (paintbrush)

NOTE: *Use pictured items and/or manipulatives if necessary. Use any of the following stimulus sentences and/or others you select from the story. The correct answers are in parentheses.*

Stimulus items:

An enormous _____. (python)

He painted toy _____. (birds)

An _____ man. (old)

It is a _____ paintbrush. (magic)

Use it _____. (carefully)

Let _____ have a boat! (us)

Liang drew _____ wind. (more)

The _____ keeled over. (boat)

Soon waves were _____ and splashing over the deck. (crashing)

Some say that he went _____ to his own village. (back)

5. Rearranging words.

What to say to the student: "I'll say some words out of order. You put them in the right order so they make sense."

EXAMPLE   " 'the paintbrush magic.' Put those words in the right order." (the magic paintbrush)

NOTE: *Use pictured items and/or manipulatives if necessary. Use any of the following stimulus words and/or others you select from the story. The correct answers are in parentheses. This word-level activity can be more difficult than some of the syllable- or phoneme-level activities because of the memory load. If your students are only able to deal with two or three words to be rearranged, add more two- and three-word samples from the story and omit the four-word level items.*

Stimulus items:

knows nobody (nobody knows)

his village own (his own village)

wide spread and far (spread far and wide)

earth the roamed painting (roamed the earth painting)

Liang instead toad a painted (Liang painted a toad instead)

instead painted he rooster a (he painted a rooster instead)

he something out left (he left something out)

I so much paint want to (I want so much to paint.)

will teach me you please (Please, will you teach me?)

ago long China in (long ago in China)

Phonological Awareness Activities at the Syllable Level

1. Syllable counting.

What to say to the student: "We're going to count syllables (or parts) of words."

> **EXAMPLE** "How many syllables do you hear in '_____'?" (stimulus word) (e.g., "How many syllables in 'paint'?") (1)

> **NOTE:** *Use pictured items and/or manipulatives if necessary. Use any of the following stimulus words and/or others you select from the story. Use any group of 10 stimulus items you select per teaching set.*

Stimulus items:

One-syllable words: paint, passed, please, placed, poor, plan, boy, but, buy, brush, birds, bans, by, been, bound, brought, bit, boat, back, to, teach, twig, toy, tools, take, toad, turned, tried, tree, day, drove, drew, drops, deer, did, drop, down, do, deck, could, keep, cut, called, came, cook, come, crane, can, cried, gave, glared, give, gold, get, jumped, joy, join, much, me, man, made, make, move, more, named, not, night, now, knew, knows, school, so, said, still, sand, slept, saw, set, sell, spread, sat, sent, sea, sank, some, soon, say, reeds, rocks, rolled, rock, roamed, fish, flew, for, friends, field, fell, full, far, his, he, him, hand, house, have, head, hands, long, life, left, large, lose, let, one, wish, was, went, will, wants, when, with, wide, were, where, which, would, word, wished, we, wind, waves, what, sure, should, thank, things, thought, think, the, that, their, then, there, they, you, and, in, a, an, art, I, at, its, are, on, of, one, as, old, it, is, earned, out, asked, eye, ink, all, up, off, earth, us, own

Two-syllable words: paintbrush, painted, parents, pictures, palace, python, pieces, painting, beggar, began, bobbing, bottom, became, teacher, table, dragon, cutting, crashing, gather, greedy, China, children, magic, money, merchants, mountains, million, something, soldiers, saying, swimming, story, splashing, river, refused, rooster, royal, fingers, finished, freedom, happened, Liang, lanterns, Liang's, listen, village, water, ago, afford, away, appeared, among, other, into, only, about, almost, ordered, instead, again, others, enough, exchange, over

Three-syllable words: delighted, gathering, marketplace, furniture, happily, wherever, whatever, enormous, firewood, accident, including, emperor, accepted, emperor's

Five-syllable words: immediately

2. Initial syllable deleting.

What to say to the student: "We're going to leave out syllables (or parts of words)."

> **EXAMPLE** "Say '_____.'" (stimulus word) "Say it again without '_____.'" (stimulus syllable) (e.g., "Say 'paintbrush.' Say it again without 'paint.'") (brush)

NOTE: *Use pictured items and/or manipulatives if necessary. Use any of the following stimulus words and/or others you select from the story. The correct answers are in parentheses.*

Stimulus items:

"Say 'children' without 'chil.'" (dren)

"Say 'refused' without 're.'" (fused)

"Say 'lanterns' without 'lan.'" (turns)

"Say 'firewood' without 'fi.'" (erwood)

"Say 'imprisoned' without 'im.'" (prisoned)

"Say 'nobody' without 'no.'" (body)

"Say 'magic' without 'mag.'" (ick)

"Say 'whatever' without 'what.'" (ever)

"Say 'fingers' without 'fing.'" (gurrs)

"Say 'gathering' without 'gath.'" (ering)

3. Final syllable deleting.

What to say to the student: "We're going to leave out syllables (or parts of words)."

> **EXAMPLE** "Say '_____.'" (stimulus word) "Say it again without '_____.'" (stimulus syllable) (e.g., "Say 'paintbrush' without 'brush.'") (paint)

NOTE: *Use pictured items and/or manipulatives if necessary. Use any of the following stimulus words and/or others you select from the story. The correct answers are in parentheses.*

Stimulus items:

"Say 'swimming' without 'ing.'" (swim)

"Say 'freedom' without 'dumb.'" (free)

"Say 'royal' without 'ul.'" (Roy)

"Say 'village' without 'udge.'" (vill)

"Say 'instead' without 'stead.'" (in)

"Say 'firewood' without 'wood.'" (fire)

"Say 'immediate' without 'lee.'" (immediate)

"Say 'Liang' without 'ang.'" (Lee)

"Say 'lanterns' without 'turns.'" (lan)

"Say 'only' without 'lee.'" (own)

4. Initial syllable adding.

What to say to the student: "Now let's add syllables (or parts) to words."

> **EXAMPLE** "Add '_____'" (stimulus syllable) "to the beginning of '_____.'" (stimulus syllable) (e.g., "Add 'paint' to the beginning of 'brush.'") (paintbrush)

NOTE: *Use pictured items and/or manipulatives if necessary. Use any of the following stimulus words and/or others you select from the story. The correct answers are in parentheses.*

Stimulus items:

"Add 'chill' to the beginning of 'drunn.'" (children)

"Add 'free' to the beginning of 'dumb.'" (freedom)

"Add 'some' to the beginning of 'thing.'" (something)

"Add 'in' to the beginning of 'cluding.'" (including)

"Add 'ex' to the beginning of 'change.'" (exchange)

"Add 'be' to the beginning of 'came.'" (became)

"Add 'gree' to the beginning of 'dee.'" (greedy)

"Add 'no' to the beginning of 'body.'" (nobody)

"Add 'splash' to the beginning of 'ing.'" (splashing)

"Add 'what' to the beginning of 'ever.'" (whatever)

5. Final syllable adding.

What to say to the student: "Now let's add syllables (or parts) to words."

> EXAMPLE "Add '_____'" (stimulus syllable) "to the end of '_____.'" (stimulus syllable) (e.g., "Add 'brush' to the end of 'paint.'") (paintbrush)

NOTE: *Use pictured items and/or manipulatives if necessary. Use any of the following stimulus words and/or others you select from the story. The correct answers are in parentheses.*

Stimulus items:

"Add 'lee' to the end of 'immediate.'" (immediately)

"Add 'ing' to the end of 'Bob.'" (bobbing)

"Add 'grrr' to the end of 'bay.'" (beggar)

"Add 'to' to the end of 'in.'" (into)

"Add 'fused' to the end of 're.'" (fused)

"Add 'dren' to the end of 'chill.'" (children)

"Add 'er' to the end of 'teach.'" (teacher)

"Add 'go' to the end of 'uh.'" (ago)

"Add 'ang' to the end of 'Lee.'" (Liang)

"Add 'place' to the end of 'market.'" (marketplace)

6. Syllable substituting.

What to say to the student: "Let's make up some new words."

> EXAMPLE "Say '_____.'" (stimulus word) "Instead of '_____'" (stimulus syllable), "say '_____.'" (stimulus syllable) (e.g., "Say 'paintbrush.' Instead of 'paint,' say 'hair.' The new word is 'hairbrush.'")

NOTE: *Use pictured items and/or manipulatives if necessary. Use of the following stimulus words and/or others you select from the story. The correct answers are in parentheses.*

Stimulus items:

"Say 'firewood.' Instead of 'wood,' say 'place.'" (fireplace)

"Say 'bobbing.' Instead of 'Bob,' say 'rob.'" (robbing)

"Say 'painting.' Instead of 'ing,' say 'er.'" (painter)

"Say 'Liang.' Instead of 'ang,' say 'roy.'" (Leroy)

"Say 'splashing.' Instead of 'splash,' say 'crash.'" (crashing)

"Say 'fingers.' Instead of 'fing,' say 'ling.'" (lingers)

"Say 'greedy.' Instead of 'dee,' say 'see.'" (greasy)

"Say 'something.' Instead of 'thing,' say 'one.'" (someone)

"Say 'cutting.' Instead of 'cut,' say 'morn.'" (morning)

"Say 'gathering.' Instead of 'ing,' say 'er.'" (gatherer)

Phonological Awareness Activities at the Phoneme Level

1. Counting sounds.

What to say to the student: "We're going to count sounds in words."

EXAMPLE   "How many sounds do you hear in this word? 'did.'" (3)

NOTE: *Use pictured items and/or manipulatives if necessary. Use any of the following stimulus words and/or others you select from the story. Be sure to give the letter sound and not the letter name. Use any group of 10 stimulus items you select per teaching set.*

Stimulus words with one sound: a, I, eye

Stimulus words with two sounds: boy, by, to, toy, day, do, joy, me, my, so, sea, say, he, were, we, the, they, you, in, an, at, on, of, as, it, is, all, up, off, earth, us, own

Stimulus words with three sounds: but, been, bit, boat, back, teach, take, toad, tree, drew, did, deck, could, keep, cut, came, cook, come, can, gave, give, get, much, man, made, make, move, not, night, knows, said, set, sell, sat, some, soon, rock, fish, flew, fell, full, his, him, have, head, long, life, lose, let, one, wish, was, will, when, with, wide, which, would, word, what, thought, that, then, and, ago, its, away, old, earned, other, over

Stimulus words with four sounds: paint, passed, please, plan, brush, beggar, brought, teacher, twig, tools, table, turned, tried, drove, drop, called, crane, cried, keeled, gather, gold, China, money, named, school, still, sand, seized, sent, reeds, river, rocks, rolled, roamed, field, hand, left, went, wished, water, wind, waves, thank, after, among, into, asked, only, again, others, enough

Stimulus words with five sounds: placed, palace, python, pieces, bottom, became, drops, greedy, jumped, magic, slept, spread, story, rooster, hands, village, wants

Stimulus words with six sounds: pictures, dragon, million, nobody, soldiers, firewood, finished, furniture, phoenix, furious, freedom, family, happily, whatever, almost, instead

Stimulus words with seven sounds: delighted, children, merchants, refused, exchange, lanterns

Stimulus words with eight sounds: paintbrush, accident

2. Sound categorization or identifying a rhyme oddity.

What to say to the student: "Guess which word I say doesn't rhyme with the other three words."

> **EXAMPLE** "Tell me which word does not rhyme with the other three: '_____,' '_____,' '_____,' '_____.'" (stimulus words) (e.g., " 'boat,' 'moat,' 'note,' 'tree.' Which word doesn't rhyme?") (tree)

> **NOTE:** *Use pictured items if necessary. Use any of the following stimulus words and/or others you select from the story. The correct answers are in parentheses.*

Stimulus items:

school, pool, stool, China (China)

paint, life, faint, taint (life)

reeds, needs, long, beads (long)

brush, rush, mush, lanterns (lanterns)

passed, mast, please, blast (please)

river, fish, wish, dish (river)

seized, pleased, left, squeezed (left)

royal, boil, dragon, foil (dragon)

village, bobbing, robbing, mobbing (village)

crashing, accident, splashing, flashing (accident)

3. Matching rhyme.

What to say to the student: "We're going to think of rhyming words."

> **EXAMPLE** "Which word rhymes with '_____'?" (stimulus word) (e.g., "Which word rhymes with 'paint': 'faint,' 'make,' 'fish,' 'move'?") (faint)

> **NOTE:** *Use pictured items if necessary. Use any of the following stimulus words and/or others you select from the story. The correct answers are in parentheses.*

Stimulus items:

day: joy, play, knows, field (play)

large: things, roamed, barge, deer (barge)

crashing: royal, phoenix, magic, splashing (splashing)

swimming: skimming, firewood, school, glaring (skimming)

brush: reeds, hush, field, named (hush)

rooster: Liang, firewood, booster, fingers (booster)

sea: joy, school, seized, me (me)

China: Dinah, soldiers, splashing, village (Dinah)

bobbing: splashing, crashing, robbing, swimming (robbing)

roamed: rolled, foamed, large, listen (foamed)

4. Producing rhyme.

What to say to the student: "Now we'll say rhyming words."

> **EXAMPLE**   "Tell me a word that rhymes with '_____.'" (stimulus word) (e.g., "Tell me a word that rhymes with 'paint.' You can make up a word if you want.") (faint, taint, maint)

> **NOTE:** *Use pictured items if necessary. Use any of the following stimulus words and/or others you select from the story (i.e., you say a word from the list below and the student is to think of a rhyming word). Use any group of 10 stimulus items you select per teaching set.*

Stimulus items:

/p/: passed, please, plan, placed, poor, pictures

/b/: boy, buy, brush, balls, bound, bit, boat, back

/t/: to, teach, teacher, twig, tools, table, toad, tree

/d/: day, did, drop, dragon, down, do, deck

/k/: cutting, cut, came, cook, crane, keeled, can, cried

/g/: gave, give, gold, get, gather, gathering

/ch/: China, children

/dz/ (as the first sound in jelly): joy, join, jumped

/m/: me, much, man, my, more, make, made, money, magic

/n/: now, not, night, knew, knows, name

/s/: so, said, still, sand, saw, set, sell, sea, splashing

/f/: fish, fingers, for, finished, full, far, fell

/v/: village

/h/: his, he, him, hand, house, have, head, hands

/r/: reeds, rocks, rolled, rock, royal, roamed

/l/: long, life, left, lost, large, let

/w/, /wh/: one, was, went, will when, with, wide, word, we, waves

/sh/: should, sugar

/voiceless th/: think, thank, things, thought

/voiced th/: the, that, their, then, they

/y/ (as the first sound in yellow): you

vowels: in, at, earned, other, of, out, up, all, and, an, us, eye

5. Sound matching (initial).

What to say to the student: "Now we'll listen for the first sound in words."

> **EXAMPLE** "Listen to this sound: / /." (stimulus sound). "Guess which word I say
> begins with that sound: '_____,' '_____,' '_____,' '_____.'"
> (stimulus words) (e.g., "Listen to this sound: /p/. Guess which word I say
> begins with that sound: 'move,' 'paint,' 'school,' 'long.'") (paint)

> **NOTE:** *Give the letter sound, not the letter name. Use pictured items if necessary. Use any
> of the following stimulus words and/or others you select from the story. The correct
> answers are in parentheses.*

Stimulus items:

/m/: join, move, teach, long (move)

/b/: Liang, hand, bobbing, children (bobbing)

/f/: village, phoenix, lanterns, splashing (phoenix)

/h/: happily, you, royal, bottom (happily)

/v/: earth, rock, soldiers, village (village)

/l/: firewood, Liang's, mountains, delighted (Liang's)

/k/: greedy, happened, keeled, tree (keeled)

/s/: swimming, crashing, bobbing, gathering (swimming)

/r/: bottom, turned, emperor, rooster (rooster)

/dz/ (as the first sound in jelly): happened, rolled, jumped, turned (jumped)

6. Sound matching (final).

What to say to the student: "Now we'll listen for the last sound in words."

> **EXAMPLE** "Listen to this sound: / /" (stimulus sound). "Guess which word I say
> ends with that sound: '_____,' '_____,' '_____,' '_____.'"
> (stimulus words) (e.g., "Listen to this sound: /k/. Guess which word I say
> ends with that sound: 'rock,' 'sell,' 'much,' 'twig.'") (rock)

> **NOTE:** *Give the letter sound, not the letter name. Use pictured items and/or manipulatives if
> necessary. Use any of the following stimulus words and/or others you select from the
> story. The correct answers are in parentheses.*

Stimulus items:

/ch/: house, teach, money, children (teach)

/n/: table, poor, python, keep (python)

/z/: Liang's, toad, man, school (Liang's)

/ng/: spread, which, thought, painting (painting)

/r/: reeds, beggar, give, teach (beggar)

/long E/: royal, emperor, exchange, immediately (immediately)

/s/: Liang, gave, phoenix, paintbrush (phoenix)

/m/: freedom, whatever, really, swimming (freedom)

/v/: enough, boat, drove, waves (drove)

/dz/ (as the first sound in jelly): please, village, happily, boy (village)

7. Identifying the initial sound in words.

What to say to the student: "I'll say a word two times. Tell me what sound is missing the second time: '_____,' '_____.'" (stimulus words)

> **EXAMPLE** "What sound do you hear in '_____'" (stimulus word) "that is missing in '_____'?" (stimulus word) (e.g., "What sound do you hear in 'can' that is missing in 'an'?") (/k/)

NOTE: *Give the letter sound, not the letter name. Use pictured items and/or manipulatives if necessary. Use any of the following stimulus words and/or others you select from the story. The correct answers are in parentheses.*

Stimulus items:

"table, able. What sound do you hear in 'table' that is missing in 'able'?" (/t/)

"far, are. What sound do you hear in 'far' that is missing in 'are'?" (/f/)

"lose, ooze. What sound do you hear in 'lose' that is missing in 'ooze'?" (/l/)

"crane, rain. What sound do you hear in 'crane' that is missing in 'rain'?" (/k/)

"made, aid. What sound do you hear in 'made' that is missing in 'aid'?" (/m/)

"twig, wig. What sound do you hear in 'twig' that is missing in 'wig'?" (/t/)

"his, is. What sound do you hear in 'his' that is missing in 'is'?" (/h/)

"school, cool. What sound do you hear in 'school' that is missing in 'cool'?" (/s/)

"their, air. What sound do you hear in 'their' that is missing in 'air'?" (/voiced th/)

"think, ink. What sound do you hear in 'think' that is missing in 'ink'?" (/voiceless th/)

8. Identifying the final sound in words.

What to say to the student: "I'll say a word two times. Tell me what sound is missing the second time: '_____,' '_____.'" (stimulus words)

> **EXAMPLE** "What sound do you hear in '_____'" (stimulus word) "that is missing in '_____'?" (stimulus word) (e.g., "What sound do you hear in 'paint' that is missing in 'pain'?") (/t/)

NOTE: *Give the letter sound, not the letter name. Use pictured items and/or manipulatives if necessary. Use any of the following stimulus words and/or others you select from the story. The correct answers are in parentheses.*

Stimulus items:

"art, are. What sound do you hear in 'art' that is missing in 'are'?" (/t/)

"story, store. What sound do you hear in 'story' that is missing in 'store'?" (/long E/)

"Liang's, Liang. What sound do you hear in 'Liang's' that is missing in 'Liang'?" (/z/)

"merchants, merchant. What sound do you hear in 'merchants' that is missing in 'merchant'?" (/s/)

"beggar, beg. What sound do you hear in 'beggar' that is missing in 'beg'?" (/r/)

"own, owe. What sound do you hear in 'own' that is missing in 'owe'?" (/n/)

"life, lie. What sound do you hear in 'life' that is missing in 'lie'?" (/f/)

"came, Kay. What sound do you hear in 'came' that is missing in 'Kay'?" (/m/)

"boat, bow. What sound do you hear in 'boat' that is missing in 'bow'?" (/t/)

"lanterns, lantern. What sound do you hear in 'lanterns' that is missing in 'lantern'?" (/z/)

9. Segmenting the initial sound in words.

What to say to the student: "Listen to the word I say and tell me the first sound you hear."

> EXAMPLE   "What's the first sound in '_____'?" (stimulus word) (e.g., "What's the first sound in 'brush'?") (/b/)

NOTE: *Give the letter sound, not the letter name. Use pictured items and/or manipulatives if necessary. Use any of the following stimulus words and/or others you select from the story. Use any group of 10 stimulus items you select per teaching set.*

Stimulus items:

/p/: paint, paintbrush, passed, please, placed, painted, poor, parents, pictures, palace, python, plan, pieces, painting

/b/: boy, but, buy, brush, beggar, birds, began, balls, by, been, bound, brought, bit, boat, bobbing, bottom, became, back

/t/: to, teach, teacher, twig, toy, tools, table, take, toad, turned, tried, tree

/d/: day, drove, drew, drops, deer, did, drop, dragon, down, do, delighted, deck

/k/: cutting, could, keep, cut, called, came, come, cook, crane, can, cried, crashing, keeled

/g/: gathering, glared, gather, gave, greedy, give, gold, get

/ch/: China, children

/dz/ (as the first sound in jelly): jumped, joy, join

/m/: magic, money, much, me, man, my, marketplace, merchants, made, make, mountains, move, more, million

/n/: named, not, night, now, knew, nobody, knows

/s/: school, so, said, still, sand, slept, saw, set, sell, something, spread, soldiers, seized, sat, sent, saying, sea, swimming, sank, story, some, soon, splashing, say

/f/: firewood, fingers, fish, flew, for, finished, friends, furniture, field, fell, phoenix, furious, freedom, full, family, far

/v/: village

/h/: his, he, him, hand, house, have, happened, head, hands, happily

/r/: reeds, river, rocks, really, refused, rooster, rolled, royal, rock, roamed

/l/: Liang, long, life, lanterns, left, Liang's, large, lose, let, listen

/w/, /wh/: one, wish, was, went, will, wants, wherever, when, with, wide, were, where, which, would, word, whatever, wished, we, water, wind, waves, what

/sh/: sure, should

/voiceless th/: thank, things, thought, think

/voiced th/: the, that, their, then, there, they

/y/ (as the first sound in yellow): you

vowels: at, and, ago, in, afford, an, away, on, of, as, old, appeared, it, enormous, after, immediately, among, other, into, asked, only, accident, everyone, about, including, almost, emperor, all, up, instead, imprisoned, off, again, accepted, enough, exchange, over, own, us

10. Segmenting the final sound in words.

What to say to the student: "Listen to the word I say and tell me the last sound you hear."

> **EXAMPLE** "What's the last sound in the word '_____'?" (stimulus word)
> (e.g., "What's the last sound in the word 'paint'?") (/t/)

NOTE: *Give the letter sound, not the letter name. Use pictured items and/or manipulatives if necessary. Use any of the following stimulus words and/or others you select from the story. Use any group of 10 stimulus items you select per teaching set.*

Stimulus items:

/p/: drop, keep, up

/t/: paint, passed, placed, but, brought, bit, boat, cut, get, almost, accident, about, went, what, thought, that, about, art, at, it, out, asked, wished

/d/: happened, head, wide, would, word, wind, and, afford, old, appeared, earned, ordered, instead, imprisoned, accepted, painted, bound, toad, turned, tried, did, delighted, could, hand, called, cried, keeled, glared, gold, made, named, said, sand, spread, seized, refused, rolled, roamed, firewood, finished, field

/k/: back, take, deck, cook, magic, make, sank, rock, thank, think, ink

/g/: twig

/ch/: teach, much, which

/dz/ (as the first sound in jelly): large, village, exchange

/m/: bottom, became, came, come, some, freedom, him

/n/: python, plan, began, been, dragon, down, crane, can, children, join, man, million, soon, listen, one, when, then, own, in, an, on, everyone, again

/ng/: Liang, swimming, something, cutting, gathering, splashing, crashing, painting, bobbing, including, among, long

/s/: parents, palace, drops, marketplace, merchants, rocks, phoenix, furious, house, wants, us, its, enormous

/z/: please, pictures, pieces, birds, balls, tools, mountains, knows, soldiers, reeds, fingers, friends, his, hands, lanterns, Liang's, lose, waves, things, others, emperor's, as, is

/f/: life, enough, off

/v/: drove, gave, give, move, have, of

/r/: poor, beggar, teacher, deer, gather, more, river, rooster, for, furniture, far, wherever, water, were, where, their, there, whatever, over, after, other, emperor

/l/: table, school, still, sell, royal, full, fell, will, all

/sh/: paintbrush, brush, fish, wish

/voiceless th/: with, earth

/long A/: day, they, away, say

/long E/: story, nobody, really, family, happily, we, sea, money, only, he

/long I/: by, my

/long O/: ago, so

/oo/: into, you, knew, flew

11. Generating words from the story beginning with a particular sound.

What to say to the student: "Let's think of words from the story that start with certain sounds."

> **EXAMPLE** "Tell me a word from the story that starts with / /." (stimulus sound) (e.g., the sound /p/) (paintbrush)

NOTE: *Give the letter sound, not the letter name. Use pictured items if necessary. Use any of the following stimulus words and/or others you select from the story. You say the sound (e.g., a voiceless /p/ sound), and the student is to say a word from the story that begins with that sound. Use any group of 10 stimulus items you select per teaching set.*

Stimulus items:

/p/: paint, paintbrush, passed, please, placed, painted, poor, parents, pictures, palace, python, plan, pieces, painting

/b/: boy, but, buy, brush, beggar, birds, began, balls, by, been, bound, brought, bit, boat, bobbing, bottom, became, back

/t/: to, teach, teacher, twig, toy, tools, table, take, toad, turned, tried, tree

/d/: day, drove, drew, drops, deer, did, drop, dragon, down, do, delighted, deck

/k/: cutting, could, keep, cut, called, came, come, cook, crane, can, cried, crashing, keeled

/g/: gathering, glared, gather, gave, greedy, give, gold, get

/ch/: China, children

/dz/ (as the first sound in jelly): jumped, joy, join

/m/: magic, money, much, me, man, my, marketplace, merchants, made, make, mountains, move, more, million

/n/: named, not, night now, knew, nobody, knows

/s/: school, so, said, still, sand, slept, saw, set, sell, something, spread, soldiers, seized, sat, sent, saying, sea, swimming, sank, story, some, soon, splashing, say

/f/: firewood, fingers, fish, flew, for, finished, friends, furniture, field, fell, phoenix, furious, freedom, full, family, far

/v/: village

/h/: his, he, him, hand, house, have, happened, head, hands, happily

/r/: reeds, river, rocks, really, refused, rooster, rolled, royal, rock, roamed

/l/: Liang, long, life, lanterns, left, Liang's, large, lose, let, listen

/w/, /wh/: one, wish, was, went, will, wants, wherever, when, with, wide, were, where, which, would, word, whatever, wished, we, water, wind, waves, what

/sh/: sure, should

/voiceless th/: thank, things, thought, think

/voiced th/: the, that, their, then, there, they

/y/ (as the first sound in yellow): you

vowels: at, and, ago, in, afford, an, away, on, of, as, old, appeared, it, enormous, after, immediately, among, other, into, asked, only, accident, everyone, about, including, almost, emperor, all, up, instead, imprisoned, off, again, accepted, enough, exchange, over, own, us

12. Blending sounds in monosyllabic words divided into onset–rime beginning with a two-consonant cluster + rime.

What to say to the student: "Now we'll put sounds together to make words."

> **EXAMPLE** "Put these sounds together to make a word: / / + / /." (stimulus sounds) "What's the word?" (e.g., "sch + ool: What's the word?") (school)

> **NOTE:** *Give the letter sound, not the letter name. Use pictured items and/or manipulatives if necessary. Use any of the following stimulus words and/or others you select from the story. The correct answers are in parentheses.*

Stimulus items:

pl + an (plan)

br + ought (brought)

tw + ig (twig)

tr + ee (tree)

cr + ane (crane)

fl + ew (flew)

cr + ied (cried)

sl + ept (slept)

dr + ove (drove)

st + ill (still)

13. Blending sounds in monosyllabic words divided into onset–rime beginning with a single consonant + rime.

What to say to the student: "Let's put sounds together to make words."

> **EXAMPLE** "Put these sounds together to make a word: / / + / /." (stimulus sounds) "What's the word?" (e.g., "/p/ + aint: What's the word?") (paint)

NOTE: *Give the letter sound, not the letter name. Use pictured items and/or manipulatives if necessary. Use any of the following stimulus words and/or others you select from the story. The correct answers are in parentheses.*

Stimulus items:

/t/ + ake (take)

/b/ + it (bit)

/dz/ (as the first sound in jelly) + oin (join)

/s/ + and (sand)

/f/ + ish (fish)

/h/ + and (hand)

/n/ + ight (night)

/r/ + eeds (reeds)

/n/ + ot (not)

/g/ + old (gold)

14. Blending sounds to form a monosyllabic word beginning with a continuant sound.

What to say to the student: "We'll put sounds together to make words."

> **EXAMPLE** "Put these sounds together to make a word: / / + / / + / /." (stimulus sounds) (e.g., /s/ /long O/) (so)

NOTE: *Give the letter sound, not the letter name. Use pictured items and/or manipulatives if necessary. Use any of the following stimulus words and/or others you select from the story. The correct answers are in parentheses.*

Stimulus items:

/l/ /long I/ /f/ (life)

/s/ /t/ /short I/ /l/ (still)

/r/ /long O/ /m/ /d/ (roamed)

/h/ /short I/ /m/ (him)

/w/ /short E/ /n/ /t/ (went)

/y/ (as the first sound in yellow) /oo/ (you)

/f/ /short I/ /sh/ (fish)

/s/ /short E/ /n/ /t/ (sent)

/r/ /ah/ /k/ (rock)

/l/ /ah/ /ng/ (long)

15. Blending sounds to form a monosyllabic word beginning with a noncontinuant sound.

What to say to the student: "We'll put sounds together to make words."

> **EXAMPLE** "Put these sounds together to make a word: / / + / / + / /." (stimulus sounds) (e.g., /p/ /l/ /short A/ /n/) (plan)

NOTE: *Give the letter sound, not the letter name. Use pictured items and/or manipulatives if necessary. Use any of the following stimulus words and/or others you select from the story. The correct answers are in parentheses.*

Stimulus items:

/b/ /r/ /short U/ /sh/ (brush)

/t/ /long E/ /ch/ (teach)

/k/ /long E/ /p/ (keep)

/b/ /short A/ /k/ (back)

/k/ /short U/ /t/ (cut)

/g/ /long A/ /v/ (gave)

/dz/ (as the first sound in jelly) /short U/ /m/ /p/ /t/ (jumped)

/p/ /l/ /long E/ /z/ (please)

/b/ /long O/ /t/ (boat)

/g/ /short E/ /t/ (get)

16. Substituting the initial sound in words.

What to say to the student: "We're going to change beginning/first sounds in words."

> **EXAMPLE**   "Say '_____.'" (stimulus word) "Instead of / /" (stimulus sound), "say / /." (stimulus sound) (e.g., "Say 'paint.' Instead of /p/, say /f/. What's your new word?") (faint)

NOTE: *Give the letter sound, not the letter name. Use pictured items and/or manipulatives if necessary. Use any of the following stimulus words and/or others you select from the story. The correct answers are in parentheses.*

Stimulus items:

"Say 'sand.' Instead of /s/, say /h/." (hand)

"Say 'river.' Instead of /r/, say /g/." (giver)

"Say 'royal.' Instead of /r/, say /s/." (soil)

"Say 'large.' Instead of /l/, say /b/." (barge)

"Say 'went.' Instead of /w/, say /b/." (bent)

"Say 'rooster.' Instead of /r/, say /b/." (booster)

"Say 'that.' Instead of /voiced th/, say /p/." (pat)

"Say 'night.' Instead of /n/, say /k/." (kite)

"Say 'flew.' Instead of /f/, say /b/." (blew)

"Say 'crashing.' Instead of /k/, say /t/." (trashing)

17. Substituting the final sound in words.

What to say to the student: "We're going to change ending/last sounds in words."

> **EXAMPLE** "Say '_____.' " (stimulus word) "Instead of / /" (stimulus sound), "say / /." (stimulus sound) (e.g., "Say 'bit.' Instead of /t/, say /n/. What's your new word?") (bin)

> **NOTE:** *Give the letter sound, not the letter name. Use pictured items and/or manipulatives if necessary. Use any of the following stimulus words and/or others you select from the story. The correct answers are in parentheses.*

Stimulus items:

"Say 'tree.' Instead of /long E/, say /oo/." (true)

"Say 'glared.' Instead of /d/, say /z/." (glares)

"Say 'plan.' Instead of /n/, say /d/." (plaid)

"Say 'cried.' Instead of /d/, say /z/." (cries)

"Say 'was.' Instead of /z/, say /n/." (one)

"Say 'gold.' Instead of /d/, say /z/." (goals)

"Say 'please.' Instead of /z/, say /t/." (pleat)

"Say 'by.' Instead of /long I/, say /long O/." (bow)

"Say 'have.' Instead of /v/, say /t/." (hat)

"Say 'waves.' Instead of /z/, say /d/." (waved)

18. Segmenting the middle sound in monosyllabic words.

What to say to the student: "Tell me the middle sound in the word I say."

> **EXAMPLE** "What's the middle sound in the word '_____'?" (stimulus word) (e.g., "What's the middle sound in the word 'his'?") (/short I/)

> **NOTE:** *Give the letter sound, not the letter name. Use pictured items and/or manipulatives if necessary. Use any of the following stimulus words and/or others you select from the story. The correct answers are in parentheses.*

Stimulus items:

long (/ah/)

deck (/short E/)

soon (/oo/)

have (/short A/)

boat (/long O/)

what (/short U/)

him (/short I/)

deck (/short E/)

cut (/short U/)

make (/long A/)

19. Substituting the middle sound in words.

What to say to the student: "We're going to change the middle sound in words."

EXAMPLE   "Say '_____.'" (stimulus word) "Instead of / /" (stimulus sound), "say / /." (stimulus sound) (e.g., "Say 'make.' Instead of /long A/, say /long I/. What's your new word?") (Mike)

NOTE: *Give the letter sound, not the letter name. Use pictured items and/or manipulatives if necessary. Use any of the following stimulus words and/or others you select from the story. The correct answers are in parentheses.*

Stimulus items:

"Say 'bit.' Instead of /short I/, say /long E/." (beat)

"Say 'not.' Instead of /ah/, say /short I/." (knit)

"Say 'made.' Instead of /long A/, say /oo/." (mood)

"Say 'rock.' Instead of /ah/, say /long A/." (rake)

"Say 'him.' Instead of /short I/, say /short U/." (hum)

"Say 'fell.' Instead of /short E/, say /short I/." (fill)

"Say 'much.' Instead of /short U/, say /short I/." (Mitch)

"Say 'bit.' Instead of /short I/, say /oo/." (boot)

"Say 'slept' Instead of /short E/, say /ah/." (slopped)

"Say 'drops.' Instead of /ah/, say /short I/." (drips)

20. Identifying all sounds in monosyllabic words.

What to say to the student: "Now tell me all the sounds you hear in the word I say."

EXAMPLE   "What sounds do you hear in the word '_____'?" (stimulus word) (e.g., "What sounds do you hear in the word 'boat'?") (/b/ /long O/ /t/)

NOTE: *Give the letter sound, not the letter name. Use pictured items and/or manipulatives if necessary. Use any of the following stimulus words and/or others you select from the story. The correct answers are in parentheses.*

Stimulus items:

not (/n/ /ah/ /t/)

get (/g/ /short E/ /t/)

drew (/d/ /r/ /oo/)

sent (/s/ /short E/ /n/ /t/)

still (/s/ /t/ /short I/ /l/)

boat (/b/ /long O/ /t/)

China (/ch/ /long I/ /n/ /short U/)
roamed (/r/ /long O/ /m/ /d/)
reeds (/r/ /long E/ /d/ /z/)
drops (/d/ /r/ /ah/ /p/ /s/)

21. Deleting sounds within words.

What to say to the student: "We're going to leave out sounds in words."

EXAMPLE "Say '_____'" (stimulus word) "without / /." (stimulus sound) (e.g., "Say 'brush' without /b/.") (rush) Say: "The word that was left—'rush'—is a real word. Sometimes, the word won't be a real word."

NOTE: *Give the letter sound, not the letter name. Use pictured items and/or manipulatives if necessary. Use any of the following stimulus words and/or others you select from the story. The correct answers are in parentheses.*

Stimulus items:
"Say 'still' without /t/." (sill)
"Say 'tried' without /r/." (tied)
"Say 'sent' without /n/." (set)
"Say 'plan' without /l/." (pan)
"Say 'left' without /f/." (let)
"Say 'wants' without /n/." (watts)
"Say 'brush' without /b/." (rush)
"Say 'twig' without /t/." (wig)
"Say 'friends' without /n/." (Fred's)
"Say 'waves' without /v/." (weighs)

22. Substituting consonants in words having a two-sound cluster.

What to say to the student: "We're going to substitute sounds in words."

EXAMPLE "Say '_____.'" (stimulus word) "Instead of / /" (stimulus sound), "say / /." (stimulus sound) (e.g., "Say 'tree.' Instead of /t/ say /f/.") (free) Say: "Sometimes, the new word will be a made-up word."

NOTE: *Give the letter sound, not the letter name. Use pictured items and/or manipulatives if necessary. Use any of the following stimulus words and/or others you select from the story. The correct answers are in parentheses.*

Stimulus items:
"Say 'please.' Instead of /p/, say /f/." (fleas)
"Say 'greedy.' Instead of /g/, say /f/." (freedy)

"Say 'swimming.' Instead of /w/, say /k/." (skimming)

"Say 'still.' Instead of /t/, say /k/." (skill)

"Say 'crashing.' Instead of /k/, say /voiceless th/." (thrashing)

"Say 'tried.' Instead of /t/, say /k/." (cried)

"Say 'flew.' Instead of /f/, say /b/." (blew)

"Say 'tools.' Instead of /l/, say /b/." (tubes)

"Say 'keeled.' Instead of /d/, say /z/." (keels)

"Say 'cried.' Instead of /k/, say /f/." (fried)

23. Phoneme reversing.

What to say to the student: "We're going to say words backward."

> **EXAMPLE** "Say the word '_____'" (stimulus word) "backward." (e.g., "Say 'take' backward.") (Kate)

> **NOTE:** *This is a difficult phoneme-level task and should only be done with older students. Give the letter sound, not the letter name. Use pictured items and/or manipulatives if necessary. Use any of the following stimulus words and/or others you select from the story. The correct answers are in parentheses.*

Stimulus items:

life (file)

sell (less)

much (chum)

let (tell)

can (knack)

but (tub)

night (tine)

make (came)

still (lits)

cut (tuck)

24. Phoneme switching.

What to say to the student: "We're going to switch the first sounds in two words."

> **EXAMPLE** "Switch the first sounds in '_____' and '_____.'" (stimulus words) (e.g., "Switch the first sounds in 'sat' and 'down.'") (dat sown)

> **NOTE:** *This is a difficult phoneme-level task and should only be done with older students. Give the letter sound, not the letter name. Use pictured items and/or manipulatives if necessary. Use any of the following stimulus words and/or others you select from the story. The correct answers are in parentheses.*

Stimulus items:

Made pictures (paid mictures)

the sea (suh thee)

sea full (fee sull)

royal family (foil ramily)

the boat (buh thoat)

he roamed (ree hoamed)

he went (we hent)

went back (bent whack)

magic paintbrush (pagic maintbrush)

Liang's hand (hiang's land)

25. Pig Latin.

What to say to the student: "We're going to speak a secret language by using words from the story. In pig Latin, you take off the first sound of a word, put it at the end of the word, and add an 'ay' sound."

> **EXAMPLE**   "Say 'boy' in pig Latin." (oybay)

> **NOTE:** *This is a difficult phoneme-level task and should only be done with older students. Use pictured items and/or manipulatives if necessary. Use any of the following stimulus words and/or others you select from the story. The correct answers are in parentheses.*

Stimulus items:

boat (oatbay)

China (inachay)

money (oneymay)

royal (oyalray)

village (illagevay)

wherever (ereverway)

cutting (uttingkay)

something (omethingsay)

bobbing (obbingbay)

splashing (plashingsay)

From Phonological Awareness into Print

> **NOTE:** *Only five examples per activity are included in this resource due to space. You are encouraged to add many more words into this section that you feel your student(s) (is) are ready to write.*

1. Substituting the initial sound or letter in words.

NOTE: *Use lined paper or copy the sheet of lined paper included in the back of this book.*

Stimulus items:

1.1 bit/fit

Task a. "Say 'bit.' Instead of /b/, say /f/. What's your new word?" (fit) "Write/copy 'bit' and 'fit.'"

Task b. "Circle the **letters** that make the words different." ([b], [f])

Task c. "What **sounds** do these letters make?" (/b/, /f/)

1.2 boat/coat

Task a. "Say 'boat.' Instead of /b/, say /k/. What's your new word?" (coat) "Write/copy 'boat' and 'coat.'"

Task b. "Circle the **letters** that make the words different." ([b], [c])

Task c. "What **sounds** do these letters make?" (/b/, /k/)

1.3 make/cake

Task a. "Say 'make.' Instead of /m/, say /k/. What's your new word?" (cake) "Write/copy 'make' and 'cake.'"

Task b. "Circle the **letters** that make the words different." ([m], [c])

Task c. "What **sounds** do these letters make?" (/m/, /k/)

1.4 rock/sock

Task a. "Say 'rock.' Instead of /r/, say /s/. What's your new word?" (sock) "Write/copy 'rock' and 'sock.'"

Task b. "Circle the **letters** that make the words different." ([r], [s])

Task c. "What **sounds** do these letters make?" (/r/, /s/)

1.5 rooster/booster

Task a. "Say 'rooster.' Instead of /r/, say /b/. What's your new word?" (booster) "Write/copy 'rooster' and 'booster.'"

Task b. "Circle the **letters** that make the words different." ([r], [b])

Task c. "What **sounds** do these letters make?" (/r/, /b/)

2. Substituting the final sound or letter in words.

NOTE: *Use lined paper or copy the sheet of lined paper included in the back of this book.*

Stimulus items:

2.1 bit/bin

Task a. "Say 'bit.' Instead of /t/, say /n/. What's your new word?" (bin) "Write/copy 'bit' and 'bin.'"

Task b. "Circle the **letters** that make the words different." ([t], [n])

Task c. "What **sounds** do these letters make?" (/t/, /n/)

2.2 him/hip

Task a. "Say 'him.' Instead of /m/, say /p/. What's your new word?" (hip) "Write/copy 'him' and 'hip.'"

Task b. "Circle the **letters** that make the words different." ([m], [p])

Task c. "What **sounds** do these letters make?" (/m/, /p/)

2.3 rock/rot

Task a. "Say 'rock.' Instead of /k/, say /t/. What's your new word?" (rot) "Write/copy 'rock' and 'rot.'"

Task b. "Circle the **letters** that make the words different." ([c], [k], [t])

Task c. "What **sounds** do these letters make?" (/k/, /t/)

2.4 waves/waved

Task a. "Say 'waves.' Instead of /z/, say /d/. What's your new word?" (waved) "Write/copy 'waves' and 'waved.'"

Task b. "Circle the **letters** that make the words different." ([s], [d])

Task c. "What **sounds** do these letters make?" (/z/, /d/)

2.5 tree/try

Task a. "Say 'tree.' Instead of /long E/, say /long I/. What's your new word?" (try) "Write/copy 'tree' and 'try.'"

Task b. "Circle the **letters** that make the words different." ([e], [e], [y])

Task c. "What **sounds** do these letters make?" (/long E/, /long I/)

3. Substituting the middle sound or letter in words.

NOTE: *Use lined paper or copy the sheet of lined paper included in the back of this book.*

Stimulus items:

3.1 but/bit

Task a. "Say 'but.' Instead of /short U/, say /short I/. What's your new word?" (bit) "Write/copy 'but' and 'bit.'"

Task b. "Circle the **letters** that make the words different." ([u], [i])

Task c. "What **sounds** do these letters make?" (/short U/, /short I/)

3.2 bit/boot

Task a. "Say 'bit.' Instead of /short I/, say /oo/. What's your new word?" (boot) "Write/copy 'bit' and 'boot.'"

Task b. "Circle the **letters** that make the words different." ([i], [o], [o])

Task c. "What **sounds** do these letters make?" (/short I/, /oo/)

3.3 bit/beat

Task a. "Say 'bit.' Instead of /short I/, say /long E/. What's your new word?" (beat) "Write/copy 'bit' and 'beat.'"

Task b. "Circle the **letters** that make the words different." ([i], [e], [a])

Task c. "What **sounds** do these letters make?" (/short I/, /long E/)

3.4 him/hum

Task a. "Say 'him.' Instead of /short I/, say /short U/. What's your new word?" (hum) "Write/copy 'him' and 'hum.'"

Task b. "Circle the **letters** that make the words different." ([i], [u])

Task c. "What **sounds** do these letters make?" (/short I/, /short U/)

3.5 not/note

Task a. "Say 'not.' Instead of /ah/, say /long O/. What's your new word?" (note) "Write/copy 'not' and 'note.'"

Task b. "Circle the **letters** that make the words different." ([o], [o], [e])

Task c. "What **sounds** do these letters make?" (/ah/, /long O/)

4. Supplying the initial sound or letter in words.

NOTE: *Use lined paper or copy the sheet of lined paper included in the back of this book.*

Stimulus items:

4.1 his/is

Task a. "Say 'his,' say 'is.' What sound did you hear in 'his' that is missing in 'is'?" (/h/) "Now we'll *change* the **letter**. Write/copy 'his' and 'is.'"

Task b. "Circle the beginning **letter** that makes the words different." ([h])

Task c. "What **sound** does this letter make?" (/h/)

4.2 twig/wig

Task a. "Say 'twig,' say 'wig.' What sound did you hear in 'twig' that is missing in 'wig'?" (/t/) "Now we'll change the **letter**. Write/copy 'twig' and 'wig.'"

Task b. "Circle the beginning **letter** that makes the words different." ([t])

Task c. "What **sound** does this letter make?" (/t/)

4.3 table/able

Task a. "Say 'table,' say 'able.' What sound did you hear in 'table' that is missing in 'able'?" (/t/) "Now we'll change the **letter**. Write/copy 'table' and 'able.'"

Task b. "Circle the beginning **letter** that makes the words different." ([t])

Task c. "What **sound** does this letter make?" (/t/)

4.4 think/ink

Task a. "Say 'think,' say 'ink.' What sound did you hear in 'think' that is missing in 'ink'?" (/voiceless th/) "Now we'll change the **letters**. Write/copy 'think' and 'ink.'"

Task b. "Circle the beginning **letters** that make the words different." ([t], [h])

Task c. "What **sound** do these letters make?" (/voiceless th/)

4.5 sand/and

Task a. "Say 'sand,' say 'and.' What sound did you hear in 'sand' that is missing in 'and'?" (/s/) "Now we'll change the **letter**. Write/copy 'sand' and 'and.'"

Task b. "Circle the beginning **letter** that makes the words different." ([s])

Task c. "What **sound** does this letter make?" (/s/)

5. Supplying the final sound or letter in words.

NOTE: *Use lined paper or copy the sheet of lined paper included in the back of this book.*

Stimulus items:

5.1 lanterns/lantern

Task a. "Say 'lanterns,' say 'lantern.' What sound did you hear in 'lanterns' that is missing in 'lantern'?" (/z/) "Now we'll *change* the **letter**. Write/copy 'lanterns' and 'lantern.'"

Task b. "Circle the ending/last **letter** that makes the words different." ([s])

Task c. "What **sound** does this letter make?" (/z/)

5.2 parents/parent

Task a. "Say 'parents,' say 'parent.' What sound did you hear in 'parents' that is missing in 'parent'?" (/s/) "Now we'll change the **letter**. Write/copy 'parents' and 'parent.'"

Task b. "Circle the ending/last **letter** that makes the words different." ([s])

Task c. "What **sound** does this letter make?" (/s/)

5.3 called/call

Task a. "Say 'called,' say 'call.' What sound did you hear in 'called' that is missing in 'call'?" (/d/) "Now we'll change the **letters**. Write/copy 'called' and 'call.'"

Task b. "Circle the ending/last **letters** that make the words different." ([e], [d])

Task c. "What **sound** do these letters make?" (/d/)

5.4 Liang's/Liang

Task a. "Say 'Liang's,' say 'Liang.' What sound did you hear in 'Liang's' that is missing in 'Liang'?" (/z/) "Now we'll change the **letter**. Write/copy 'Liang's' and 'Liang.'"

Task b. "Circle the ending/last **letter** that makes the word different." (['s])

Task c. "What **sound** does this letter make?" (/z/)

5.5 greedy/greed

Task a. "Say 'greedy,' say 'greed.' What sound did you hear in 'greedy' that is missing in 'greed'?" (/long E/) "Now we'll change the **letter**. Write/copy 'greedy' and 'greed.'"

Task b. "Circle the ending/last **letter** that makes the words different." ([y])

Task c. "What **sound** does this letter make?" (/long E/)

6. Switching the first sound and letter in words (ADVANCED).

NOTE: *Use lined paper or copy the sheet of lined paper included in the back of this book.*

Stimulus items:

6.1 he went

Task a. "Say 'he,' say 'went.' What sound do you hear at the beginning of 'he'?" (/h/) "What sound do you hear at the beginning of 'went'?" (/w/) "Switch the first sounds in those words." (we hent) "Now we'll change the **letters**. Write/copy 'he went' and 'we hent.'"

Task b. "Circle the beginning **letters** that change the words." ([h], [w])

Task c. "What **sounds** do those letters make?" (/h/, /w/)

6.2 went back

Task a. "Say 'went,' say 'back.' What sound do you hear at the beginning of 'went'?" (/w/) "What sound do you hear at the beginning of 'back'?" (/b/) "Switch the first sounds in those words." (bent wack) "Now we'll change the **letters**. Write/copy 'went back' and 'bent wack.'"

Task b. "Circle the beginning **letters** that change the words." ([w], [b])

Task c. "What **sounds** do those letters make?" (/w/, /b/)

6.3 Liang's hand

Task a. "Say 'Liang's,' say 'hand.' What sound do you hear at the beginning of 'Liang's'?" (/l/) "What sound do you hear at the beginning of 'hand'?" (/h/) "Switch the first sounds in those words." (hiang's land) "Now we'll change the **letters**. Write/copy 'Liang's hand' and 'hiang's Land.'"

Task b. "Circle the beginning **letters** that change the words." ([L], [h])

Task c. "What **sounds** do those letters make?" (/l/, /h/)

6.4 join him

Task a. "Say 'join,' say 'him.' What sound do you hear at the beginning of 'join'?" (/dz/, as in the first sound in jelly) "What sound do you hear at the beginning of 'him'?" (/h/) "Switch the first sounds in those words." (hoin jim) "Now we'll change the **letters**. Write/copy 'join him' and 'hoin jim.'"

Task b. "Circle the beginning **letters** that change the words." ([j], [h])

Task c. "What **sounds** do those letters make?" (/dz/, /h/)

6.5 made pictures

Task a. "Say 'made,' say 'pictures.' What sound do you hear at the beginning of 'made'?" (/m/) "What sound do you hear at the beginning of 'pictures'?" (/p/) "Switch the first sounds in those words." (pade mictures) "Now we'll change the **letters**. Write/copy 'made pictures' and 'pade mictures.'"

Task b. "Circle the beginning **letters** that change the words." ([m], [p])

Task c. "What **sounds** do those letters make?" (/m/, /p/)

CHAPTER 10

Phonological Awareness Activities to Use with *Mice Squeak, We Speak*

Text version used for selection of stimulus items:

Shaprio, A., and DePaola, T. (Illustrator). (2000). *Mice Squeak, We Speak*. New York: Puffin Books/Penguin Putnam Books for Young Readers.

Phonological Awareness Activities at the Word Level

1. Counting words.

What to say to the student: "We're going to count words."

> **EXAMPLE** "How many words do you hear in this sentence (or phrase)? 'cats purr?'" (2)

> **NOTE:** *Use pictured items and/or manipulatives if necessary. Use any of the following stimulus phrases or sentences and/or others you select from the story. The correct answers are in parentheses.*

Stimulus items:

lions roar (2)

owls hoot (2)

But I speak! (3)

crickets creak (2)

monkeys chatter (2)

But I say! (3)

coyotes howl (2)

But I talk! (3)

Mice squeak, we speak. (4)

a poem by Arnold Shapiro (5)

2. Identifying the missing word from a list.

What to say to the student: "Listen to the words I say. I'll say them again. You tell me which word I leave out."

EXAMPLE "Listen to the words I say: 'purr,' 'dogs,' 'doves.' I'll say them again. Tell me which one I leave out: 'purr,' 'dogs.'" (doves)

NOTE: *Use pictured items and/or manipulatives if necessary. Use any of the following stimulus words and/or others you select from the story. The correct answers are in parentheses.*

Stimulus set #1	Stimulus set #2
mice, sheep	mice (sheep)
growl, talk	talk (growl)
crickets, we	we (crickets)
horses, flies, frogs	horses, flies (frogs)
monkeys, sheep, cats	monkeys, sheep (cats)
lions, say, bears	lions, bears (say)
chatter, growl, squeak	growl, squeak (chatter)
speak, frogs, squeal	speak, squeal (frogs)
roar, monkeys, flies	roar, flies (monkeys)
snore, chickens, moo, neigh	snore, moo, neigh (chickens)

3. Identifying the missing word in a phrase or sentence.

What to say to the student: "Listen to the sentence I read. Tell me which word is missing the second time I read the sentence."

EXAMPLE "'mice squeak.' Listen again and tell me which word I leave out: 'mice _____.'" (squeak)

NOTE: *Use pictured items and/or manipulatives if necessary. Use any of the following stimulus sentences and/or others you select from the story. The correct answers are in parentheses.*

Stimulus items:

Cats purr. Cats _____. (purr)

Parrots squawk. Parrots _____. (squawk)

Bees buzz. _____ buzz. (bees)

But I speak! But _____ speak! (I)

Coyotes howl. _____ howl. (Coyotes)

Frogs croak. Frogs _____. (croak)

But I say! But I _____! (say)

Mice squeak, we speak. Mice _____, we speak. (squeak)

But I talk! _____ I talk! (But)

A poem by Arnold Shapiro. A _____ by Arnold Shapiro. (poem)

4. Supplying the missing word as an adult reads.

What to say to the student: "I want you to help me read the story. You fill in the words I leave out."

> **EXAMPLE**   "Mice _____." (squeak)

> **NOTE:** *Use pictured items and/or manipulatives if necessary. Use any of the following stimulus sentences and/or others you select from the story. The correct answers are in parentheses.*

Stimulus items:

Cats _____. (purr)

Lions _____. (roar)

But I _____! (speak)

_____ chatter. (Monkeys)

_____ quack. (Ducks)

But _____ say! (I)

Chickens _____. (cluck)

_____ I talk! (But)

Mice squeak, we _____. (speak)

A poem _____ Arnold Shapiro. (by)

5. Rearranging words.

What to say to the student: "I'll say some words out of order. You put them in the right order so they make sense."

> **EXAMPLE**   " 'squeak mice.' Put those words in the right order." (mice squeak)

> **NOTE:** *Use pictured items and/or manipulatives if necessary. Use any of the following stimulus words and/or others you select from the story. The correct answers are in parentheses. This word-level activity can be more difficult than some of the syllable- or phoneme-level activities because of the memory load. If your students are only able to deal with two or three words to be rearranged, add more two- and three-word samples from the story and omit the four-word level items.*

Stimulus items:

neigh horses (Horses neigh.)

coo doves (Doves coo.)

but speak I. (But I speak.)

squeal pigs (Pigs squeal.)

hum flies (Flies hum.)

say I but (But I say.)

screech bats (Bats screech.)

squeak mice we speak (Mice squeak, we speak.)

I talk but (But I talk.)

poem a Shapiro Michael by (a poem by Michael Shapiro)

Phonological Awareness Activities at the Syllable Level

1. Syllable counting.

What to say to the student: "We're going to count syllables (or parts) of words."

> **EXAMPLE** "How many syllables do you hear in '_____'?" (stimulus word) (e.g., "How many syllables do you hear in 'mice'?") (1)

NOTE: *Use pictured items and/or manipulatives if necessary. Use any of the following stimulus words and/or others you select from the story. Use any group of 10 stimulus items you select per teaching set.*

Stimulus items:

One-syllable words: pure, pigs, bears, baa, but, bats, bees, buzz, by, talk, ducks, doves, dogs, cats, creak, cows, quack, coo, cluck, croak, growl, mice, moo, neigh, squeak, snore, say, screech, squawk, roar, flies, frogs, hoot, hum, howl, we, sheep, I

Two-syllable words: parrots, poem, crickets, chatter, chickens, monkeys, horses, lions, Arnold

Three-syllable words: coyotes, Shapiro

2. Initial syllable deleting.

What to say to the student: "We're going to leave out syllables (or parts of words)."

> **EXAMPLE** "Say '_____.'" (stimulus word) "Say it again without '_____.'" (stimulus syllable) (e.g., "Say 'bullfrogs.' Say it again without 'bull.'") (frogs)

NOTE: *Use pictured items and/or manipulatives if necessary. Use any of the following stimulus words and/or others you select from the story. The correct answers are in parentheses.*

Stimulus items:

"Say 'chatter' without 'chat.'" (er)

"Say 'parrots' without 'pear.'" (uts)

"Say 'crickets' without 'crick.'" (uts)

"Say 'coyotes' without 'kai.'" (oaties)

"Say 'chickens' without 'chick.'" (ens)

"Say 'lions' without 'lie.'" (uns)

"Say 'poem' without 'po.'" (em)

"Say 'monkeys' without 'mung.'" (keys)

"Say 'snoring' without 'snore.'" (ing)

"Say 'bumblebees' without 'bum.'" (bulbees)

3. Final syllable deleting.

What to say to the student: "We're going to leave out syllables (or parts of words)."

> EXAMPLE   "Say '_____.'" (stimulus word) "Say it again without '_____.'"
> (stimulus syllable) (e.g., "Say 'bullfrogs' without 'frogs.'") (bull)

> **NOTE:** *Use pictured items and/or manipulatives if necessary. Use any of the following stimulus words and/or others you select from the story. The correct answers are in parentheses.*

Stimulus items:

"Say 'chatter' without 'er.'" (chat)

"Say 'parrots' without 'uts.'" (pear)

"Say 'crickets' without 'uts.'" (crick)

"Say 'coyotes' without 'tease.'" (kai-oh)

"Say 'chickens' without 'ens.'" (chick)

"Say 'lions' without 'uns.'" (lie)

"Say 'poem' without 'em.'" (po)

"Say 'monkeys' without 'keys.'" (mung)

"Say 'snoring' without 'ing.'" (snore)

"Say 'bumblebees' without 'bees.'" (bumble)

4. Initial syllable adding.

What to say to the student: "Now let's add syllables (or parts) to words."

> EXAMPLE   "Add '_____'" (stimulus syllable) "to the beginning of '_____.'"
> (stimulus syllable) (e.g., "Add 'bull' to the beginning of 'frogs.'")
> (bullfrogs)

> **NOTE:** *Use pictured items and/or manipulatives if necessary. Use any of the following stimulus words and/or others you select from the story. The correct answers are in parentheses.*

Stimulus items:

"Add 'chat' to the beginning of 'er.'" (chatter)

"Add 'pear' to the beginning of 'uts.'" (parrots)

"Add 'crick' to the beginning of 'uts.'" (crickets)

"Add 'kai' to the beginning of 'oaties.'" (coyotes)

"Add 'chick' to the beginning of 'ens.'" (chickens)

"Add 'lie' to the beginning of 'uns.'" (lions)

"Add 'po' to the beginning of 'em.'" (poem)

"Add 'mung' to the beginning of 'keys.'" (monkeys)

"Add 'snore' to the beginning of 'ing.'" (snoring)

"Add 'bum' to the beginning of 'bulbees.'" (bumblebees)

5. Final syllable adding.

What to say to the student: "Now let's add syllables (or parts) to words."

> **EXAMPLE** "Add '_____'" (stimulus syllable) "to the end of '_____.'" (stimulus syllable) (e.g., "Add 'frogs' to the end of 'bull.'") (bullfrogs)

> **NOTE:** *Use pictured items and/or manipulatives if necessary. Use any of the following stimulus words and/or others you select from the story. The correct answers are in parentheses.*

Stimulus items:

"Add 'er' to the end of 'chat.'" (chatter)

"Add 'uts' to the end of 'pear.'" (parrots)

"Add 'uts' to the end of 'crick.'" (crickets)

"Add 'tease' to the end of 'kai-oh.'" (coyotes)

"Add 'ens' to the end of 'chick.'" (chickens)

"Add 'uns' to the end of 'lie.'" (lions)

"Add 'em' to the end of 'po.'" (poem)

"Add 'keys' to the end of 'mung.'" (monkeys)

"Add 'ing' to the end of 'snore.'" (snoring)

"Add 'bees' to the end of 'bumble.'" (bumblebees)

6. Syllable substituting.

What to say to the student: "Let's make up some new words."

> **EXAMPLE** "Say '_____.'" (stimulus word) "Instead of '_____'" (stimulus syllable), "say '_____.'" (stimulus syllable) (e.g., "Say 'bullfrogs.' Instead of 'bull,' say 'leap.' The new word is 'leapfrogs.'")

> **NOTE:** *Use pictured items and/or manipulatives if necessary. Use of the following stimulus words and/or others you select from the story. The correct answers are in parentheses.*

Stimulus items:

"Say 'chatter.' Instead of 'er,' say 'ing.'" (chatting)

"Say 'parrots.' Instead of 'pear,' say 'care.'" (carrots)

"Say 'crickets.' Instead of 'crick,' say 'tick.'" (tickets)

"Say 'chickens.' Instead of 'chick,' say 'sick.'" (sickens)

"Say 'snoring.' Instead of 'snore,' say 'bore.'" (boring)

Sourcebook users are encouraged to add stimulus items into this activity from curriculum materials they may be using with *Mice Squeak, We Speak.*

Phonological Awareness Activities at the Phoneme Level

1. Counting sounds.

What to say to the student: "We're going to count sounds in words."

> **EXAMPLE**   "How many sounds do you hear in this word: 'we'?" (2)

> **NOTE:** *Use pictured items and/or manipulatives if necessary. Use any of the following stimulus words and/or others you select from the story. Be sure to give the letter sound and not the letter name. Use any group of 10 stimulus items you select per teaching set.*

Stimulus words with two sounds: purr, by, coo, moo, neigh, say, we

Stimulus words with three sounds: buzz, mice, hoot, hum, sheep, bees

Stimulus words with four sounds: pigs, poem, bears, ducks, doves, dogs, cats, creak, quack, cluck, croak, chatter, speak, flies

Stimulus words with five sounds: squeak, squeal, screech, squawk, frogs, lions

Stimulus words with six sounds: coyotes, chickens, monkeys, parrots

Stimulus words with seven sounds: crickets

2. Sound categorization or identifying a rhyme oddity.

What to say to the student: "Guess which word I say doesn't rhyme with the other three words."

> **EXAMPLE**   "Tell me which word does not rhyme with the other three: '_____,' '_____,' '_____,' '_____.'" (stimulus words) (e.g., " 'bats,' 'cats,' 'rats,' 'screech.' Which word doesn't rhyme?") (screech)

> **NOTE:** *Use pictured items if necessary. Use any of the following stimulus words and/or others you select from the story. The correct answers are in parentheses.*

Stimulus items:

mice, ice, rice, chatter (chatter)

flies, tries, frogs, lies (frogs)

coo, neigh, moo, brew (neigh)

buzz, fuzz, mice, was (mice)

cats, spoke, choke, croak (cats)

hum, mum, howl, gum (howl)

chatter, horses, scatter, splatter (horses)

quack, cats, bats, gnats (quack)

bears, pears, squeak, chairs (squeak)

sheep, cheap, weep, we (we)

3. Matching rhyme.

What to say to the student: "We're going to think of rhyming words."

> **EXAMPLE** "Which word rhymes with '_____'?" (stimulus word) (e.g., "Which word rhymes with 'mice': 'neigh,' 'growl,' 'hum,' 'rice'?") (rice)

NOTE: *Use pictured items if necessary. Use any of the following stimulus words and/or others you select from the story. The correct answers are in parentheses.*

Stimulus items:

neigh: growl, roar, squeak, play (play)

chatter: crickets, lions, patter, squeak (patter)

hoot: screech, boot, owls, purr (boot)

ducks: bucks, hum, flies, neigh (bucks)

bears: cats, squawk, pears, owls (pears)

doves: moo, croak, cows, gloves (gloves)

pigs: wigs, chickens, lions, snore (wigs)

roar: chatter, more, growl, coyotes (more)

speak: neigh, squeak, chatter, coo (squeak)

neigh: hay, lions, doves, howl (hay)

4. Producing rhyme.

What to say to the student: "Now we'll say rhyming words."

> **EXAMPLE** "Tell me a word that rhymes with '_____.'" (stimulus word) (e.g., "Tell me a word that rhymes with 'mice.' You can make up a word if you want.") (rice or twice)

NOTE: *Use pictured items if necessary. Use any of the following stimulus words and/or others you select from the story (i.e., you say a word from the list below and the student is to think of a rhyming word). Use any group of 10 stimulus items you select per teaching set.*

Stimulus items:

/p/: purr, pigs, parrots

/b/: bears, baa, but, bats, bees, buzz, by

/t/: talk

/d/: ducks, doves, dogs

/k/: cats, crickets, creak, cows, quack, coo, croak

/g/: growl

/ch/: chatter, chickens

/m/: mice, moo

/n/: neigh

/s/: squeak, speak, snore, squeal, say, screech

/f/: flies, frogs

/h/: hoot, hum, howl, horses

/r/: roar

/l/: lions

/w/, /wh/: we

/sh/: sheep

vowels: owls, I

5. Sound matching (initial).

What to say to the student: "Now we'll listen for the first sound in words."

> **EXAMPLE**   "Listen to this sound: / /." (stimulus sound). "Guess which word I say begins with that sound: '_____,' '_____,' '_____,' '_____.'" (stimulus words) (e.g., "Listen to this sound: /m/. Guess which word I say begins with that sound: 'neigh,' 'mice,' 'squeak,' 'growl.'") (mice)

NOTE: *Give the letter sound, not the letter name. Use pictured items if necessary. Use any of the following stimulus words and/or others you select from the story. The correct answers are in parentheses.*

Stimulus items:

/ch/: baa, chickens, crickets, doves (chickens)

/s/: hum, growl, snore, croak (snore)

/f/: lions, frogs, talk, bats (frogs)

/h/: neigh, speak, howl, coyotes (howl)

/sh/: sheep, chatter, we, ducks (sheep)

/l/: cats, lions, owls, I (lions)

/k/: growl, roar, crickets, flies (crickets)

/d/: doves, purr, talk, snore (doves)

/r/: ducks, chatter, roar, say (roar)

/t/: growl, talk, neigh, howl (talk)

6. Sound matching (final).

What to say to the student: "Now we'll listen for the last sound in words."

> **EXAMPLE** "Listen to this sound: / /." (stimulus sound) "Guess which word I say ends with that sound: '_____,' '_____,' '_____,' '_____.'" (stimulus words) (e.g., "Listen to this sound: /k/. Guess which word I say ends with that sound: 'sheep,' 'hum,' 'mice,' 'squeak.'") (squeak)

NOTE: *Give the letter sound, not the letter name. Use pictured items and/or manipulatives if necessary. Use any of the following stimulus words and/or others you select from the story. The correct answers are in parentheses.*

Stimulus items:

/t/: squeak, hum, screech, hoot (hoot)

/ch/: screech, owls, pigs, squeal (screech)

/z/: poem, pigs, creak, sheep (pigs)

/p/: talk, hoot, sheep, hum (sheep)

/m/: poem, chatter, frogs, flies (poem)

/long A/: hum, neigh, coo, we (neigh)

/s/: roar, say, parrots, pigs (parrots)

/r/: growl, by, bats, purr (purr)

/oo/: we, coo, doves, chatter (coo)

/l/: howl, poem, Arnold, pigs (howl)

7. Identifying the initial sound in words.

What to say to the student: "I'll say a word two times. Tell me what sound is missing the second time: '_____,' '_____.'" (stimulus words)

> **EXAMPLE** "What sound do you hear in '_____'" (stimulus word) "that is missing in '_____'?" (stimulus word) (e.g., "What sound do you hear in 'mice' that is missing in 'ice'") (/m/)

NOTE: *Give the letter sound, not the letter name. Use pictured items and/or manipulatives if necessary. Use any of the following stimulus words and/or others you select from the story. The correct answers are in parentheses.*

Stimulus items:

"speak, peak. What sound do you hear in 'speak' that is missing in 'peak'?" (/s/)

"cluck, luck. What sound do you hear in 'cluck' that is missing in 'luck'?" (/k/)

"moo, ooh. What sound do you hear in 'moo' that is missing in 'ooh'?" (/m/)

"roar, or. What sound do you hear in 'roar' that is missing in 'or'?" (/r/)

"flies, lies. What sound do you hear in 'flies' that is missing in 'lies'?" (/f/)

"hum, um. What sound do you hear in 'hum' that is missing in 'um'?" (/h/)

"crickets, rickets. What sound do you hear in 'crickets' that is missing in 'rickets'?" (/k/)

"snore, nor. What sound do you hear in 'snore' that is missing in 'nor'?" (/s/)

"howl, owl. What sound do you hear in 'howl' that is missing in 'owl'?" (/h/)

"creak, reek. What sound do you hear in 'creak' that is missing in 'reek'?" (/k/)

8. Identifying the final sound in words.

What to say to the student: "I'll say a word two times. Tell me what sound is missing the second time: '_____,' '_____.'" (stimulus words)

> **EXAMPLE** "What sound do you hear in '_____'" (stimulus word) "that is missing in '_____'?" (stimulus word) (e.g., "What sound do you hear in 'dogs' that is missing in 'dog'?") (/z/)

> **NOTE:** *Give the letter sound, not the letter name. Use pictured items and/or manipulatives if necessary. Use any of the following stimulus words and/or others you select from the story. The correct answers are in parentheses.*

Stimulus items:

"sheep, she. What sound do you hear in 'sheep' that is missing in 'she'?" (/p/)

"hoot, who. What sound do you hear in 'hoot' that is missing in 'who'?" (/t/)

"pigs, pig. What sound do you hear in 'pigs' that is missing in 'pig'?" (/z/)

"hum, huh?. What sound do you hear in 'hum' that is missing in 'huh'?" (/m/)

"chatter, chat. What sound do you hear in 'chatter' that is missing in 'chat'?" (/r/)

"flies, fly. What sound do you hear in 'flies' that is missing in 'fly'?" (/z/)

"croak, crow. What sound do you hear in 'croak' that is missing in 'crow'?" (/k/)

"parrots, parrot. What sound do you hear in 'parrots' that is missing in 'parrot'?" (/s/)

"monkeys, monkey. What sound do you hear in 'monkeys' that is missing in 'monkey'?" (/z/)

"mice, my. What sound do you hear in 'mice' that is missing in 'my'?" (/s/)

9. Segmenting the initial sound in words.

What to say to the student: "Listen to the word I say and tell me the first sound you hear."

> **EXAMPLE** "What's the first sound in '_____'?" (stimulus word) (e.g., "What's the first sound in 'dogs'?") (/d/)

> **NOTE:** *Give the letter sound, not the letter name. Use pictured items and/or manipulatives if necessary. Use any of the following stimulus words and/or others you select from the story. Use any group of 10 stimulus items you select per teaching set.*

Stimulus items:

/p/: purr, pigs, parrots, poem

/b/: bears, baa, but, bats, bees, buzz, by

/t/: talk

/d/: ducks, doves, dogs

/k/: cats, crickets, creak, cows, quack, coo, cluck, coyotes, croak

/g/: growl

/ch/: chatter, chickens

/m/: mice, monkeys, moo

/n/: neigh

/s/: squeak, speak, snore, squeal, say, screech, squawk

/f/: flies, frogs

/h/: hoot, horses, hum, howl

/r/: roar

/l/: lions

/w/, /wh/: we

/sh/: sheep, Shapiro

vowels: I

10. Segmenting the final sound in words.

What to say to the student: "Listen to the word I say and tell me the last sound you hear."

> **EXAMPLE**   "What's the last sound in the word '_____'?" (stimulus word)
> (e.g., "What's the last sound in the word 'dogs'?") (/z/)

> **NOTE:** *Give the letter sound, not the letter name. Use pictured items and/or manipulatives if necessary. Use any of the following stimulus words and/or others you select from the story. Use any group of 10 stimulus items you select per teaching set.*

Stimulus items:

/p/: sheep

/t/: but, hoot

/d/: Arnold

/k/: squeak, speak, talk, creak, quack, clock, croak, squawk

/ch/: screech

/m/: poem, hum

/s/: mice, parrots, bats, ducks, cats, crickets

/z/: pigs, bears, bees, buzz, doves, dogs, cows, coyotes, chickens, monkeys, flies, frogs, horses, lions, owls

/r/: purr, chatter, snore, roar

/l/: growl, squeal, howl

/long A/: neigh, say

/long E/: we

/long I/: by
/oo/: coo, moo
/ah/: baa

11. Generating words from the story beginning with a particular sound.

What to say to the student: "Let's think of words from the story that start with certain sounds."

> **EXAMPLE** "Tell me a word from the story that starts with / /." (stimulus sound)
> (e.g., the sound /p/) (purr)

> **NOTE:** *Give the letter sound, not the letter name. Use pictured items if necessary. Use any of the following stimulus words and/or others you select from the story. You say the sound (e.g., a voiceless /p/ sound), and the student is to say a word from the story that begins with that sound. Use any group of 10 stimulus items you select per teaching set.*

Stimulus items:

/p/: purr, pigs, parrots, poem
/b/: bears, baa, but, bats, bees, buzz, by
/t/: talk
/d/: ducks, doves, dogs
/k/: cats, crickets, creak, cows, quack, coo, cluck, coyotes, croak
/g/: growl
/ch/: chatter, chickens
/m/: mice, monkeys, moo
/n/: neigh
/s/: squeak, speak, snore, squeal, say, screech, squawk
/f/: flies, frogs
/h/: hoot, horses, hum, howl
/r/: roar
/l/: lions
/w/, /wh/: we
/sh/: sheep, Shapiro

vowels: I

12. Blending sounds in monosyllabic words divided into onset–rime beginning with a two-consonant cluster + rime.

What to say to the student: "Now we'll put sounds together to make words."

> **EXAMPLE** "Put these sounds together to make a word: / / + / /." (stimulus sounds)
> "What's the word?" (e.g., "fl + ip: What's the word?") (flip)

NOTE: *Give the letter sound, not the letter name. Use pictured items and/or manipulatives if necessary. Use any of the following stimulus words and/or others you select from the story. The correct answers are in parentheses.*

Stimulus items:

cr + eak (creak)

sp + eak (speak)

fl + ies (flies)

qu + ack (quack)

cl + uck (cluck)

gr + owl (growl)

sn + ore (snore)

cr + oak (croak)

Sourcebook users are encouraged to add stimulus items into this activity from curriculum materials they may be using with *Mice Squeak, We Speak.*

13. Blending sounds in monosyllabic words divided into onset/rime beginning with a single consonant + rime.

What to say to the student: "Let's put sounds together to make words."

> **EXAMPLE** "Put these sounds together to make a word: / / + / /." (stimulus sounds)
> "What's the word?" (e.g., "/d/ + ogs: What's the word?") (dogs)

NOTE: *Give the letter sound, not the letter name. Use pictured items and/or manipulatives if necessary. Use any of the following stimulus words and/or others you select from the story. The correct answers are in parentheses.*

Stimulus items:

/p/ + urr (purr)

/d/ + ucks (ducks)

/k/ + ats (cats)

/m/ + ice (mice)

/s/ + ay (say)

/h/ + oot (hoot)

/sh/ + eep (sheep)

/b/ + ats (bats)

/n/ + eigh (neigh)

/p/ + igs (pigs)

14. Blending sounds to form a monosyllabic word beginning with a continuant sound.

What to say to the student: "We'll put sounds together to make words."

> **EXAMPLE** "Put these sounds together to make a word: / / + / / + / /."
> (stimulus sounds) (e.g., /s/ /long A/) (say)

NOTE: *Give the letter sound, not the letter name. Use pictured items and/or manipulatives if necessary. Use any of the following stimulus words and/or others you select from the story. The correct answers are in parentheses.*

Stimulus items:

/h/ /oo/ /t/ (hoot)
/w/ /long E/ (we)
/f/ /l/ /long I/ /z/ (flies)
/s/ /p/ /long E/ /k/ (speak)
/f/ /r/ /ah/ /g/ /z/ (frogs)
/h/ /short U/ /m/ (hum)
/sh/ /long E/ /p/ (sheep)
/s/ /k/ /r/ /long E/ /ch/ (screech)
/l/ /long I/ /short U/ /n/ /z/ (lions)
/m/ /long I/ /s/ (mice)

15. Blending sounds to form a monosyllabic word beginning with a noncontinuant sound.

What to say to the student: "We'll put sounds together to make words."

> **EXAMPLE** "Put these sounds together to make a word: / / + / / + / /." (stimulus sounds) (e.g., /d/ /ah/ /g/ /z/) (dogs)

NOTE: *Give the letter sound, not the letter name. Use pictured items and/or manipulatives if necessary. Use any of the following stimulus words and/or others you select from the story. The correct answers are in parentheses.*

Stimulus items:

/p/ /short I/ /g/ /z/ (pigs)
/b/ /short A/ /t/ /s/ (bats)
/d/ /short U/ /v/ /z/ (doves)
/d/ /ah/ /g/ /z/ (dogs)
/k/ /r/ /long E/ /k/ (creak)
/b/ /long E/ /z/ (bees)
/d/ /short U/ /k/ /s/ (ducks)
/k/ /short A/ /t/ /s/ (cats)
/p/ /r/ (purr)
/k/ /r/ /long O/ /k/ (croak)

16. Substituting the initial sound in words.

What to say to the student: "We're going to change beginning/first sounds in words."

> **EXAMPLE** "Say '_____.'" (stimulus word) "Instead of / /" (stimulus sound), "say / /." (stimulus sound) (e.g., "Say 'dogs.' Instead of /d/, say /h/. What's your new word?") (hogs)

> **NOTE:** *Give the letter sound, not the letter name. Use pictured items and/or manipulatives if necessary. Use any of the following stimulus words and/or others you select from the story. The correct answers are in parentheses.*

Stimulus items:

"Say 'mice.' Instead of /m/, say /r/." (rice)

"Say 'cats.' Instead of /k/, say /h/." (hats)

"Say 'growl.' Instead of /g/, say /p/." (prowl)

"Say 'chatter.' Instead of /ch/, say /b/." (batter)

"Say 'croak.' Instead of /k/, say /b/." (broke)

"Say 'bears.' Instead of /b/, say /ch/." (chairs)

"Say 'buzz.' Instead of /b/, say /f/." (fuzz)

"Say 'by.' Instead of /b/, say /p/." (pie)

"Say 'moo.' Instead of /m/, say /b/." (boo)

"Say 'sheep.' Instead of /sh/, say /p/." (peep)

17. Substituting the final sound in words.

What to say to the student: "We're going to change ending/last sounds in words."

> **EXAMPLE** "Say '_____.'" (stimulus word) "Instead of / /" (stimulus sound), "say / /." (stimulus sound) (e.g., "Say 'sheep.' Instead of /p/, say /t/. What's your new word?") (sheet)

> **NOTE:** *Give the letter sound, not the letter name. Use pictured items and/or manipulatives if necessary. Use any of the following stimulus words and/or others you select from the story. The correct answers are in parentheses.*

Stimulus items:

"Say 'hum.' Instead of /m/, say /t/." (hut)

"Say 'hoot.' Instead of /t/, say /p/." (hoop)

"Say 'screech.' Instead of /ch/, say /n/." (screen)

"Say 'squeal.' Instead of /l/, say /k/." (squeak)

"Say 'coo.' Instead of /oo/, say /long E/." (key)

"Say 'bees.' Instead of /z/, say /t/." (beet)

"Say 'by.' Instead of /long I/, say /oo/." (boo)

"Say 'squeal.' Instead of /l/, say /z/." (squeeze)

"Say 'creak.' Instead of /k/, say /p/." (creep)

"Say 'flies.' Instead of /z/, say /r/." (flier)

18. Segmenting the middle sound in monosyllabic words.

What to say to the student: "Tell me the middle sound in the word I say."

> **EXAMPLE** "What's the middle sound in the word '_____'?" (stimulus word) (e.g., "What's the middle sound in the word 'bat'?") (/short A/)

> **NOTE:** *Give the letter sound, not the letter name. Use pictured items and/or manipulatives if necessary. Use any of the following stimulus words and/or others you select from the story. The correct answers are in parentheses.*

Stimulus items:

but (/short U/)

hoot (/oo/)

mice (/long I/)

sheep (/long E/)

talk (/ah/)

lions (/short U/)

bees (long E/)

buzz (/short U/)

frogs (/ah/)

hum (/short U/)

19. Substituting the middle sound in words.

What to say to the student: "We're going to change the middle sound in words."

> **EXAMPLE** "Say '_____.'" (stimulus word) "Instead of / /" (stimulus sound), "say / /." (stimulus sound) (e.g., "Say 'bat.' Instead of /short A/, say /short I/. What's your new word?") (bit)

> **NOTE:** *Give the letter sound, not the letter name. Use pictured items and/or manipulatives if necessary. Use any of the following stimulus words and/or others you select from the story. The correct answers are in parentheses.*

Stimulus items:

"Say 'bees.' Instead of /long E/, say /short U/." (buzz)

"Say 'hum.' Instead of /short U/, say /short I/." (him)

"Say 'hum.' Instead of /short U/, say /short A/." (ham)

"Say 'mice.' Instead of /long I/, say /oo/." (moose)

"Say 'sheep.' Instead of /long E/, say /ah/." (shop)

"Say 'hoot.' Instead of /oo/, say /ah/." (hot)

"Say 'but.' Instead of /short U/, say /short I/." (bit)

"Say 'pig.' Instead of /short I/, say /short U/." (pug)

"Say 'buzz.' Instead of /short U/, say /short I/." (biz)

"Say 'dove.' Instead of /short U/, say /long I/." (dive)

20. Identifying all sounds in monosyllabic words.

What to say to the student: "Now tell me all the sounds you hear in the word I say."

> EXAMPLE   "What sounds do you hear in the word '_____'?" (stimulus word)
> (e.g., "What sounds do you hear in the word 'hum'?") (/h/ /short
> U/ /m/)

NOTE: *Give the letter sound, not the letter name. Use pictured items and/or manipulatives if necessary. Use any of the following stimulus words and/or others you select from the story. The correct answers are in parentheses.*

Stimulus items:

hoot (/h/ /oo/ /t/)

pigs (/p/ /short I/ /g/ /z/)

screech (/s/ /k/ /r/ /long E/ /ch/)

mice (/m/ /long I/ /s/)

cluck (/k/ /l/ /short U/ /k/)

doves (/d/ /short U/ /v/ /z/)

quack (/k/ /w/ /short A/ /k/)

flies (/f/ /l/ /long I/ /z/)

creak (/k/ /r/ /long E/ /k/)

croak (/k/ /r/ /long O/ /k/)

21. Deleting sounds within words.

What to say to the student: "We're going to leave out sounds in words."

> EXAMPLE   "Say '_____'" (stimulus word) "without / /." (stimulus sound) (e.g.,
> "Say 'bats' without /t/.") (bass) Say "The word that is left—'bass'—is a real
> word. Sometimes, the word won't be a real word."

NOTE: *Give the letter sound, not the letter name. Use pictured items and/or manipulatives if necessary. Use any of the following stimulus words and/or others you select from the story. The correct answers are in parentheses.*

Stimulus items:

"Say 'doves' without /v/." (does)

"Say 'speak' without /p/." (seek)

"Say 'snore' without /n/." (sore)

"Say 'frogs' without /r/." (fogs)

"Say 'lions' without /short U/." (lines)

"Say 'quack' without /w/." (kack)

"Say 'crickets' without /r/." (kickets)

"Say 'squeal' without /w/." (skeel)

"Say 'growl' without /r/." (gowl)

"Say 'cats' without /t/." (Cass)

22. Substituting consonants in words having a two-sound cluster.

What to say to the student: "We're going to substitute sounds in words."

> **EXAMPLE**   "Say '_____.'" (stimulus word) "Instead of / /" (stimulus sound), "say / /." (stimulus sound) (e.g., "Say 'pigs.' Instead of /g/, say /t/.") (pits) Say: "Sometimes, the new word will be a made-up word."

> **NOTE:** *Give the letter sound, not the letter name. Use pictured items and/or manipulatives if necessary. Use any of the following stimulus words and/or others you select from the story. The correct answers are in parentheses.*

Stimulus items:

"Say 'bats.' Instead of /s/, say /r/." (batter)

"Say 'cats.' Instead of /t/, say /p/." (caps)

"Say 'creak.' Instead of /k/, say /g/." (Greek)

"Say 'snore.' Instead of /n/, say /t/." (store)

"Say 'cluck.' Instead of /k/, say /p/." (pluck)

"Say 'speak.' Instead of /p/, say /n/." (sneak)

"Say 'pigs.' Instead of /g/, say /b/." (pibs)

"Say 'croak.' Instead of /r/, say /l/." (cloak)

"Say 'frogs.' Instead of /g/, say /d/." (frauds)

"Say 'howl.' Instead of /l/, say /s/." (house)

23. Phoneme reversing.

What to say to the student: "We're going to say words backward."

> **EXAMPLE**   "Say the word '_____'" (stimulus word) "backward." (e.g., "Say 'buzz' backward.") (zubb)

NOTE: *This is a difficult phoneme-level task and should only be done with older students. Give the letter sound, not the letter name. Use pictured items and/or manipulatives if necessary. Use any of the following stimulus words and/or others you select from the story. The correct answers are in parentheses.*

Stimulus items:

moo (oom)

but (tub)

mice (sime)

sheep (peesh)

speak (keeps)

cats (stack)

by (I'b)

purr (rupp)

pigs (sgip)

croak (cork)

24. Phoneme switching.

What to say to the student: "We're going to switch the first sounds in two words."

EXAMPLE "Switch the first sounds in '_____' and '_____.'" (stimulus words) (e.g., "Switch the first sounds in 'lions' and 'roar.'") (rions loar)

NOTE: *This is a difficult phoneme-level task and should only be done with older students. Give the letter sound, not the letter name. Use pictured items and/or manipulatives if necessary. Use any of the following stimulus words and/or others you select from the story. The correct answers are in parentheses.*

Stimulus items:

cats purr (pats curr)

sheep baa (beep shaw)

monkeys chatter (chunkies matter)

cows moo (mows coo)

doves coo (cuvs doo)

horses neigh (norses hay)

coyotes howl (hoyotes cowl)

frogs croak (crogs froak)

poem by (boem pie)

dogs growl (gogs drowl)

25. Pig Latin.

What to say to the student: "We're going to speak a secret language by using words from the story. In pig Latin, you take off the first sound of a word, put it at the end of the word, and add an 'ay' sound."

> **EXAMPLE** "Say 'dogs' in pig Latin." (ogsday)

> **NOTE:** *This is a difficult phoneme-level task and should only be done with older students. Use pictured items and/or manipulatives if necessary. Use any of the following stimulus words and/or others you select from the story. The correct answers are in parentheses.*

Stimulus items:

pigs (igspay)

doves (ovesday)

chatter (atterchay)

monkeys (onkeysmay)

frogs (rogsfay)

hoot (oothay)

lions (ionslay)

crickets (ricketskay)

parrots (arrotspay)

horses (orseshay)

From Phonological Awareness Into Print

> **NOTE:** *Only five examples per activity are included in this resource due to space. You are encouraged to add many more words into this section that you feel your student(s) are ready to write.*

1. Substituting the initial sound or letter in words.

> **NOTE:** *Use lined paper or copy the sheet of lined paper included in the back of this book.*

Stimulus items:

1.1 hats/cats

Task a. "Say 'hats.' Instead of /h/, say /k/. What's your new word?" (cats) "Write/copy 'hats' and 'cats.'"

Task b. "Circle the **letters** that make the words different." ([h], [c])

Task c. "What **sounds** do these letters make?" (/h/, /k/)

1.2 ducks/bucks

Task a. "Say 'ducks.' Instead of /d/, say /b/. What's your new word?" (bucks) "Write/copy 'ducks' and 'bucks.'"

Task b. "Circle the **letters** that make the words different." ([d], [b])

Task c. "What **sounds** do these letters make?" (/d/, /b/)

1.3 bats/rats

Task a. "Say 'bats.' Instead of /b/, say /r/. What's your new word?" (rats) "Write/copy 'bats' and 'rats.'"

Task b. "Circle the **letters** that make the words different." ([b], [r])

Task c. "What **sounds** do these letters make?" (/b/, /r/)

1.4 chatter/batter

Task a. "Say 'chatter.' Instead of /ch/, say /b/. What's your new word?" (batter) "Write/copy 'chatter' and 'batter.'"

Task b. "Circle the **letters** that make the words different." ([c], [h], [b])

Task c. "What **sounds** do these letters make?" (/ch/, /b/)

1.5 say/pay

Task a. "Say 'say.' Instead of /s/, say /p/. What's your new word?" (pay) "Write/copy 'say' and 'pay.'"

Task b. "Circle the **letters** that make the words different." ([s], [p])

Task c. "What **sounds** do these letters make?" (/s/, /p/)

2. Substituting the final sound or letter in words.

NOTE: *Use lined paper or copy the sheet of lined paper included in the back of this book.*

Stimulus items:

2.1 but/bus

Task a. "Say 'but.' Instead of /t/, say /s/. What's your new word?" (bus) "Write/copy 'but' and 'bus.'"

Task b. "Circle the **letters** that make the words different." ([t], [s])

Task c. "What **sounds** do these letters make?" (/t/, /s/)

2.2 bees/beep

Task a. "Say 'bees.' Instead of /z/, say /p/. What's your new word?" (beep) "Write/copy 'bees' and 'beep.'"

Task b. "Circle the **letters** that make the words different." ([s], [p])

Task c. "What **sounds** do these letters make?" (/z/, /p/)

2.3 hoot/hoop

Task a. "Say 'hoot.' Instead of /t/, say /p/. What's your new word?" (hoop) "Write/copy 'hoot' and 'hoop.'"

Task b. "Circle the **letters** that make the words different." ([t], [p])

Task c. "What **sounds** do these letters make?" (/t/, /p/)

2.4 sheep/sheet

Task a. "Say 'sheep.' Instead of /p/, say /t/. What's your new word?" (sheet) "Write/copy 'sheep' and 'sheet.'"

Task b. "Circle the **letters** that make the words different." ([p], [t])

Task c. "What **sounds** do these letters make?" (/p/, /t/)

2.5 hum/hub

Task a. "Say 'hum.' Instead of /m/, say /b/. What's your new word?" (hub) "Write/copy 'hum' and 'hub.'"

Task b. "Circle the **letters** that make the words different." ([m], [b])

Task c. "What **sounds** do these letters make?" (/m/, /b/)

3. Substituting the middle sound or letter in words.

NOTE: *Use lined paper or copy the sheet of lined paper included in the back of this book.*

Stimulus items:

3.1 hoot/hut

Task a. "Say 'hoot.' Instead of /oo/, say /short U/. What's your new word?" (hut) "Write/copy 'hoot' and 'hut.'"

Task b. "Circle the **letters** that make the words different." ([o], [o], [u])

Task c. "What **sounds** do these letters make?" (/oo/, /short U/)

3.2 but/bit

Task a. "Say 'but.' Instead of /short U/, say /short I/. What's your new word?" (bit) "Write/copy 'but' and 'bit.'"

Task b. "Circle the **letters** that make the words different." ([u], [i])

Task c. "What **sounds** do these letters make?" (/short U/, /short I/)

3.3 hum/ham

Task a. "Say 'hum.' Instead of /short U/, say /short A/. What's your new word?" (ham) "Write/copy 'hum' and 'ham.'"

Task b. "Circle the **letters** that make the words different." ([u], [a])

Task c. "What **sounds** do these letters make?" (/short U/, /short A/)

3.4 sheep/shop

Task a. "Say 'sheep.' Instead of /long E/, say /ah/. What's your new word?" (shop) "Write/copy 'sheep' and 'shop.'"

Task b. "Circle the **letters** that make the words different." ([e], [e], [o])

Task c. "What **sounds** do these letters make?" (/long E/, /ah/)

3.5 hoot/heat

Task a. "Say 'hoot.' Instead of /oo/, say /long E/. What's your new word?" (heat) "Write/copy 'hoot' and 'heat.'"

Task b. "Circle the **letters** that make the words different." ([o], [o], [e], [a])

Task c. "What **sounds** do these letters make?" (/oo/, /long E/)

4. Supplying the initial sound or letter in words.

NOTE: *Use lined paper or copy the sheet of lined paper included in the back of this book.*

Stimulus items:

4.1 cluck/luck
Task a. "Say 'cluck,' say 'luck.' What sound did you hear in 'cluck' that is missing in 'luck'?" (/k/) "Now we'll *change* the **letter**. Write/copy 'cluck' and 'luck.'"

Task b. "Circle the beginning **letter** that makes the words different." ([c])

Task c. "What **sound** does this letter make?" (/k/)

4.2 mice/ice
Task a. "Say 'mice,' say 'ice.' What sound did you hear in 'mice' that is missing in 'ice'?" (/m/) "Now we'll change the **letter**. Write/copy 'mice' and 'ice.'"

Task b. "Circle the beginning **letter** that makes the words different." ([m])

Task c. "What **sound** does this letter make?" (/m/)

4.3 speak/peak
Task a. "Say 'speak,' say 'peak.' What sound did you hear in 'speak' that is missing in 'peak'?" (/s/) "Now we'll change the **letter**. Write/copy 'speak' and 'peak.'"

Task b. "Circle the beginning **letter** that makes the words different." ([s])

Task c. "What **sound** does this letter make?" (/s/)

4.4 flies/lies
Task a. "Say 'flies,' say 'lies.' What sound did you hear in 'flies' that is missing in 'lies'?" (/f/) "Now we'll change the **letter**. Write/copy 'flies' and 'lies.'"

Task b. "Circle the beginning **letter** that makes the words different." ([f])

Task c. "What **sound** does this letter make?" (/f/)

4.5 howl/owl
Task a. "Say 'howl,' say 'owl.' What sound did you hear in 'howl' that is missing in 'owl'?" (/h/) "Now we'll change the **letter**. Write/copy 'howl' and 'owl.'"

Task b. "Circle the beginning **letter** that makes the words different." ([h])

Task c. "What **sound** does this letter make?" (/h/)

5. Supplying the final sound or letter in words.

NOTE: *Use lined paper or copy the sheet of lined paper included in the back of this book.*

Stimulus items:

5.1 bats/bat
Task a. "Say 'bats,' say 'bat.' What sound did you hear in 'bats' that is missing in 'bat'?" (/s/) "Now we'll *change* the **letter**. Write/copy 'bats' and 'bat.'"

Task b. "Circle the ending/last **letter** that makes the words different." ([s])

Task c. "What **sound** does this letter make?" (/s/)

5.2 howl/how

Task a. "Say 'howl,' say 'how.' What sound did you hear in 'howl' that is missing in 'how'?" (/l/) "Now we'll change the **letter**. Write/copy 'howl' and 'how.'"

Task b. "Circle the ending/last **letter** that makes the words different." ([l])

Task c. "What **sound** does this letter make?" (/l/)

5.3 pigs/pig

Task a. "Say 'pigs,' say 'pig.' What sound did you hear in 'pigs' that is missing in 'pig'?" (/z/) "Now we'll change the **letter**. Write/copy 'pigs' and 'pig.'"

Task b. "Circle the ending/last **letter** that makes the words different." ([s])

Task c. "What **sound** does this letter make?" (/z/)

5.4 ducks/duck

Task a. "Say 'ducks,' say 'duck.' What sound did you hear in 'ducks' that is missing in 'duck'?" (/s/) "Now we'll change the **letter**. Write/copy 'ducks' and 'duck.'"

Task b. "Circle the ending/last **letter** that makes the word different." ([s])

Task c. "What **sound** does this letter make?" (/s/)

5.5 bees/bee

Task a. "Say 'bees,' say 'bee.' What sound did you hear in 'bees' that is missing in 'bee'?" (/z/) "Now we'll change the **letter**. Write/copy 'bees' and 'bee.'"

Task b. "Circle the ending/last **letter** that makes the words different." ([s])

Task c. "What **sound** does this letter make?" (/z/)

6. Switching the first sound and letter in words (ADVANCED).

NOTE: *Use lined paper or copy the sheet of lined paper included in the back of this book.*

Stimulus items:

6.1 frogs croak

Task a. "Say 'frogs,' say 'croak.' What sound do you hear at the beginning of 'frogs'?" (/f/) "What sound do you hear at the beginning of 'croak'?" (/k/) "Switch the first sounds in those words." (crogs froak) "Now we'll change the **letters**. Write/copy 'frogs croak' and 'crogs froak.'"

Task b. "Circle the beginning **letters** that change the words." ([f], [c])

Task c. "What **sounds** do those letters make?" (/f/, /k/)

6.2 sheep baa

Task a. "Say 'sheep,' say 'baa.' What sound do you hear at the beginning of 'sheep'?" (/sh/) "What sound do you hear at the beginning of 'baa'?" (/b/) "Switch the first sounds in those words." (beep shaa) "Now we'll change the **letters**. Write/copy 'sheep baa' and 'beep shaa.'"

Task b. "Circle the beginning **letters** that change the words." ([s], [h], [b])

Task c. "What **sounds** do those letters make?" (/sh/, /b/)

6.3 cats purr

    Task a. "Say 'cats,' say 'purr.' What sound do you hear at the beginning of 'cats'?" (/k/) "What sound do you hear at the beginning of 'purr'?" (/p/) "Switch the first sounds in those words." (pats curr) "Now we'll change the **letters**. Write/copy 'cats purr' and 'pats curr.'"

    Task b. "Circle the beginning **letters** that change the words." ([c], [p])

    Task c. "What **sounds** do those letters make?" (/k/, /p/)

6.4 lions roar

    Task a. "Say 'lions,' say 'roar.' What sound do you hear at the beginning of 'lions'?" (/l/) "What sound do you hear at the beginning of 'roar'?" (/r/) "Switch the first sounds in those words." (rions loar) "Now we'll change the **letters**. Write/copy 'lions roar' and 'rions loar.'"

    Task b. "Circle the beginning **letters** that change the words." ([l], [r])

    Task c. "What **sounds** do those letters make?" (/l/, /r/)

6.5 but talk

    Task a. "Say 'but,' say 'talk.' What sound do you hear at the beginning of 'but'?" (/b/) "What sound do you hear at the beginning of 'talk'?" (/t/) "Switch the first sounds in those words." (tut balk) "Now we'll change the **letters**. Write/copy 'but talk' and 'tut balk.'"

    Task b. "Circle the beginning **letters** that change the words." ([b], [t])

    Task c. "What **sounds** do those letters make?" (/b/, /t/)

CHAPTER 11
Phonological Awareness Activities to Use with *Miss Bindergarten Gets Ready for Kindergarten*

Text version used for selection of stimulus items:

Slate, J., and Wolff, A. (Illustrator). (1996). *Miss Bindergarten Gets Ready for Kindergarten.* New York: The Penguin Group.

Phonological Awareness Activities at the Word Level

1. Counting words.

What to say to the student: "We're going to count words."

> **EXAMPLE** "How many words do you hear in this sentence (or phrase): 'first day'?" (2)

> **NOTE:** *Use pictured items and/or manipulatives if necessary. Use any of the following stimulus phrases or sentences and/or others you select from the story. The correct answers are in parentheses.*

Stimulus items:

Zach Blair (2)

marches in (2)

right on (2)

pedals her bike (3)

packs her bunny (3)

looks out the window (4)

Fetter fights his sweater. (4)

Lindo looks out the window. (5)

Jessie Sike pedals her bike. (5)

Ian Lowe says "I won't go!" (6)

2. Identifying the missing word from a list.

What to say to the student: "Listen to the words I say. I'll say them again. You tell me which word I leave out."

> **EXAMPLE**   "Listen to the words I say: 'climbs right on.' I'll say them again. Tell me which one I leave out: 'climbs right.'" (on)

> **NOTE:** *Use pictured items and/or manipulatives if necessary. Use any of the following stimulus words and/or others you select from the story. The correct answers are in parentheses.*

Stimulus set #1	Stimulus set #2
Jessie, shoe	shoe (Jessie)
Wanda, Raffie	Wanda (Raffie)
Tommy, vroom, Noah	vroom, Noah (Tommy)
bunny, Tuttle, Gwen	Tuttle, Gwen (bunny)
fights, sweater, Christopher	fights, Christopher (sweater)
marches, Lenny, Patricia	marches, Lenny (Patricia)
friend, kindergarten, hops,	friend, hops (kindergarten)
Zach, Packer, rushes, friend	Packer, rushes, friend (Zach)
Bonn, hello, kangaroo, Lister	Bonn, hello, kangaroo (Lister)
gorilla, McGunny, Lindo, Kiki	McGunny, Lindo, Kiki (gorilla)

3. Identifying the missing word in a phrase or sentence.

What to say to the student: "Listen to the sentence I read. Tell me which word is missing the second time I read the sentence."

> **EXAMPLE**   "'gets ready for.' Listen again and tell me which word I leave out: 'gets ready _____.'" (for)

> **NOTE:** *Use pictured items and/or manipulatives if necessary. Use any of the following stimulus sentences and/or others you select from the story. The correct answers are in parentheses.*

Stimulus items:

her bunny. her _____. (bunny)

gets ready. _____ready. (gets)

I won't go. I _____ go. (won't)

pedals her bike. _____ her bike. (pedals)

hugs good-bye. hugs good-_____. (bye)

is the first one off. is the _____ one off. (first)

Ursula Crewe ties her shoe. Ursula Crew ties her _____. (shoe)

Zach Blair finds his chair. _____ Blair finds his chair. (Zach)

Jessie Sike pedals her bike. Jessie Sike _____ her bike. (pedals)

Ophelia Nye hugs good-bye. Ophelia Nye _____ good-bye. (hugs)

4. Supplying the missing word as an adult reads.

What to say to the student: "I want you to help me read the story. You fill in the words I leave out."

> EXAMPLE   "Miss _____." (Bindergarten)

NOTE: *Use pictured items and/or manipulatives if necessary. Use any of the following stimulus sentences and/or others you select from the story. The correct answers are in parentheses.*

Stimulus items:

hugs _____. (good-bye)

gets ready for _____. (kindergarten)

jumps a _____. (puddle)

Fran Lister _____ her sister. (kisses)

Ian Lowe says, "I _____ go!" (won't)

Kiki Wongs hops _____. (along)

Noah Bonn climbs right _____. (on)

Matty Lindo _____ out the window. (looks)

Sara von Hoff is the first one _____. (off)

Miss _____ is ready for kindergarten. (Bindergarten)

5. Rearranging words.

What to say to the student: "I'll say some words out of order. You put them in the right order so they make sense."

> EXAMPLE   " 'one first off.' Put those words in the right order." (first one off)

NOTE: *Use pictured items and/or manipulatives if necessary. Use any of the following stim- ulus words and/or others you select from the story. The correct answers are in pa- rentheses. This word-level activity can be more difficult than some of the syllable- or phoneme-level activities because of the memory load. If your students are only able to deal with two or three words to be rearranged, add more two- and three-word samples from the story and omit the four-word level items.*

Stimulus items:

high back fives (high-fives back)

her pedals bike (pedals her bike)

puddle a jumps (jumps a puddle)

to rushes dress (rushes to dress)

fights sweater his (fights his sweater)

Densel her pencil bites. (Densel bites her pencil.)

around Yolanda Pound looks. (Yolanda Pound looks around.)

in Chin Wanda marches. (Wanda Chin marches in.)

"Vroom" Lenny says Loome. ("Vroom," says Lenny Loome.)

packs Gwen McGunny bunny her. (Gwen McGunny packs her bunny.)

Phonological Awareness Activities at the Syllable Level

1. Syllable counting.

What to say to the student: "We're going to count syllables (or parts) of words."

> **EXAMPLE** "How many syllables do you hear in '_____'?" (stimulus word)
> (e.g., "How many syllables in 'Densel'?") (2)

> **NOTE:** *Use pictured items and/or manipulatives if necessary. Use any of the following stimulus words and/or others you select from the story. Use any group of 10 stimulus items you select per teaching set.*

Stimulus items:

One-syllable words: packs, Pound, pig, bike, bye, Bonn, back, bites, Blair, teeth, ties, dress, dog, Krupp, cools, climbs, Crewe, cat, Gwen, go, gets, good, Chin, chair, jumps, Mack, Miss, Moose, Nye, Sike, sneaks, Fran, finds, fights, first, five, friend, frog, fun, Hess, Heath, hops, hugs, Huff, right, Roe, looks, Lowe, Loome, wakes, Wong, won't, Wend, shoe, Zach, broom, off, yells

Two-syllable words: pedals, Packer, puddle, pencil, Brenda, brushes, Beaker, bunny, began, beaver, begun, Tommy, Tuttle, tiger, Danny, Densel, kisses, Kiki, cracker, Quentin, cocoa, Jessie, Matty, Moko, marches, morning, monkey, Noah, sneaker, sister, sweater, Sara, squirrel, Fetter, Vicky, Henry, hello, ready, rushes, Raffie, Lister, Lenny, Lindo, lion, Wanda, zebra, Ian, window, Adam, ready, along, around

Three-syllable words: Patricia, Christopher, kangaroo, gorilla, McGunny, Yolanda, Ophelia, iguana, Emily, elephant, Ursula

Four-syllable words: Bindergarten, kindergarten, alligator

2. Initial syllable deleting.

What to say to the student: "We're going to leave out syllables (or parts of words)."

> **EXAMPLE** "Say '_____.'" (stimulus word) "Say it again without '_____.'"
> (stimulus syllable) (e.g., "Say 'morning.' Say it again without 'morn.'") (ing)

> **NOTE:** *Use pictured items and/or manipulatives if necessary. Use any of the following stimulus words and/or others you select from the story. The correct answers are in parentheses.*

Stimulus items:

"Say 'monkey' without 'mun.'" (key)

"Say 'sister' without 'sis.'" (-ter)

"Say 'sneaker' without 'sneak.'" (-er)

"Say 'Quentin' without 'quent.'" (in)

"Say 'Moko' without 'mo.'" (ko)

"Say 'began' without 'be.'" (-gan)

"Say 'marches' without 'march.' " (-ez)

"Say 'gorilla' without 'gore.' " (-illa)

"Say 'cracker' without 'crack.' " (-er)

"Say 'kangaroo' without 'kang.' " (-aroo)

3. Final syllable deleting.

What to say to the student: "We're going to leave out syllables (or parts of words)."

> **EXAMPLE** "Say '_____.' " (stimulus word) "Say it again without '_____.' " (stimulus syllable) (e.g., "Say 'morning' without 'ing.' ") (morn)

> **NOTE:** *Use pictured items and/or manipulatives if necessary. Use any of the following stimulus words and/or others you select from the story. The correct answers are in parentheses.*

Stimulus items:

"Say 'cracker' without '-er.' " (crack)

"Say 'Noah' without '-uh.' " (no)

"Say 'began' without 'gan.' " (be)

"Say 'Lister' without '-er.' " (list)

"Say 'sneaker' without '-er.' " (sneak)

"Say 'kangaroo' without 'roo.' " (kanga)

"Say 'Moko' without 'ko.' " (moe)

"Say 'Beaker' without '-er.' " (beak)

"Say 'Kiki' without 'key.' " (key)

"Say 'Henry' without 'ree.' " (hen)

4. Initial syllable adding.

What to say to the student: "Now let's add syllables (or parts) to words."

> **EXAMPLE** "Add '_____' " (stimulus syllable) "to the beginning of '_____.' " (stimulus syllable) (e.g., "Add 'morn' to the beginning of 'ing.' ") (morning)

> **NOTE:** *Use pictured items and/or manipulatives if necessary. Use any of the following stimulus words and/or others you select from the story. The correct answers are in parentheses.*

Stimulus items:

"Add 'moe' to the beginning of 'koe.' " (Moko)

"Add 'be' to the beginning of 'gan.' " (began)

"Add 'gore' to the beginning of 'illa.' " (gorilla)

"Add 'hen' to the beginning of 'ree.' " (Henry)

"Add 'bren' to the beginning of 'duh.'" (Brenda)

"Add 'sweat' to the beginning of 'er.'" (sweater)

"Add 'lynn' to the beginning of 'doe.'" (Lindo)

"Add 'pack' to the beginning of '-er.'" (Packer)

"Add 'bin' to the beginning of 'dergarten.'" (Bindergarten)

"Add 'kin' to the beginning of 'dergarten.'" (kindergarten)

5. Final syllable adding.

What to say to the student: "Now let's add syllables (or parts) to words."

> **EXAMPLE** "Add '_____'" (stimulus syllable) "to the end of '_____.'" (stimulus syllable) (e.g., "Add 'ing' to the end of 'cut.'") (cutting)

NOTE: *Use pictured items and/or manipulatives if necessary. Use any of the following stimulus words and/or others you select from the story. The correct answers are in parentheses.*

Stimulus items:

"Add 'koe' to the end of 'moe.'" (Moko)

"Add 'er' to the end of 'beak.'" (Beaker)

"Add 'sul' to the end of 'pen.'" (pencil)

"Add 'ee' to the end of 'bun.'" (bunny)

"Add 'us' to the end of 'rhineosser.'" (rhinoceros)

"Add 'doe' to the end of 'lynn.'" (Lindo)

"Add 'yuh' to the end of 'ofeel.'" (Ophelia)

"Add 'ree' to the end of 'hen.'" (Henry)

"Add 'er' to the end of 'fett.'" (Fetter)

"Add 'gun' to the end of 'be.'" (begun)

6. Syllable substituting.

What to say to the student: "Let's make up some new words."

> **EXAMPLE** "Say '_____.'" (stimulus word) "Instead of '_____'" (stimulus syllable), "say '_____.'" (stimulus syllable) (e.g., "Say 'morning.' Instead of 'morn,' say 'bake.' The new word is 'baking.'")

NOTE: *Use pictured items and/or manipulatives if necessary. Use of the following stimulus words and/or others you select from the story. The correct answers are in parentheses.*

Stimulus items:

"Say 'bunny.' Instead of 'bun,' say 'fun.'" (funny)

"Say 'Packer.' Instead of 'pack,' say 'back.'" (backer)

"Say 'Lindo.' Instead of 'doe,' say 'dee.'" (Lindy)

"Say 'Tommy.' Instead of 'Tom,' say 'Dan.'" (Danny)

"Say 'brushes.' Instead of 'brush,' say 'march.'" (marches)

"Say 'Brenda.' Instead of 'Bren,' say 'Juan.'" (Wanda)

"Say 'Densel.' Instead of 'zel,' say 'knee.'" (Denny)

"Say 'sneaker.' Instead of '-er,' say '-ing.'" (sneaking)

"Say 'bindergarten.' Instead of 'bin,' say 'kin.'" (kindergarten)

"Say 'Lister.' Instead of 'lis,' say 'sis.'" (sister)

Phonological Awareness Activities at the Phoneme Level

1. Counting sounds.

What to say to the student: "We're going to count sounds in words."

> **EXAMPLE**   "How many sounds do you hear in this word: 'dog'?" (3)

> **NOTE:** *Use pictured items and/or manipulatives if necessary. Use any of the following stimulus words and/or others you select from the story. Be sure to give the letter sound and not the letter name. Use any group of 10 stimulus items you select per teaching set.*

Stimulus words with two sounds: bye, to, day, go, Nye, now, high, Roe, Lowe, shoe

Stimulus words with three sounds: pig, bike, Bonn, back, teeth, ties, dog, Crewe, cat, good, Chin, miss, Mack, moose, Noah, Sike, says, Von, Heath, his, Hess, Huff, right, Zach, Ian,

Stimulus words with four sounds: packs, Packer, Pound, Beaker, bunny, bites, Tommy, Tuttle, tiger, Danny, dress, Krupp, cools, cocoa, Kiki, gets, Gwen, Jessie, Moko, Matty, first, Fran, fights, Fetter, fives, find, fun's, frog, vroom, Vicky, hops, hugs, ready, Raffie, Lenny, looks, lion, wakes, won't, Wend

Stimulus words with five sounds: pedals, kisses, climbs, cracker, jumps, sneaker, sister, sweater, sneaks, finds, rushes, Lindo, Wanda, window, Emily

2. Sound categorization or identifying a rhyme oddity.

What to say to the student: "Guess which word I say does not rhyme with the other three words."

> **EXAMPLE**   "Tell me which word does not rhyme with the other three: '_____,' '_____,' '_____,' '_____.'" (stimulus words) (e.g., "Roe,' 'so,' 'show,' 'her.' Which word doesn't rhyme?") (her)

> **NOTE:** *Use pictured items if necessary. Use any of the following stimulus words and/or others you select from the story. The correct answers are in parentheses.*

Stimulus items:

Wend, Loome, bend, send (Loome)

eye, Fetter, Nye, sigh (Fetter)

cup, Krupp, pup, Densel (Densel)

Vicky, sneaker, Beaker, seeker (Vicky)

sister, rhinoceros, Lister, blister (rhinoceros)

Raffie, Sike, bike, hike (Raffie)

Benny, penny, Lenny, Wanda (Wanda)

Crewe, knew, gorilla, Sue (gorilla)

Tuttle, puddle, jumps, subtle (jumps)

Fran, McGunny, Dan, Stan (McGunny)

3. Matching rhyme.

What to say to the student: "We're going to think of rhyming words."

> **EXAMPLE** "Which word rhymes with '_____'?" (stimulus word) (e.g., "Which word rhymes with 'dog': 'friend,' 'fog,' 'gorilla,' 'Mack'?") (fog)

NOTE: *Use pictured items if necessary. Use any of the following stimulus words and/or others you select from the story. The correct answers are in parentheses.*

Stimulus items:

Benny: fights, hello, Lenny, Fran (Lenny)

taffy: kindergarten, Raffie, Wanda, Von (Raffie)

when: Christopher, cocoa, Gwen, jumps (Gwen)

Wong: song, hippopotamus, rushes, zebra (song)

Sue: Jessie, sweater, Crewe, Krupp (Crewe)

picky: Noah, morning, Vicky, Lindo (Vicky)

sister: Bindergarten, McGunny, Loome, Lister (Lister)

tiki: Kiki, cracker, Sara, kangaroo (Kiki)

puddle: Henry, Tuttle, Densel, Quentin (Tuttle)

sweater: Lister, Wanda, Fetter, gorilla (Fetter)

4. Producing rhyme.

What to say to the student: "Now we'll say rhyming words."

> **EXAMPLE** "Tell me a word that rhymes with '_____.'" (stimulus word) (e.g., "Tell me a word that rhymes with 'shoe.' You can make up a word if you want.") (boo, too)

NOTE: *Use pictured items if necessary. Use any of the following stimulus words and/or others you select from the story (i.e., you say a word from the list below and the student is to think of a rhyming word). Use any group of 10 stimulus items you select per teaching set.*

Stimulus items:

/p/ packs, pedals, Patricia, Packer, puddle, pencil, Pound, pig

/b/ Bindergarten, Brenda, Brushes, beaker, bunny, bike, bye, Bonn, back, bites, Blair, begun, beaver

/t/: teeth, to, Tommy, ties, tiger

/d/: day, Danny, dress, Densel, dog

/k/: kindergarten, Krupp, Christopher, cools, cocoa, kisses, Kiki, climbs, cracker, Quentin, Crewe, cat, kangaroo

/g/: gets, Gwen, go, good, gorilla

/ch/: Chin, chair

/dz/ (as in gem): Jessie, jumps, jaguar

/m/: Miss, Moko, McGunny, Matty, Mack, marches, morning, moose, monkey

/n/: Nye, Noah, now

/s/: sneaker, sister, sweater, says, Sike, sneaks, Sara, says, squirrel

/z/: Zach, zebra

/f/: for, first, finds, Fran, Fetter, fights, fives, friend, find, fun's, frog

/v/: vroom, Von, Vicky

/h/: Heath, her, his, Hess, Henry, hops, hugs, high, Huff, hello, hippopotamus

/r/: ready, rushes, right, Raffie, rhinoceros, Roe

/l/: Lister, Lowe, Lenny, Loome, Lindo, looks, lion

/w/, /wh/: wakes, won't, Wong, Wend, one, Wanda, wolf

/sh/: shoe

/voiceless th/: three, thank

/voiced th/: then, they

/y/ (as in yellow): yells, Yolanda, yak

/short A/: alligator

/short U/: of, up, along, a, around, other

/short E/: Emily, elephant

/short I/: iguana, it, is

/long E/: Ian

/long I/: I

/long O/: oh, Ophelia

5. Sound matching (initial).

What to say to the student: "Now we'll listen for the first sound in words."

> **EXAMPLE** "Listen to this sound: / /." (stimulus sound). "Guess which word I say begins with that sound: '_____,' '_____,' '_____,' '_____.'" (stimulus words) (e.g., "Listen to this sound: /f/. Guess which word I say begins with that sound: 'sweater,' 'Fran,' 'hugs,' 'Roe.'") (Fran)

NOTE: *Give the letter sound, not the letter name. Use pictured items if necessary. Use any of the following stimulus words and/or others you select from the story. The correct answers are in parentheses.*

Stimulus items:

/b/: Jessie, Raffie, Bindergarten, Crewe (Bindergarten)

/k/: gorilla, Wanda, rushes, Christopher (Christopher)

/n/: Noah, Kiki, cracker, Henry (Noah)

/dz/ (as in gem): McGunny, lion, Jessie, wakes (Jessie)

/h/: morning, Huff, rhinoceros, sneaker (Huff)

/long O/: around, kindergarten, Ophelia, Yolanda (Ophelia)

/r/: Densel, Raffie, kisses, bunny (Raffie)

/y/ (as in yellow): teeth, hippopotamus, Yolanda, Wanda, Xavier (Yolanda)

/t/: Brenda, Tuttle, Beaker, Lindo (Tuttle)

/p/: Hess, Moko, squirrel, Patricia (Patricia)

6. Sound matching (final).

What to say to the student: "Now we'll listen for the last sound in words."

> **EXAMPLE** "Listen to this sound: / /" (stimulus sound). "Guess which word I say ends with that sound: '_____,' '_____,' '_____,' '_____.'" (stimulus words) (e.g., "Listen to this sound: /k/. Guess which word I say ends with that sound: 'hops,' 'Mack,' 'Lister,' 'Fran.'") (Mack)

> **NOTE:** *Give the letter sound, not the letter name. Use pictured items and/or manipulatives if necessary. Use any of the following stimulus words and/or others you select from the story. The correct answers are in parentheses.*

Stimulus items:

/n/: sneaks, around, almost, kindergarten (kindergarten)

/voiceless th/: Heath, pencil, Lister, marches (Heath)

/z/: elephant, pedals, Zach, Christopher (pedals)

/f/: Bindergarten, rushes, Huff, Xavier (Huff)

/t/: Mack, Blair, Ursula, elephant (elephant)

/long E/: Quentin, McGunny, Ian, morning (McGunny)

/k/: sweater, Krupp, pencil, Sike (Sike)

/m/: vroom, Tuttle, window, Yolanda (vroom)

/long O/: Wend, Beaker, Lindo, Lister (Lindo)

/g/: Ophelia, Noah, window, pig (pig)

7. Identifying the initial sound in words.

What to say to the student: "I'll say a word two times. Tell me what sound is missing the second time: '_____,' '_____.'" (stimulus words)

> **EXAMPLE** "What sound do you hear in '_____'" (stimulus word) "that is missing in '_____'?" (stimulus word) (e.g., "What sound do you hear in 'his' that is missing in 'is'?") (/h/)

NOTE: *Give the letter sound, not the letter name. Use pictured items and/or manipulatives if necessary. Use any of the following stimulus words and/or others you select from the story. The correct answers are in parentheses.*

Stimulus items:

"chair, air. What sound do you hear in 'chair' that is missing in 'air'?" (/ch/)

"brushes, rushes. What sound do you hear in 'brushes' that is missing in 'rushes'?" (/b/)

"Chin, in. What sound do you hear in 'chin' that is missing in 'in'?" (/ch/)

"Fran, ran. What sound do you hear in 'Fran' that is missing in 'ran'?" (/f/)

"vroom, room. What sound do you hear in 'vroom' that is missing in 'room'?" (/v/)

"climbs, limes. What sound do you hear in 'climbs' that is missing in 'limes'?" (/k/)

"Quent, went. What sound do you hear in 'Quent' that is missing in 'went'?" (/k/)

"marches, arches. What sound do you hear in 'marches' that is missing in 'arches'?" (/m/)

"along, long. What sound do you hear in 'along' that is missing in 'long'?" (/uh/)

"Vicky, icky. What sound do you hear in 'Vicky' that is missing in 'icky'?" (/v/)

8. Identifying the final sound in words.

What to say to the student: "I'll say a word two times. Tell me what sound is missing the second time: '_____,' '_____.'" (stimulus words)

> **EXAMPLE**   "What sound do you hear in '_____'" (stimulus word) "that is missing in '_____'?" (stimulus word) (e.g., "What sound do you hear in 'Wend' that is missing in 'when'?") (/d/)

NOTE: *Give the letter sound, not the letter name. Use pictured items and/or manipulatives if necessary. Use any of the following stimulus words and/or others you select from the story. The correct answers are in parentheses.*

Stimulus items:

"gets, get. What sound do you hear in 'gets' that is missing in 'get'?" (/s/)

"Vicky, Vick. What sound do you hear in 'Vicky' that is missing in 'Vick'?" (/long E/)

"moose, moo. What sound do you hear in 'moose' that is missing in 'moo'?" (/s/)

"Lenny, Len. What sound do you hear in 'Lenny' that is missing in 'Len'?" (/long E/)

"climbs, climb. What sound do you hear in 'climbs' that is missing in 'climb'?" (/z/)

"sneaker, sneak. What sound do you hear in 'sneaker' that is missing in 'sneak'?" (/r/)

"Noah, no. What sound do you hear in 'Noah' that is missing in 'no'?" (/uh/)

"Sike, sigh. What sound do you hear in 'Sike' that is missing in 'sigh'?" (/k/)

"Danny, Dan. What sound do you hear in 'Danny' that is missing in 'Dan'?" (/long E/)

"hops, hop. What sound do you hear in 'hops' that is missing in 'hop'?" (/s/)

9. Segmenting the initial sound in words.

What to say to the student: "Listen to the word I say and tell me the first sound you hear."

EXAMPLE   "What's the first sound in '_____'?" (stimulus word) (e.g., "What's the first sound in 'cat'?") (/k/)

NOTE: *Give the letter sound, not the letter name. Use pictured items and/or manipulatives if necessary. Use any of the following stimulus words and/or others you select from the story. Use any group of 10 stimulus items you select per teaching set.*

Stimulus items:

/p/: packs, pedals, Patricia, Packer, puddle, pencil, Pound, pig

/b/: Bindergarten, Brenda, Brushes, beaker, bunny, bike, bye, Bonn, back, bites, Blair, begun, beaver

/t/: teeth, to, Tommy, ties, tiger

/d/: day, Danny, dress, Densel, dog

/k/: kindergarten, Krupp, Christopher, cools, cocoa, kisses, Kiki, climbs, cracker, Quentin, Crewe, cat, kangaroo

/g/: gets, Gwen, go, good, gorilla

/ch/: Chin, chair

/dz/ (as in gem): Jessie, jumps, jaguar

/m/: Miss, Moko, McGunny, Matty, Mack, marches, morning, moose, monkey

/n/: Nye, Noah, now

/s/: sneaker, sister, sweater, says, Sike, sneaks, Sara, says, squirrel

/z/: Zach, zebra

/f/: for, first, finds, Fran, Fetter, fights, fives, friend, find, fun's, frog

/v/: vroom, Von, Vicky

/h/: Heath, her, his, Hess, Henry, hops, hugs, high, Huff, hello, hippopotamus

/r/: ready, rushes, right, Raffie, rhinoceros, Roe

/l/: Lister, Lowe, Lenny, Loome, Lindo, looks, lion

/w/, /wh/: wakes, won't, Wong, Wend, one, Wanda, wolf

/sh/: shoe

/voiceless th/: three, thank

/voiced th/: then, they

/y/ (as in yellow): yells, Yolanda, yak

/short A/: alligator

/short U/: of, up, along, a, around, other

/short E/: Emily, elephant

/short I/: iguana, it, is

/long E/: Ian

/long I/: I

/long O/: oh, Ophelia

10. Segmenting the final sound in words.

What to say to the student: "Listen to the word I say and tell me the last sound you hear."

> **EXAMPLE** "What's the last sound in the word '_____'?" (stimulus word)
> (e.g., "What's the last sound in the word 'cat'?") (/t/)

> **NOTE:** *Give the letter sound, not the letter name. Use pictured items and/or manipulatives if necessary. Use any of the following stimulus words and/or others you select from the story. Use any group of 10 stimulus items you select per teaching set.*

Stimulus items:

/p/: Krupp, up

/t/: it, first, won't, out, right, almost, cat, elephant, newt

/d/: and, good, Wend, Friend, Pound, around

/k/: Sike, bike, Mack, back, Zach, yak

/g/: dog, frog, pig

/m/: Loome, vroom

/n/: Bindergarten, kindergarten, Fran, Gwen, Ian, Bonn, on, Quentin, Vonn, one, Chin, in, begun, lion

/ng/: Wong, along, morning

/s/: Miss, gets, wakes, Hess, dress, packs, fights, hops, looks, sneaks, jumps, bites, hippopotamus, moose, rhinoceros

/z/: is, brushes, finds, his, rushes, cools, kisses, says, pedals, climbs, hugs, fives, ties, marches, yells, funs

/v/: of

/r/: paper, brother, butcher, together, Mister, sister, four, Hopper for, her, Christopher, Beaker, sneaker, Lister, sister, Fetter, sweater, Packer, Cracker, Blair, chair

/l/: Densel, pencil, Tuttle, puddle, all

/voiceless th/: Heath, teeth

/long A/: day

/long E/: ready, Danny, Emily, McGunny, bunny, Henry, Jessie, Kiki, Lenny, Matty, Raffie, Tommy, Vicky

/long I/: I, Nye, bye, high

/long O/: oh, Moko, cocoa, Lowe, go, Lindo, window, Roe, hello

/oo/: to, Crewe, shoe, kangaroo

/uh/: the, Noah, Ophelia, Patricia, Sara, Ursula, Wanda, Yolanda, gorilla

11. Generating words from the story beginning with a particular sound.

What to say to the student: "Let's think of words from the story that start with certain sounds."

> **EXAMPLE** "Tell me a word from the story that starts with / /." (stimulus sound)
> (e.g., the sound /b/) (bunny)

NOTE: *Give the letter sound, not the letter name. Use pictured items if necessary. Use any of the following stimulus words and/or others you select from the story. You say the sound (e.g., a voiceless /p/ sound), and the student is to say a word from the story that begins with that sound. Use any group of 10 stimulus items you select per teaching set.*

Stimulus items:

/p/: packs, pedals, Patricia, Packer, puddle, pencil, Pound, pig

/b/: Bindergarten, Brenda, Brushes, beaker, bunny, bike, bye, Bonn, back, bites, Blair, begun, beaver

/t/: teeth, to, Tommy, ties, tiger

/d/: day, Danny, dress, Densel, dog

/k/: kindergarten, Krupp, Christopher, cools, cocoa, kisses, Kiki, climbs, cracker, Quentin, Crewe, cat, kangaroo

/g/: gets, Gwen, go, good, gorilla

/ch/: Chin, chair

/dz/ (as in gem): Jessie, jumps, jaguar

/m/: Miss, Moko, McGunny, Matty, Mack, marches, morning, moose, monkey

/n/: Nye, Noah, now

/s/: sneaker, sister, sweater, says, Sike, sneaks, Sara, squirrel

/z/: Zach, zebra

/f/: for, first, finds, Fran, Fetter, fights, fives, friend, find, fun's, frog

/v/: vroom, Von, Vicky

/h/: Heath, her, his, Hess, Henry, hops, hugs, high, Huff, hello, hippopotamus

/r/: ready, rushes, right, Raffie, rhinoceros, Roe

/l/: Lister, Lowe, Lenny, Loome, Lindo, looks, lion

/w/, /wh/: wakes, won't, Wong, Wend, one, Wanda, wolf

/sh/: shoe

/voiceless th/: three, thank

/voiced th/: then, they

/y/ (as in yellow): yells, Yolanda, yak

/short A/: alligator

/short U/: of, up, along, a, around, other

/short E/: Emily, elephant

/short I/: iguana, it, is

/long E/: Ian

/long I/: I

/long O/: oh, Ophelia

12. Blending sounds in monosyllabic words divided into onset/rime beginning with a two-consonant cluster + rime.

What to say to the student: "Now we'll put sounds together to make words."

> **EXAMPLE** "Put these sounds together to make a word: / / + / /." (stimulus sounds) "What's the word?" (e.g., "fl + ip: What's the word?") (flip)

> **NOTE:** *Give the letter sound, not the letter name. Use pictured items and/or manipulatives if necessary. Use any of the following stimulus words and/or others you select from the story. The correct answers are in parentheses.*

Stimulus items:

bl + air (Blair)

kr + up (Krupp)

kl + I'm (climb)

fr + end (friend)

kr + oo (Crewe)

gw + en (Gwen)

fr + end (friend)

vr + oom (vroom)

fr + og (frog)

sn + eeks (sneaks)

13. Blending sounds in monosyllabic words divided into onset/rime beginning with a single consonant + rime.

What to say to the student: "Let's put sounds together to make words."

> **EXAMPLE** "Put these sounds together to make a word: / / + / /." (stimulus sounds) "What's the word?" (e.g., "/g/ + ood: What's the word?") (good)

> **NOTE:** *Give the letter sound, not the letter name. Use pictured items and/or manipulatives if necessary. Use any of the following stimulus words and/or others you select from the story. The correct answers are in parentheses.*

Stimulus items:

/l/ + owe (Lowe)

/h/ + ess (Hess)

/b/ + ike (bike)

/v/ + room (vroom)

/k/ + at (cat)

/f/ + rog (frog)

/g/ + ets (gets)

/m/ + iss (miss)

/t/ + eeth (teeth)

/h/ + ops (hops)

14. Blending sounds to form a monosyllabic word beginning with a continuant sound.

What to say to the student: "We'll put sounds together to make words."

> **EXAMPLE** "Put these sounds together to make a word: / / + / / + / /." (stimulus sounds) (e.g., /m/ /ah/ /m/) (mom)

> **NOTE:** *Give the letter sound, not the letter name. Use pictured items and/or manipulatives if necessary. Use any of the following stimulus words and/or others you select from the story. The correct answers are in parentheses.*

Stimulus items:

/n/ /ow/ (now)

/v/ /r/ /oo/ /m/ (vroom)

/l/ /oo/ /m/ (Loome)

/s/ /n/ /long E/ /k/ (sneak)

/f/ /r/ /short A/ /n/ (Fran)

/h/ /short U/ /g/ /z/ (hugs)

/n/ /long I/ (Nye)

/h/ /long E/ /voiceless th/ (Heath)

/m/ /short A/ /k/ (Mack)

/w/ /long A/ /k/ /s/ (wakes)

15. Blending sounds to form a monosyllabic word beginning with a noncontinuant sound.

What to say to the student: "We'll put sounds together to make words."

> **EXAMPLE** "Put these sounds together to make a word: / / + / / + / /." (stimulus sounds) (e.g., /d/ /ah/ /g/) (dog)

> **NOTE:** *Give the letter sound, not the letter name. Use pictured items and/or manipulatives if necessary. Use any of the following stimulus words and/or others you select from the story. The correct answers are in parentheses.*

Stimulus items:

/ch/ /short I/ /n/ (chin)

/t/ /long E/ /voiceless th/ (teeth)

/b/ /long I/ /k/ (bike)

/g/ /long O/ (go)

/b/ /ah/ /n/ (Bonn)

/dz/ (as in gem) /uh/ /m/ /p/ /s/ (jumps)

/k/ /l/ /long I/ /m/ /z/ (climbs)

/b/ /short A/ /k/ (back)

/d/ /r/ /short E/ /s/ (dress)

/p/ /ow/ /n/ /d/ (Pound)

16. Substituting the initial sound in words.

What to say to the student: "We're going to change beginning/first sounds in words."

> **EXAMPLE** "Say '_____.'" (stimulus word) "Instead of / /" (stimulus sound), "say / /." (stimulus sound) (e.g., "Say 'chin.' Instead of /ch/, say /voiceless th/. What's your new word?") (thin)

> **NOTE:** *Give the letter sound, not the letter name. Use pictured items and/or manipulatives if necessary. Use any of the following stimulus words and/or others you select from the story. The correct answers are in parentheses.*

Stimulus items:

"Say 'jumps.' Instead of /dz/ (as in gem), say /b/." (bumps)

"Say 'hugs.' Instead of /h/, say /p/." (pugs)

"Say 'bunny.' Instead of /b/, say /f/." (funny)

"Say 'Bonn.' Instead of /b/, say /v/." (Vonn)

"Say 'Tuttle.' Instead of /t/, say /sh/." (shuttle)

"Say 'Danny.' Instead of /d/, say /n/." (nanny)

"Say 'right.' Instead of /r/, say /s/." (sight)

"Say 'meat.' Instead of /m/, say /b/." (beat)

"Say 'shoe.' Instead of /sh/, say /b/." (boo)

"Say 'Wanda.' Instead of /w/, say /f/." (Fonda)

17. Substituting the final sound in words.

What to say to the student: "We're going to change ending/last sounds in words."

> **EXAMPLE** "Say '_____.'" (stimulus word) "Instead of / /" (stimulus sound), "say / /." (stimulus sound) (e.g., "Say 'back.' Instead of /k/, say /t/. What's your new word?") (bat)

> **NOTE:** *Give the letter sound, not the letter name. Use pictured items and/or manipulatives if necessary. Use any of the following stimulus words and/or others you select from the story. The correct answers are in parentheses.*

Stimulus items:

"Say 'dog.' Instead of /g/, say /t/." (dot)

"Say 'Mack.' Instead of /k/, say /t/." (mat)

"Say 'jumps.' Instead of /s/, say /t/." (jumped)

"Say 'cracker.' Instead of /r/, say /s/." (cracks)

"Say 'bike.' Instead of /k/, say /t/." (bite)

"Say 'Heath.' Instead of /voiceless th/, say /p/." (heap)

"Say 'hello.' Instead of /long O/, say /p/." (help)

"Say 'right.' Instead of /t/, say /m/." (rhyme)

"Say 'Wend.' Instead of /d/, say /t/." (went)

"Say 'pedals.' Instead of /z/, say /d/." (peddled)

18. Segmenting the middle sound in monosyllabic words.

What to say to the student: "Tell me the middle sound in the word I say."

EXAMPLE "What's the middle sound in the word '_____'?" (stimulus word)
(e.g., "What's the middle sound in the word 'back'?") (/short A/)

NOTE: *Give the letter sound, not the letter name. Use pictured items and/or manipulatives if necessary. Use any of the following stimulus words and/or others you select from the story. The correct answers are in parentheses.*

Stimulus items:

packs (/short A/)

cat (/short A/)

dog (/ah/)

toes (/long O/)

Von (/ah/)

Hess (/short E/)

teeth (/long E/)

Sike (/long I/)

ties (/long I/)

bike (/long I/)

19. Substituting the middle sound in words.

What to say to the student: "We're going to change the middle sound in words."

EXAMPLE "Say '_____.'" (stimulus word) "Instead of / /" (stimulus sound),
"say / /." (stimulus sound) (e.g., "Say 'cat.' Instead of /short A/, say /uh/.
What's your new word?") (cut)

NOTE: *Give the letter sound, not the letter name. Use pictured items and/or manipulatives if necessary. Use any of the following stimulus words and/or others you select from the story. The correct answers are in parentheses.*

Stimulus items:

"Say 'Crewe.' Instead of /r/, say /l/." (clue)

"Say 'ties.' Instead of /long I/, say /long O/." (toes)

"Say 'Wend.' Instead of /short E/, say /ah/." (wand)

"Say 'right.' Instead of /long I/, say /long O/." (wrote)

"Say 'Von.' Instead of /ah/, say /long I/." (vine)

"Say 'bite.' Instead of /long I/, say /ah/." (bought)

"Say 'dog.' Instead of /ah/, say /short I/." (dig)

"Say 'hops.' Instead of /ah/, say /short I/." (hips)

"Say 'right.' Instead of /long I/, say /long A/." (rate)

"Say 'chin.' Instead of /short I/, say /long A/." (chain)

20. Identifying all sounds in monosyllabic words.

What to say to the student: "Now tell me all the sounds you hear in the word I say."

> EXAMPLE   "What sounds do you hear in the word '_____'?" (stimulus word) (e.g., "What sounds do you hear in the word 'dog'?") (/d/ /ah/ /g/)

NOTE: *Give the letter sound, not the letter name. Use pictured items and/or manipulatives if necessary. Use any of the following stimulus words and/or others you select from the story. The correct answers are in parentheses.*

Stimulus items:

ties (/t/ /long I/ /z/)

fives (/f/ /long I/ /v/ /z/)

miss (/m/ /short I/ /s/)

Heath (/h/ /long E/ /voiceless th/)

Nye (/n/ /long I/)

shoe (/sh/ /oo/)

Lowe (/l/ /long O/)

jumps (/dz/ (as in gem) /uh/ /m/ /p/ /s/)

Bonn (/b/ /ah/ /n/)

hugs (/h/ /uh/ /g/ /z/)

21. Deleting sounds within words.

What to say to the student: "We're going to leave out sounds in words."

> EXAMPLE   "Say '_____'" (stimulus word) "without / /." (stimulus sound) (e.g., "Say 'slid' without /l/.") (sid) Say: "The word that is left—'sid'—is a real word. Sometimes, the word won't be a real word."

NOTE: *Give the letter sound, not the letter name. Use pictured items and/or manipulatives if necessary. Use any of the following stimulus words and/or others you select from the story. The correct answers are in parentheses.*

Stimulus items:

"Say 'Fran' without /r/." (fan)

"Say 'sneaker' without /n/." (seeker)

"Say 'friend' without /r/." (fend)

"Say 'Blair' without /l/." (bear)

"Say 'Krupp' without /r/." (cup)

"Say 'vroom' without /v/." (room)

"Say 'sneaks' without /n/." (seeks)

"Say 'sweater' without /w/." (setter)

"Say 'Gwen' without /g/." (when)

"Say 'Crewe' without /r/." (coo)

22. Substituting consonants in words having a two-sound cluster.

What to say to the student: "We're going to substitute sounds in words."

> **EXAMPLE** "Say '_____.'" (stimulus word) "Instead of / /" (stimulus sound), "say / /." (stimulus sound) (e.g., "Say 'stop.' Instead of /t/, say /l/.") (slop) Say: "Sometimes, the new word will be a made-up word."

NOTE: *Give the letter sound, not the letter name. Use pictured items and/or manipulatives if necessary. Use any of the following stimulus words and/or others you select from the story. The correct answers are in parentheses.*

Stimulus items:

"Say 'dress.' Instead of /d/, say /p/." (press)

"Say 'Fran.' Instead of /r/, say /l/." (flan)

"Say 'Krupp.' Instead of /k/, say /g/." (grupp)

"Say 'brushes.' Instead of /r/, say /l/." (blushes)

"Say 'climbs.' Instead of /l/, say /r/." (crimes)

"Say 'Crewe.' Instead of /r/, say /l/." (clue)

"Say 'Gwen.' Instead of /w/, say /l/." (Glen)

"Say 'sneaker.' Instead of /n/, say /l/." (sleeker)

"Say 'vroom.' Instead of /v/, say /b/." (broom)

"Say 'sneak.' Instead of /n/, say /p/." (speak)

23. Phoneme reversing.

What to say to the student: "We're going to say words backward."

> **EXAMPLE** "Say the word '_____'" (stimulus word) "backward." (e.g., "Say 'bone' backward.") (nobe)

NOTE: *This is a difficult phoneme-level task and should only be done with older students. Give the letter sound, not the letter name. Use pictured items and/or manipulatives if necessary. Use any of the following stimulus words and/or others you select from the story. The correct answers are in parentheses.*

Stimulus items:

    back (cab)

    right (tire)

    cat (tack)

    to (oot)

    Von (nov)

    all (law)

    Bonn (nob)

    Mack (cam)

    pack (cap)

    day (aid)

24. Phoneme switching.

What to say to the student: "We're going to switch the first sounds in two words."

> **EXAMPLE**   "Switch the first sounds in '_____' and '_____.'" (stimulus words)
> (e.g., "Switch the first sounds in 'pedals' and 'bike.'") (bedals pike)

NOTE: *This is a difficult phoneme-level task and should only be done with older students. Give the letter sound, not the letter name. Use pictured items and/or manipulatives if necessary. Use any of the following stimulus words and/or others you select from the story. The correct answers are in parentheses.*

Stimulus items:

    Noah Bonn (Boah Nonn)

    her teeth (ter heeth)

    first day (dirst fay)

    gets ready (rets geddy)

    kisses sister (sisses kister)

    Danny Hess (Hanny Dess)

    Henry Fetter (Fenry Hetter)

    packs bunny (backs punny)

    high fives (figh hives)

    Bindergarten Kindergarten (Kindergarten Bindergarten)

25. Pig Latin.

What to say to the student: "We're going to speak a secret language by using words from the story. In pig Latin, you take off the first sound of a word, put it at the end of the word, and add an 'ay' sound."

> **EXAMPLE**   "Say 'dog' in pig Latin." (ogday)

NOTE: *This is a difficult phoneme-level task and should only be done with older students. Use pictured items and/or manipulatives if necessary. Use any of the following stimulus words and/or others you select from the story. The correct answers are in parentheses.*

Stimulus items:

Lister (isterlay)

Wend (endway)

ready (eddyray)

Raffie (affieray)

Packer (ackerpay)

Hoff (offhay)

Zach (ackzay)

chair (airchay)

marches (archesmay)

Bindergarten (indergartenbay)

From Phonological Awareness into Print

NOTE: *Only five examples per activity are included in this resource due to space. You are encouraged to add many more words into this section that you feel your student(s) is(are) ready to write.*

1. Substituting the initial sound or letter in words.

NOTE: *Use lined paper or copy the sheet of lined paper included in the back of this book.*

Stimulus items:

1.1 pig/big

Task a. "Say 'pig.' Instead of /p/, say /b/. What's your new word?" (big) "Write/copy 'pig' and 'big.'"

Task b. "Circle the **letters** that make the words different." ([p], [b])

Task c. "What **sounds** do these letters make?" (/p/, /b/)

1.2 hops/pops

Task a. "Say 'hops.' Instead of /h/, say /p/. What's your new word?" (pops) "Write/copy 'hops' and 'pops.'"

Task b. "Circle the **letters** that make the words different." ([h], [p])

Task c. "What **sounds** do these letters make?" (/h/, /p/)

1.3 bunny/funny

Task a. "Say 'bunny.' Instead of /b/, say /f/. What's your new word?" (funny) "Write/copy 'bunny' and 'funny.'"

Task b. "Circle the **letters** that make the words different." ([b], [f])

Task c. "What **sounds** do these letters make?" (/b/, /f/)

1.4 Wong/song

Task a. "Say 'Wong.' Instead of /w/, say /s/. What's your new word?" (song) "Write/copy 'Wong' and 'song.'"

Task b. "Circle the **letters** that make the words different." ([w], [s])

Task c. "What **sounds** do these letters make?" (/w/, /s/)

1.5 Bindergarten/kindergarten

Task a. "Say 'Bindergarten.' Instead of /b/, say /k/. What's your new word?" (kindergarten) "Write/copy 'Bindergarten' and 'kindergarten.'"

Task b. "Circle the **letters** that make the words different." ([b], [k])

Task c. "What **sounds** do these letters make?" (/b/, /k/)

2. Substituting the final sound or letter in words.

NOTE: *Use lined paper or copy the sheet of lined paper included in the back of this book.*

Stimulus items:

2.1 cat/cab

Task a. "Say 'cat.' Instead of /t/, say /b/. What's your new word?" (cab) "Write/copy 'cat' and 'cab.'"

Task b. "Circle the **letters** that make the words different." ([t], [b])

Task c. "What **sounds** do these letters make?" (/t/, /b/)

2.2 ties/tied

Task a. "Say 'ties.' Instead of /z/, say /d/. What's your new word?" (tied) "Write/copy 'ties' and 'tied.'"

Task b. "Circle the **letters** that make the words different." ([s], [d])

Task c. "What **sounds** do these letters make?" (/z/, /d/)

2.3 dog/dot

Task a. "Say 'dog.' Instead of /g/, say /t/. What's your new word?" (dot) "Write/copy 'dog' and 'dot.'"

Task b. "Circle the **letters** that make the words different." ([g], [t])

Task c. "What **sounds** do these letters make?" (/g/, /t/)

2.4 Heath/heap

Task a. "Say 'heath.' Instead of /voiceless th/, say /p/. What's your new word?" (heap) "Write/copy 'heath' and 'heap.'"

Task b. "Circle the **letters** that make the words different." ([t], [h], [p])

Task c. "What **sounds** do these letters make?" (/voiceless th/, /p/)

2.5 jumps/jumped

Task a. "Say 'jumps.' Instead of /s/, say /t/. What's your new word?" (jumped) "Write/copy 'jumps' and 'jumped.'"

Task b. "Circle the **letters** that make the words different." ([s], [e], [d])

Task c. "What **sounds** do these letters make?" (/s/, /t/)

3. Substituting the middle sound or letter in words.

NOTE: *Use lined paper or copy the sheet of lined paper included in the back of this book.*

Stimulus items:

3.1 bike/bake

Task a. "Say 'bike.' Instead of /long I/, say /long A/. What's your new word?" (bake) "Write/copy 'bike' and 'bake.'"

Task b. "Circle the **letters** that make the words different." ([i], [a])

Task c. "What **sounds** do these letters make?" (/long I/, /long A/)

3.2 Miss/moss

Task a. "Say 'miss.' Instead of /short I/, say /ah/. What's your new word?" (moss) "Write/copy 'miss' and 'moss.'"

Task b. "Circle the **letters** that make the words different." ([i], [o])

Task c. "What **sounds** do these letters make?" (/short I/, /ah/)

3.3 Von/van

Task a. "Say 'von.' Instead of /ah/, say /short A/. What's your new word?" (van) "Write/copy 'von' and 'van.'"

Task b. "Circle the **letters** that make the words different." ([o], [a])

Task c. "What **sounds** do these letters make?" (/ah/, /short A/)

3.4 Wend/wand

Task a. "Say 'wend.' Instead of /short E/, say /ah/. What's your new word?" (wand) "Write/copy 'wend' and 'wand.'"

Task b. "Circle the **letters** that make the words different." ([e], [a])

Task c. "What **sounds** do these letters make?" (/short E/, /ah/)

3.5 Mack/Mick

Task a. "Say 'mack.' Instead of /short A/, say /short I/. What's your new word?" (mick) "Write/copy 'mack' and 'mick.'"

Task b. "Circle the **letters** that make the words different." ([a], [i])

Task c. "What **sounds** do these letters make?" (/short A/, /short I/)

4. Supplying the initial sound or letter in words.

NOTE: *Use lined paper or copy the sheet of lined paper included in the back of this book.*

Stimulus items:

4.1 Von/on

Task a. "Say 'von,' say 'on.' What sound did you hear in 'von' that is missing in 'on'?" (/v/) "Now we'll change the **letter.** Write/copy 'von' and 'on.'"

Task b. "Circle the beginning **letter** that makes the words different." ([v])

Task c. "What **sound** does this letter make?" (/v/)

4.2 his/is

Task a. "Say 'his,' say 'is.' What sound did you hear in 'his' that is missing in 'is'?" (/h/) "Now we'll change the **letter.** Write/copy 'his' and 'is.'"

Task b. "Circle the beginning **letter** that makes the words different." ([h])

Task c. "What **sound** does this letter make?" (/h/)

4.3 Wend/end

Task a. "Say 'wend,' say 'end.' What sound did you hear in 'wend' that is missing in 'end'?" (/w/) "Now we'll change the **letter.** Write/copy 'wend' and 'end.'"

Task b. "Circle the beginning **letter** that makes the words different." ([w])

Task c. "What **sound** do these letters make?" (/w/)

4.4 Lowe/owe

Task a. "Say 'lowe,' say 'owe.' What sound did you hear in 'lowe' that is missing in 'owe'?" (/l/) "Now we'll change the **letter.** Write/copy 'lowe' and 'owe.'"

Task b. "Circle the beginning **letter** that makes the words different." ([l])

Task c. "What **sound** does this letter make?" (/l/)

4.5 chair/air

Task a. "Say 'chair,' say 'air.' What sound did you hear in 'chair' that is missing in 'air'?" (/ch/) "Now we'll change the **letter.** Write/copy 'chair' and 'air.'"

Task b. "Circle the beginning **letters** that make the words different." ([c], [h])

Task c. "What **sound** do these letters make?" (/ch/)

5. Supplying the final sound or letter in words.

NOTE: *Use lined paper or copy the sheet of lined paper included in the back of this book.*

Stimulus items:

5.1 ties/tie

Task a. "Say 'ties,' say 'tie.' What sound did you hear in 'ties' that is missing in 'tie'?" (/z/) "Now we'll change the **letter.** Write/copy 'ties' and 'tie.'"

Task b. "Circle the ending/last **letter** that makes the words different." ([s])

Task c. "What **sound** does this letter make?" (/z/)

5.2 looks/look

Task a. "Say 'looks,' say 'look.' What sound did you hear in 'looks' that is missing in 'look'?" (/s/) "Now we'll change the **letter.** Write/copy 'looks' and 'look.'"

Task b. "Circle the ending/last **letter** that makes the words different." ([s])

Task c. "What **sound** does this letter make?" (/s/)

5.3 Lindo/lind

Task a. "Say 'lindo,' say 'lind.' What sound did you hear in 'lindo' that is missing in 'lind'?" (/long O/) "Now we'll change the **letter.** Write/copy 'lindo' and 'lind.'"

Task b. "Circle the ending/last **letter** that make the words different." ([o])

Task c. "What **sound** does this letter make?" (/long O/)

5.4 teeth/tee

Task a. "Say 'teeth,' say 'tee.' What sound did you hear in 'teeth' that is missing in 'tee'?" (/voiceless th/) "Now we'll change the **letter.** Write/copy 'teeth' and 'tee.'"

Task b. "Circle the ending/last **letters** that make the word different." ([t], [h])

Task c. "What **sound** do these letters make?" (/voiceless th/)

5.5 Matty/Matt

Task a. "Say 'matty,' say 'matt.' What sound did you hear in 'matty' that is missing in 'matt'?" (/long E/) "Now we'll change the **letter.** Write/copy 'matty' and 'matt.'"

Task b. "Circle the ending/last **letter** that makes the words different." ([y])

Task c. "What **sound** does this letter make?" (/long E/)

6. Switching the first sound and letter in words (ADVANCED).

NOTE: *Use lined paper or copy the sheet of lined paper included in the back of this book.*

Stimulus items:

6.1 packs bunny

Task a. "Say 'packs,' say 'bunny.' What sound do you hear at the beginning of 'packs'?" (/p/) "What sound do you hear at the beginning of 'bunny'?" (/b/) "Switch the first sounds in those words." (backs punny) "Now we'll change the **letters.** Write/copy 'packs bunny' and 'backs punny.'"

Task b. "Circle the beginning **letters** that change the words." ([p], [b])

Task c. "What **sounds** do those letters make?" (/p/, /b/)

6.2 Kiki Wong

Task a. "Say 'kiki' say 'wong.' What sound do you hear at the beginning of 'kiki'?" (/k/) "What sound do you hear at the beginning of 'wong'?" (/w/) "Switch the first sounds in those words." (wiki kong) "Now we'll change the **letters.** Write/copy 'kiki wong' and 'wiki kong.'"

Task b. "Circle the beginning **letters** that change the words." ([k], [w])

Task c. "What **sounds** do those letters make?" (/k/, /w/)

6.3 Matty Lindo

Task a. "Say 'matty,' say 'lindo.' What sound do you hear at the beginning of 'matty'?" (/m/) "What sound do you hear at the beginning of 'lindo'?" (/l/) "Switch the first sounds in those words." (latty mindo) "Now we'll change the **letters.** Write/copy 'matty lindo' and 'latty mindo.'"

Task b. "Circle the beginning **letters** that change the words." ([l], [m])

Task c. "What **sounds** do those letters make?" (/l/, /m/)

6.4 high fives

Task a. "Say 'high,' say 'fives.' What sound do you hear at the beginning of 'high'?" (/h/) "What sound do you hear at the beginning of 'fives'?" (/f/) "Switch the first sounds in those words." (figh hives) "Now we'll change the **letters.** Write/copy 'high fives' and 'figh hives.'"

Task b. "Circle the beginning **letters** that change the words." ([h], [f])

Task c. "What **sounds** do those letters make?" (/h/, /f/)

6.5 Bindergarten kindergarten

Task a. "Say 'bindergarten,' say 'kindergarten' What sound do you hear at the beginning of 'bindergarten'?" (/b/) "What sound do you hear at the beginning of 'kindergarten'?" (/k/) "Switch the first sounds in those words." (kindergarten bindergarten). "Now we'll change the **letters.** Write/copy 'bindergarten kindergarten' and 'kindergarten bindergarten.'"

Task b. "Circle the beginning **letters** that change the words." ([m], [k])

Task c. "What **sounds** do those letters make?" (/b/, /k/)

CHAPTER

12

Phonological Awareness Activities to Use with *The Garden*

Text version used for selection of stimulus items:

Lobel, L. (1971, 1972). *The Garden* from *Frog and Toad Together*. HarperCollins Publishers.

Phonological Awareness Activities at the Word Level

1. Counting words.

What to say to the student: "We're going to count words."

> **EXAMPLE** "How many words do you hear in this sentence (or phrase): 'my great-grandmother'?" (3)

> **NOTE:** *Use pictured items and/or manipulatives if necessary. Use any of the following stimulus phrases or sentences and/or others you select from the story. The correct answers are in parentheses.*

Stimulus items:

    flower seeds (2)

    Start growing! (2)

    a fine garden (3)

    in the ground (3)

    shouting too much (3)

    for a few days (4)

    Toad felt very tired. (4)

    Look at your garden. (4)

    Toad read a long story. (5)

    Toad read poems to his seeds. (6)

2. Identifying the missing word from a list.

What to say to the student: "Listen to the words I say. I'll say them again. You tell me which word I leave out."

> **EXAMPLE** "Listen to the words I say: 'toad,' 'seeds,' 'rain.' I'll say them again. Tell me which one I leave out: 'toad,' 'seeds.'" (rain)

> **NOTE:** *Use pictured items and/or manipulatives if necessary. Use any of the following stimulus words and/or others you select from the story. The correct answers are in parentheses.*

Stimulus set #1	Stimulus set #2
dark, ground	dark (ground)
grow, drat	drat (grow)
candles, garden, down	candles, down (garden)
frog, running, seeds	running, seeds (frog)
flower, fine, frightened	flower, frightened (fine)
window, hard, story	window, hard (story)
walking, much, noise, shouted	much, noise, shouted (walking)
night, stopped, shine, poems	night, shine, poems (stopped)
frog, very, little, home	frog, very, home (little)
loudly, shall, music, plants	loudly, shall, music (plants)

3. Identifying the missing word in a phrase or sentence.

What to say to the student: "Listen to the sentence I read. Tell me which word is missing the second time I read the sentence."

> **EXAMPLE** "'Toad read poems.' Listen again and tell me which word I leave out: '_____ read poems.'" (toad)

> **NOTE:** *Use pictured items and/or manipulatives if necessary. Use any of the following stimulus sentences and/or others you select from the story. The correct answers are in parentheses.*

Stimulus items:

His garden. His _____. (garden)

How soon? _____ soon? (how)

A fine garden. A _____ garden. (fine)

Toad ran home. Toad ran _____. (home)

Now seeds, start growing! Now seeds, _____ growing! (start)

You were right, frog. You were right, _____. (frog)

You are shouting too much. You are _____ too much. (shouting)

Toad walked up and down. Toad _____ up and down. (walked)

He planted the flower seeds. He planted _____ flower seeds. (the)

It was very hard work. _____ was very hard work. (It)

4. Supplying the missing word as an adult reads.

What to say to the student: "I want you to help me read the story. You fill in the words I leave out."

> **EXAMPLE**   "Toad ran _____." (home)

> **NOTE:** *Use pictured items and/or manipulatives if necessary. Use any of the following stimulus sentences and/or others you select from the story. The correct answers are in parentheses.*

Stimulus items:

Start _____! (growing)

Frog was in his _____. (garden)

He _____ asleep. (fell)

Let the _____ shine on them. (sun)

Let the rain _____ on them. (fall)

Soon your _____ will start to grow. (seeds)

My seeds are _____ to grow. (afraid)

I will _____ the seeds a story. (read)

Toad sang songs to his _____. (seeds)

And now you will have a nice _____ too. (garden)

5. Rearranging words.

What to say to the student: "I'll say some words out of order. You put them in the right order so they make sense."

> **EXAMPLE**   " 'garden a nice.' Put those words in the right order." (a nice garden)

> **NOTE:** *Use pictured items and/or manipulatives if necessary. Use any of the following stimulus words and/or others you select from the story. The correct answers are in parentheses. This word-level activity can be more difficult than some of the syllable- or phoneme-level activities because of the memory load. If your students are only able to deal with two or three words to be rearranged, add more two- and three-word samples from the story and omit the four-word level items.*

Stimulus items:

growing start. (Start growing.)

down up and (up and down)

home toad ran. (Toad ran home.)

leave alone them. (Leave them alone.)

not will seeds my grow. (My seeds will not grow.)

at your look garden. (Look at your garden.)

work it was hard very. (It was very hard work.)

toad music played seeds for his. (Toad played music for his seeds.)

poems toad seeds to his read. (Toad read poems to his seeds.)

tired then felt toad very. (Then toad felt very tired.)

Phonological Awareness Activities at the Syllable Level

1. Syllable counting.

What to say to the student: "We're going to count syllables (or parts) of words."

> **EXAMPLE** "How many syllables do you hear in '_____'?" (stimulus word)
> (e.g., "How many syllables do you hear in 'plant'?") (1)

> **NOTE:** *Use pictured items and/or manipulatives if necessary. Use any of the following stimulus words and/or others you select from the story. Use any group of 10 stimulus items you select per teaching set.*

Stimulus items:

One-syllable words: plant, put, path, poor, played, by, but, be, toad, times, to, too, tired, down, did, days, drat, dark, day, do, came, quite, close, course, cried, ground, grow, green, my, much, must, most, nice, now, not, noise, night, next, said, some, seeds, start, sun, soon, sang, songs, still, stopped, ran, rain, read, right, frog, fine, few, for, fall, felt, fell, his, have, he, hard, had, here, how, home, head, whole, looked, leave, let, long, look, last, was, what, work, wish, will, walked, with, wake, were, shine, shall, the, them, this, these, that, then, they, you, yes, in, a, it, is, I, are, and, asked, up, at, all, of, on, out

Two-syllable words: planted, poems, being, candles, coming, garden, growing, music, story, running, flower, frightened, loudly, little, very, walking, window, shouted, shouting, story, again, afraid, alone, asleep

2. Initial syllable deleting.

What to say to the student: "We're going to leave out syllables (or parts of words)."

> **EXAMPLE** "Say '_____.'" (stimulus word) "Say it again without '_____.'"
> (stimulus syllable) (e.g., "Say 'loudly.' Say it again without 'loud.'") (Lee)

> **NOTE:** *Use pictured items and/or manipulatives if necessary. Use any of the following stimulus words and/or others you select from the story. The correct answers are in parentheses.*

Stimulus items:

"Say 'window' without 'win.'" (dough)

"Say 'walking' without 'walk.'" (ing)

"Say 'candles' without 'can.'" (dulls)

"Say 'little' without 'lit.'" (ul)

"Say 'being' without 'be.'" (ing)

"Say 'afraid' without 'uh.'" (frayed)

"Say 'music' without 'mew.'" (zic)

"Say 'poems' without 'po.'" (ums)

"Say 'flower' without 'flau.'" (er)

"Say 'very' without 'ver.'" (ee)

3. Final syllable deleting.

What to say to the student: "We're going to leave out syllables (or parts of words)."

> **EXAMPLE** "Say '_____.'" (stimulus word) "Say it again without '_____.'" (stimulus syllable) (e.g., "Say 'loudly' without 'lee.'") (loud)

> **NOTE:** *Use pictured items and/or manipulatives if necessary. Use any of the following stimulus words and/or others you select from the story. The correct answers are in parentheses.*

Stimulus items:

"Say 'garden' without 'dun.'" (gar)

"Say 'being' without 'ing.'" (be)

"Say 'flower' without 'er.'" (flau)

"Say 'music' without 'zic.'" (mew)

"Say 'shouting' without 'ing.'" (shout)

"Say 'alone' without 'lone.'" (uh)

"Say 'window' without 'dough.'" (win)

"Say 'coming' without 'ing.'" (come)

"Say 'story' without 'ee.'" (store)

"Say 'running' without 'ing.'" (run)

4. Initial syllable adding.

What to say to the student: "Now let's add syllables (or parts) to words."

> **EXAMPLE** "Add '_____'" (stimulus syllable) "to the beginning of '_____.'" (stimulus syllable) (e.g., "Add 'loud' to the beginning of 'Lee.'") (loudly)

> **NOTE:** *Use pictured items and/or manipulatives if necessary. Use any of the following stimulus words and/or others you select from the story. The correct answers are in parentheses.*

Stimulus items:

"Add 'gar' to the beginning of 'dun.'" (garden)

"Add 'grow' to the beginning of 'ing.'" (growing)

"Add 'uh' to the beginning of 'sleep.'" (asleep)

"Add 'shout' to the beginning of 'ing.'" (shouting)

"Add 'can' to the beginning of 'dulls.'" (candles)

"Add 'mew' to the beginning of 'zic.'" (music)

"Add 'po' to the beginning of 'ums.'" (poems)

"Add 'uh' to the beginning of 'gen.'" (again)

"Add 'shout' to the beginning of 'ud.'" (shouted)

"Add 'come' to the beginning of 'ing.'" (coming)

5. Final syllable adding.

What to say to the student: "Now let's add syllables (or parts) to words."

EXAMPLE "Add '_____'" (stimulus syllable) "to the end of '_____.'" (stimulus syllable) (e.g., "Add 'Lee' to the end of 'loud.'") (loudly)

NOTE: *Use pictured items and/or manipulatives if necessary. Use any of the following stimulus words and/or others you select from the story. The correct answers are in parentheses.*

Stimulus items:

"Add 'dulls' to the end of 'can.'" (candles)

"Add 'ing' to the end of 'walk.'" (walking)

"Add 'dough' to the end of 'win.'" (window)

"Add 'tend' to the end of 'fry.'" (frightened)

"Add 'sleep' to the end of 'uh.'" (asleep)

"Add 'ing' to the end of 'run.'" (running)

"Add 'ers' to the end of 'flau.'" (flowers)

"Add 'ud' to the end of 'shout.'" (shouted)

"Add 'dun' to the end of 'gar.'" (garden)

"Add 'dough' to the end of 'win.'" (window)

6. Syllable substituting.

What to say to the student: "Let's make up some new words."

EXAMPLE "Say '_____.'" (stimulus word) "Instead of '_____'" (stimulus syllable), "say '_____.'" (stimulus syllable) (e.g., "Say 'loudly.' Instead of 'loud,' say 'friend.' The new word is 'friendly.'")

NOTE: *Use pictured items and/or manipulatives if necessary. Use any of the following stimulus words and/or others you select from the story. The correct answers are in parentheses.*

Stimulus items:

"Say 'running.' Instead of 'run,' say 'wish.'" (wishing)

"Say 'candles.' Instead of 'dulls,' say 'Dee.'" (candy)

"Say 'running.' Instead of 'ing,' say 'er.'" (runner)

"Say 'shouted.' Instead of 'shout,' say 'pout.'" (pouted)

"Say 'walking.' Instead of 'walk,' say 'talk.'" (talking)

"Say 'poems.' Instead of 'ums,' say 'zee.'" (posie)

"Say 'window.' Instead of 'dough,' say 'ter.'" (winter)

"Say 'asleep.' Instead of 'sleep,' say 'wear.'" (aware)

"Say 'flower.' Instead of 'flau,' say 'pow.'" (power)

"Say 'alone.' Instead of 'lone,' say 'frayed.'" (afraid)

Phonological Awareness Activities at the Phoneme Level

1. Counting sounds.

What to say to the student: "We're going to count sounds in words."

EXAMPLE "How many sounds do you hear in this word? 'toad.'" (3)

NOTE: *Use pictured items and/or manipulatives if necessary. Use any of the following stimulus words and/or others you select from the story. Be sure to give the letter sound and not the letter name. Use any group of 10 stimulus items you select per teaching set.*

Stimulus words with one sound: *a*

Stimulus words with two sounds: by, be, to, too, day, do, my, he, the, they, you, it, is, in, up, at, all, are, of, on

Stimulus words with three sounds: put, path, but, toad, down, did, days, came, grow, much, nice, night, said, some, sun, soon, sang, ran, rain, read, right, fine, few, fall, fell, his, have, had, home, head, whole, leave, let, long, was, what, work, wish, will, with, wake, shine, shall, them, this, these, that, then, yes, and

Stimulus words with four sounds: played, times, drat, quite, close, cried, green, must, most, seeds, songs, still, frog, felt, looked, little, last, went, world, asked, again, alone

Stimulus words with five sounds: plant, poems, next, stopped, window, story, afraid, asleep

Stimulus words with six sounds: plants, candles, music

Stimulus words with seven sounds: frightened

2. Sound categorization or identifying a rhyme oddity.

What to say to the student: "Guess which word I say doesn't rhyme with the other three words."

EXAMPLE "Tell me which word doesn't rhyme with the other three words: '_____,' '_____,' '_____,' '_____.'" (stimulus words) (e.g., "'nice,' 'ice,' 'read,' 'rice.' Which word doesn't rhyme?") (read)

NOTE: *Use pictured items if necessary. Use any of the following stimulus words and/or others you select from the story. The correct answers are in parentheses.*

Stimulus items:

noise, boys, toys, frog (frog)

fine, line, green, mine (green)

flower, toad, power, sour (toad)

looked, cooked, booked, window (window)

work, shouted, pouted, grouted (work)

frog, stopped, log, jog (stopped)

nice, roam, home, gnome (nice)

flowers, powers, music, showers (music)

must, much, rust, trust (much)

ground, round, poems, found (poems)

3. Matching rhyme.

What to say to the student: "We're going to think of rhyming words."

> **EXAMPLE**   "Which word rhymes with '_____'?" (stimulus word) (e.g., "Which word rhymes with 'toad': 'days,' 'must,' 'ground,' 'load'?") (load)

> **NOTE:** *Use pictured items if necessary. Use any of the following stimulus words and/or others you select from the story. The correct answers are in parentheses.*

Stimulus items:

sang: rang, much, seeds, leave (rang)

look: stopped, walked, book, rain (book)

loudly: flower, proudly, shouting, work (proudly)

walking: frightened, again, talking, world (talking)

story: glory, looked, being, long (glory)

garden: flower, again, music, pardon (pardon)

much: ground, such, times, to (such)

frightened: window, shouted, lightened, walking (lightened)

frog: log, read, alone, right (log)

flower: music, power, afraid, story (power)

4. Producing rhyme.

What to say to the student: "Now we'll say rhyming words."

> **EXAMPLE**   "Tell me a word that rhymes with '_____.'" (stimulus word) (e.g., "Tell me a word that rhymes with 'frog.' You can make up a word if you want.") (dog, log, sog)

> **NOTE:** *Use pictured items if necessary. Use any of the following stimulus words and/or others you select from the story (i.e., you say a word from the list below and the student is to think of a rhyming word). Use any group of 10 stimulus items you select per teaching set.*

Stimulus items:

/p/: plant, put, path, played

/b/: by, but, be, being

/t/: toad, times, to

/d/: down, did, days, drat, dark, day, do

/k/: came, close, candles, cried

/g/: grow, green, ground

/m/: my, much, must, most

/n/: nice, now, not, night

/s/: said, some, seeds, sun, sang, songs, still

/f/: frog, fine, for, fall, felt, fell

/v/: very

/h/: his, have, he, hard, had, how, home, head

/r/: ran, rain, read, right

/l/: let, look, last

/w/, /wh/: was, wish, will, went, wake

/sh/: shine, shouting, shouted

/voiced th/: the, them, that, then

/y/ (as in yellow): you, yes

vowels: is, are, and, on, out

5. Sound matching (initial).

What to say to the student: "Now we'll listen for the first sound in words."

> **EXAMPLE** "Listen to this sound: / /." (stimulus sound). "Guess which word I say begins with that sound: '_____,' '_____,' '_____,' '_____.'" (stimulus words) (e.g., "Listen to this sound: /p/. Guess which word I say begins with that sound: 'frog,' 'poor,' 'days,' 'ground.'") (poor)

NOTE: *Give the letter sound, not the letter name. Use pictured items if necessary. Use any of the following stimulus words and/or others you select from the story. The correct answers are in parentheses.*

Stimulus items:

/m/: came, music, toad, green (music)

/d/: drat, came, rain, still (drat)

/p/: dark, poems, flower, very (poems)

/h/: days, seeds, home, alone (home)

/v/: frog, shine, head, very (very)

/l/: loudly, music, flower, walking (loudly)

/k/: little, much, candles, stopped (candles)

/s/: they, songs, nice, music (songs)

/voiced th/: that, home, story, asked (that)

/r/: head, asleep, loudly, running (running)

6. Sound matching (final).

What to say to the student: "Now we'll listen for the last sound in words."

> **EXAMPLE** "Listen to this sound: / /" (stimulus sound). "Guess which word I say ends with that sound: '_____,' '_____,' '_____,' '_____.'" (stimulus words) (e.g., "Listen to this sound: /g/. Guess which word I say ends with that sound: 'frog,' 'be,' 'the,' 'ran.'") (frog)

> **NOTE:** *Give the letter sound, not the letter name. Use pictured items and/or manipulatives if necessary. Use any of the following stimulus words and/or others you select from the story. The correct answers are in parentheses.*

Stimulus items:

/k/: work, some, what, toad (work)

/n/: head, garden, yes, much (garden)

/z/: fine, head, plants, was (was)

/ng/: walking, plants, frog, seeds (walking)

/r/: course, wish, candles, flower (flower)

/long O/: path, window, have, my (window)

/s/: plants, running, grow, still (plants)

/long E/: fine, sang, loudly, whole (loudly)

/v/: poor, seeds, little, leave (leave)

/l/: and, fine, shall, came (shall)

7. Identifying the initial sound in words.

What to say to the student: "I'll say a word two times. Tell me what sound is missing the second time: '_____,' '_____.'" (stimulus words)

> **EXAMPLE** "What sound do you hear in '_____'" (stimulus word) "that is missing in '_____'?" (stimulus word) (e.g., "What sound do you hear in 'toad' that is missing in 'owed'?") (/t/)

> **NOTE:** *Give the letter sound, not the letter name. Use pictured items and/or manipulatives if necessary. Use any of the following stimulus words and/or others you select from the story. The correct answers are in parentheses.*

Stimulus items:

"came, aim. What sound do you hear in 'came' that is missing in 'aim'?" (/k/)

"still, till. What sound do you hear in 'still' that is missing in 'till'?" (/s/)

"leave, eave. What sound do you hear in 'leave' that is missing in 'eave'?" (/l/)

"ran, an. What sound do you hear in 'ran' that is missing in 'an'?" (/r/)

"afraid, frayed. What sound do you hear in 'afraid' that is missing in 'frayed'?" (/short U/)

"shouting, outing. What sound do you hear in 'shouting' that is missing in 'outing'?" (/sh/)

"will, ill. What sound do you hear in 'will' that is missing in 'ill'?" (/w/)

"nice, ice. What sound do you hear in 'nice' that is missing in 'ice'?" (/n/)

"these, ease. What sound do you hear in 'these' that is missing in 'ease'?" (/voiced th/)

"had, add. What sound do you hear in 'had' that is missing in 'add'?" (/h/)

8. Identifying the final sound in words.

What to say to the student: "I'll say a word two times. Tell me what sound is missing the second time: '_____,' '_____.'" (stimulus words)

> **EXAMPLE** "What sound do you hear in '_____'" (stimulus word) "that is missing in '_____'?" (stimulus word) (e.g., "What sound do you hear in 'toad' that is missing in 'toe'?") (/d/)

NOTE: *Give the letter sound, not the letter name. Use pictured items and/or manipulatives if necessary. Use any of the following stimulus words and/or others you select from the story. The correct answers are in parentheses.*

Stimulus items:

"start, star. What sound do you hear in 'start' that is missing in 'star'?" (/t/)

"story, store. What sound do you hear in 'story' that is missing in 'store'?" (/long E/)

"candles, candle. What sound do you hear in 'candles' that is missing in 'candle'?" (/z/)

"plants, plant. What sound do you hear in 'plants' that is missing in 'plant'?" (/s/)

"looked, look. What sound do you hear in 'looked' that is missing in 'look'?" (/t/)

"window, wind. What sound do you hear in 'window' that is missing in 'wind'?" (/long O/)

"played, play. What sound do you hear in 'played' that is missing in 'play'?" (/d/)

"shine, shy. What sound do you hear in 'shine' that is missing in 'shy'?" (/n/)

"rain, ray. What sound do you hear in 'rain' that is missing in 'ray'?" (/n/)

"seeds, seed. What sound do you hear in 'seeds' that is missing in 'seed'?" (/z/)

9. Segmenting the initial sound in words.

What to say to the student: "Listen to the word I say and tell me the first sound you hear."

> **EXAMPLE** "What's the first sound in '_____'?" (stimulus word) (e.g., "What's the first sound in 'toad'?") (/t/)

NOTE: *Give the letter sound, not the letter name. Use pictured items and/or manipulatives if necessary. Use any of the following stimulus words and/or others you select from the story. Use any group of 10 stimulus items you select per teaching set.*

Stimulus items:

/p/: plant, planted, put, path, poor, poems, played, plants

/b/: by, but, be, being

/t/: toad, times, to, too, tired

/d/: down, did, days, drat, dark, day, do

/k/: came, quite, close, course, candles, cried, coming

/g/: garden, ground, growing, grow, green

/m/: my, much, must, music, most

/n/: nice, now, not, noise, night, next

/s/: said, some, seeds, start, sun, soon, story, sang, songs, still, stopped

/f/: frog, fine, flower, few, for, fall, frightened, felt, fell

/v/: very

/h/: his, have, he, hard, had, here, how, home, head

/r/: ran, running, rain, read, right

/l/: loudly, looked, leave, let, long, look, little, last

/w/, /wh/: was, working, what, work, wish, will, walked, window, went, with, world, wake, were

/sh/: shouted, shouting, shine, shall

/voiced th/: the, them, this, these, that, them, they

/y/ (as in yellow): you, yes, your

vowels: in, a, it, is, and, asked, up, at, again, all, afraid, of, alone, on, out, asleep

10. Segmenting the final sound in words.

What to say to the student: "Listen to the word I say and tell me the last sound you hear."

> **EXAMPLE** "What's the last sound in the word '_____'?" (stimulus word)
> (e.g., "What's the last sound in the word 'frog'?") (/g/)

NOTE: *Give the letter sound, not the letter name. Use pictured items and/or manipulatives if necessary. Use any of the following stimulus words and/or others you select from the story. Use any group of 10 stimulus items you select per teaching set.*

Stimulus items:

/p/: up, asleep

/t/: what, it, but, plant, asked, quite, start, walked, not, put, looked, at, let, that, night, out, drat, must, went, next, must, felt, last, stopped, right

/d/: toad, said, hard, had, ground, and, planted, did, head, shouted, afraid, started, read, played, cried, frightened, world, tired

/k/: work, dark, music, wake, look

/g/: frog

/ch/: much

/m/: came, some, them, home

/n/: in, garden, fine, soon, ran, down, again, alone, rain, on, then, green

/ng/: walking, growing, running, shouting, long, sang, being, coming

/s/: yes, nice, close, this, course, plants

/z/: was, his, is, seeds, times, noise, these, days, candles, songs

/v/: have, of, leave

/r/: here, are, flower, poor, for, your, were

/l/: will, all, fall, still, shall, whole, fell, little

/sh/: wish

/voiceless th/: path, with

/long A/: they, day

/long E/: he, very, be, loudly, story

/long I/: by, my

/long O/: grow, window

/short U/: the

/oo/: you, few, to, too, do

11. Generating words from the story beginning with a particular sound.

What to say to the student: "Let's think of words from the story that start with certain sounds."

EXAMPLE "Tell me a word from the story that starts with / /." (stimulus sound) (e.g., the sound /t/) (toad)

NOTE: *Give the letter sound, not the letter name. Use pictured items if necessary. Use any of the following stimulus words and/or others you select from the story. You say the sound (e.g., a voiceless /p/ sound), and the student is to say a word from the story that begins with that sound. Use any group of 10 stimulus items you select per teaching set.*

Stimulus items:

/p/: plant, planted, put, path, poor, poems, played, plants

/b/: by, but, be, being

/t/: toad, times, to, too, tired

/d/: down, did, days, drat, dark, day, do

/k/: came, quite, close, course, candles, cried, coming

/g/: garden, ground, growing, grow, green

/m/: my, much, must, music, most

/n/: nice, now, not, noise, night, next

/s/: said, some, seeds, start, sun, soon, story, sang, songs, still, stopped

/f/: frog, fine, flower, few, for, fall, frightened, felt, fell

/v/: very

/h/: his, have, he, hard, had, here, how, home, head

/r/: ran, running, rain, read, right

/l/: loudly, looked, leave, let, long, look, little, last

/w/, /wh/: was, working, what, work, wish, will, walked, window, went, with, world, wake, were

/sh/: shouted, shouting, shine, shall

/voiced th/: the, them, this, these, that, they

/y/ (as in yellow): you, yes, your

vowels: in, a, it, is, and, asked, up, at, again, all, afraid, of, alone, on, out, asleep

12. Blending sounds in monosyllabic words divided into onset–rime beginning with a two-consonant cluster + rime.

What to say to the student: "Now we'll put sounds together to make words."

> **EXAMPLE** "Put these sounds together to make a word (/ / + / /)." (stimulus sounds) "What's the word?" (e.g., "fr + og: What's the word?") (frog)

> **NOTE:** *Give the letter sound, not the letter name. Use pictured items and/or manipulatives if necessary. Use any of the following stimulus words and/or others you select from the story. The correct answers are in parentheses.*

Stimulus items:

st + ill (still)

kw + ite (quite)

st + opped (stopped)

cl + ose (close)

gr + ound (ground)

st + art (start)

cr + ied (cried)

gr + een (green)

pl + ant (plant)

gr + ow (grow)

13. Blending sounds in monosyllabic words divided into onset–rime beginning with a single consonant + rime.

What to say to the student: "Let's put sounds together to make words."

> **EXAMPLE** "Put these sounds together to make a word: / / + / /." (stimulus sounds) "What's the word?" (e.g., "/t/ + oad: What's the word?") (toad)

> **NOTE:** *Give the letter sound, not the letter name. Use pictured items and/or manipulatives if necessary. Use any of the following stimulus words and/or others you select from the story. The correct answers are in parentheses.*

Stimulus items:

/t/ + imes (times)

/s/ + eeds (seeds)

/d/ + ays (days)

/s/ + ang (sang)

/h/ + ome (home)

/voiced th/ + ese (these)

/m/ + ust (must)

/l/ + ooked (looked)

/w/ + ish (wish)

/voiced th/ + at (that)

14. Blending sounds to form a monosyllabic word beginning with a continuant sound.

What to say to the student: "We'll put sounds together to make words."

> **EXAMPLE** "Put these sounds together to make a word (/ / + / / + / /)." (stimulus sounds) (e.g., /n/ /long I/ /s/) (nice)

NOTE: *Give the letter sound, not the letter name. Use pictured items and/or manipulatives if necessary. Use any of the following stimulus words and/or others you select from the story. The correct answers are in parentheses.*

Stimulus items:

/l/ /long E/ /v/ (leave)

/s/ /short U/ /n/ (sun)

/r/ /long A/ /n/ (rain)

/h/ /long O/ /m/ (home)

/w/ /short I/ /voiceless th/ (with)

/y/ (as in yellow) /short E/ /s/ (yes)

/h/ /short E/ /d/ (head)

/s/ /oo/ /n/ (soon)

/voiced th/ /short E/ /m/ (them)

/m/ /short U/ /s/ /t/ (must)

15. Blending sounds to form a monosyllabic word beginning with a noncontinuant sound.

What to say to the student: "We'll put sounds together to make words."

> **EXAMPLE** "Put these sounds together to make a word (/ / + / / + / /)." (stimulus sounds) (e.g., /t/ /long O/ /d/) (toad)

NOTE: *Give the letter sound, not the letter name. Use pictured items and/or manipulatives if necessary. Use any of the following stimulus words and/or others you select from the story. The correct answers are in parentheses.*

Stimulus items:

/b/ /long I/ (by)

/t/ /long I/ /m/ /z/ (times)

/k/ /long A/ /m/ (came)

/t/ /oo/ (to)

/b/ /short U/ /t/ (but)

/d/ /long A/ /z/ (days)

/p/ /l/ /short A /n/ /t/ (plant)

/d/ /short I/ /d/ (did)

/p/ /short A/ /voiceless th/ (path)

/d/ /oo/ (do)

16. Substituting the initial sound in words.

What to say to the student: "We're going to change beginning/first sounds in words."

> EXAMPLE "Say '_____.'" (stimulus word) "Instead of / /" (stimulus sound), "say / /." (stimulus sound) (e.g., "Say 'toad.' Instead of /t/, say /l/. What's your new word?") (load)

NOTE: *Give the letter sound, not the letter name. Use pictured items and/or manipulatives if necessary. Use any of the following stimulus words and/or others you select from the story. The correct answers are in parentheses.*

Stimulus items:

"Say 'times.' Instead of /t/, say /l/." (limes)

"Say 'came.' Instead of /k/, say /s/." (same)

"Say 'tired.' Instead of /t/, say /f/." (fired)

"Say 'sang.' Instead of /s/, say /b/." (bang)

"Say 'must.' Instead of /m/, say /d/." (dust)

"Say 'songs.' Instead of /s/, say /t/." (tongs)

"Say 'that.' Instead of /voiced th/, say /k/." (cat)

"Say 'walking.' Instead of /w/, say /t/." (talking)

"Say 'cried.' Instead of /k/, say /f/." (fried)

"Say 'shine.' Instead of /sh/, say /m/." (mine)

17. Substituting the final sound in words.

What to say to the student: "We're going to change ending/last sounds in words."

> EXAMPLE "Say '_____.'" (stimulus word) "Instead of / /" (stimulus sound), "say / /." (stimulus sound) (e.g., "Say 'toad.' Instead of /d/, say /z/. What's your new word?") (toes)

NOTE: *Give the letter sound, not the letter name. Use pictured items and/or manipulatives if necessary. Use any of the following stimulus words and/or others you select from the story. The correct answers are in parentheses.*

Stimulus items:

"Say 'my.' Instead of /long I/, say /long E/." (me)

"Say 'frightened.' Instead of /d/, say /z/." (frightens)

"Say 'some.' Instead of /m/, say /n/." (sun)

"Say 'times.' Instead of /z/, say /d/." (timed)

"Say 'was.' Instead of /z/, say /n/." (one)

"Say 'fine.' Instead of /n/, say /t/." (fight)

"Say 'window.' Instead of /long O/, say /long E/." (windy)

"Say 'to.' Instead of /oo/, say /long I/." (tie)

"Say 'leave.' Instead of /v/, say /n/." (lean)

"Say 'course.' Instead of /s/, say /t/." (court)

18. Segmenting the middle sound in monosyllabic words.

What to say to the student: "Tell me the middle sound in the word I say."

> **EXAMPLE** "What's the middle sound in the word '_____'?" (stimulus word) (e.g., "What's the middle sound in the word 'toad'?") (/long O/)

> **NOTE:** *Give the letter sound, not the letter name. Use pictured items and/or manipulatives if necessary. Use any of the following stimulus words and/or others you select from the story. The correct answers are in parentheses.*

Stimulus items:

but (/short U/)

let (/short E/)

much (/short U/)

came (/long A/)

nice (/long I/)

plant (/short A/)

soon (/oo/)

head (/short E/)

right (/long I/)

not (/ah/)

19. Substituting the middle sound in words.

What to say to the student: "We're going to change the middle sound in words."

> **EXAMPLE** "Say '_____.'" (stimulus word) "Instead of / /" (stimulus sound), "say / /." (stimulus sound) (e.g., "Say 'toad.' Instead of /long O/, say /short E/. What's your new word?") (Ted)

> **NOTE:** *Give the letter sound, not the letter name. Use pictured items and/or manipulatives if necessary. Use any of the following stimulus words and/or others you select from the story. The correct answers are in parentheses.*

Stimulus items:

"Say 'but.' Instead of /short U/, say /short E/." (bet)

"Say 'right.' Instead of /long I/, say /long O/." (wrote)

"Say 'not.' Instead of /ah/, say /short E/." (net)

"Say 'came.' Instead of /long A/, say /short U/." (come)

"Say 'put.' Instead of /ew/ as in (wood), say /short I/." (pit)

"Say 'these.' Instead of /long E/, say /long O/." (those)

"Say 'wish.' Instead of /short I/, say /ah/." (wash)

"Say 'will.' Instead of /short I/, say /ah/." (wall)

"Say 'was.' Instead of /short U/, say /short I/." (wiz)

"Say 'fine.' Instead of /long I/, say /long O/." (phone)

20. Identifying all sounds in monosyllabic words.

What to say to the student: "Now tell me all the sounds you hear in the word I say."

> **EXAMPLE** "What sounds do you hear in the word '_____'?" (stimulus word)
> (e.g., "What sounds do you hear in the word 'toad'?")
> (/t/ /long O/ /d/)

NOTE: *Give the letter sound, not the letter name. Use pictured items and/or manipulatives if necessary. Use any of the following stimulus words and/or others you select from the story. The correct answers are in parentheses.*

Stimulus items:

did (/d/ /short I/ /d/)

too (/t/ /oo/)

times (/t/ /long I/ /m/ /z/)

came (/k/ /long A/ /m/)

quite (/k/ /w/ /long I/ /t/)

drat (/d/ /r/ /short A/ /t/)

few (/f/ /y/ (as in yellow) /oo/)

grow (/g/ /r/ /long O/)

songs (/s/ /ah/ /ng/ /z/)

much (/m/ /short U/ /ch/)

21. Deleting sounds within words.

What to say to the student: "We're going to leave out sounds in words."

> **EXAMPLE** "Say '_____'" (stimulus word) "without / /." (stimulus sound) (e.g.,
> "Say 'grow' without /r /.") (go) Say: "The word that is left—'go'—is a real
> word. Sometimes, the word won't be a real word."

NOTE: *Give the letter sound, not the letter name. Use pictured items and/or manipulatives if necessary. Use any of the following stimulus words and/or others you select from the story. The correct answers are in parentheses.*

Stimulus items:

"Say 'plants' without /l/." (pants)

"Say 'stopped' without /t/." (sopped)

"Say 'quite' without /w/." (kite)

"Say 'growing' without /r/." (going)

"Say 'frog' without /r/." (fog)

"Say 'afraid' without /f/." (arrayed)

"Say 'must' without /s/." (mutt)

"Say 'still' without /t/." (sill)

"Say 'window' without /n/." (widow)

"Say 'times' without /m/." (ties)

22. Substituting consonants in words having a two-sound cluster.

What to say to the student: "We're going to substitute sounds in words."

> **EXAMPLE**   "Say '_____.'" (stimulus word) "Instead of / /" (stimulus sound), "say / /." (stimulus sound) (e.g., "Say 'cried.' Instead of /k/, say /f/.") (fried) Say: "Sometimes, the new word will be a made-up word."

NOTE: *Give the letter sound, not the letter name. Use pictured items and/or manipulatives if necessary. Use any of the following stimulus words and/or others you select from the story. The correct answers are in parentheses.*

Stimulus items:

"Say 'drat.' Instead of /d/, say /b/." (brat)

"Say 'green.' Instead of /g/, say /p/." (preen)

"Say 'grow.' Instead of /g/, say /voiceless th/." (throw)

"Say 'stopped.' Instead of /t/, say /l/." (slopped)

"Say 'flower.' Instead of /f/, say /p/." (plower)

"Say 'went.' Instead of /n/, say /s/." (west)

"Say 'frightened.' Instead of /d/, say /z/." (frightens)

"Say 'times.' Instead of /z/, say /d/." (timed)

"Say 'still.' Instead of /t/, say /p/." (spill)

"Say 'most.' Instead of /s/, say /p/." (moped)

23. Phoneme reversing.

What to say to the student: "We're going to say words backward."

> **EXAMPLE**   "Say the word '_____'" (stimulus word) "backward." (e.g., "Say the word 'toad' backward.") (dote)

NOTE: *This is a difficult phoneme-level task and should only be done with older students. Give the letter sound, not the letter name. Use pictured items and/or manipulatives if necessary. Use any of the following stimulus words and/or others you select from the story. The correct answers are in parentheses.*

Stimulus items:

but (tub)

did (did)

these (zeethe)

let (tell)

much (chum)

nice (sign)

still (lits)

fell (leff)

fine (knife)

shine (nishe)

24. Phoneme switching.

What to say to the student: "We're going to switch the first sounds in two words."

> **EXAMPLE**   "Switch the first sounds in '_____' and '_____.'" (stimulus words) (e.g., "Switch the first sounds in 'toad' and 'ran.'") (road tan)

> **NOTE:** *This is a difficult phoneme-level task and should only be done with older students. Give the letter sound, not the letter name. Use pictured items and/or manipulatives if necessary. Use any of the following stimulus words and/or others you select from the story. The correct answers are in parentheses.*

Stimulus items:

now seeds (sow needs)

toad walked (woad talked)

his garden (gis harden)

toad came (code tame)

fine garden (gine farden)

will not (nill watt)

came running (rame cunning)

too much (moo touch)

next day (dext nay)

read poems (ped roems)

25. Pig Latin.

What to say to the student: "We're going to speak a secret language by using words from the story. In pig Latin, you take off the first sound of a word, put it at the end of the word, and add an 'ay' sound."

> **EXAMPLE**   "Say 'toad' in pig Latin." (oadtay)

> **NOTE:** *This is a difficult phoneme-level task and should only be done with older students. Use pictured items and/or manipulatives if necessary. Use any of the following stimulus words and/or others you select from the story. The correct answers are in parentheses.*

Stimulus items:

frog (rogfay)

next (extnay)

played (layedpay)

times (imestay)

soon (oonsay)

world (urldway)

fine (inefay)

little (ittlelay)

shouting (outingshay)

frightened (rightenedfay)

From Phonological Awareness into Print

NOTE: *Only five examples per activity are included in this resource due to space. You are encouraged to add many more words into this section that you feel your student(s) is(are) ready to write.*

1. Substituting the initial sound or letter in words.

NOTE: *Use lined paper or copy the sheet of lined paper included in the back of this book.*

Stimulus items:

1.1 too/boo

Task a. "Say 'too.' Instead of /t/, say /b/. What's your new word?" (boo) "Write/copy 'too' and 'boo.'"

Task b. "Circle the **letters** that make the words different." ([t], [b])

Task c. "What **sounds** do these letters make?" (/t/, /b/)

1.2 but/rut

Task a. "Say 'but.' Instead of /b/, say /r/. What's your new word?" (rut) "Write/copy 'but' and 'rut.'"

Task b. "Circle the **letters** that make the words different." ([b], [r])

Task c. "What **sounds** do these letters make?" (/b/, /r/)

1.3 sun/fun

Task a. "Say 'sun.' Instead of /s/, say /f/. What's your new word?" (fun) "Write/copy 'sun' and 'fun.'"

Task b. "Circle the **letters** that make the words different." ([s], [f])

Task c. "What **sounds** do these letters make?" (/s/, /f/)

1.4 must/rust

Task a. "Say 'must.' Instead of /m/, say /r/. What's your new word?" (rust) "Write/ copy 'must' and 'rust.'"

Task b. "Circle the **letters** that make the words different." ([m], [r])

Task c. "What **sounds** do these letters make?" (/m/, /r/)

1.5 shouting/pouting

Task a. "Say 'shouting.' Instead of /sh/, say /p/. What's your new word?" (pouting) "Write/copy 'shouting' and 'pouting.'"

Task b. "Circle the **letters** that make the words different." ([s], [h], [p])

Task c. "What **sounds** do these letters make?" (/sh/, /p/)

2. Substituting the final sound or letter in words.

NOTE: *Use lined paper or copy the sheet of lined paper included in the back of this book.*

Stimulus items:

2.1 much/mush

Task a. "Say 'much.' Instead of /ch/, say /sh/. What's your new word?" (mush) "Write/ copy 'much' and 'mush.'"

Task b. "Circle the **letters** that make the words different." ([c], [h], [s], [h])

Task c. "What **sounds** do these letters make?" (/ch/, /sh/)

2.2 ran/rat

Task a. "Say 'ran.' Instead of /n/, say /t /. What's your new word?" (rat) "Write/copy 'ran' and 'rat.'"

Task b. "Circle the **letters** that make the words different." ([n], [t])

Task c. "What **sounds** do these letters make?" (/n/, /t/)

2.3 came/cane

Task a. "Say 'came.' Instead of /m/, say /n/. What's your new word?" (cane) "Write/ copy 'came' and 'cane.'"

Task b. "Circle the **letters** that make the words different." ([m], [n])

Task c. "What **sounds** do these letters make?" (/m/, /n/)

2.4 frightened/frightens

Task a. "Say 'frightened.' Instead of /d/, say /z/. What's your new word?" (frightens) "Write/copy 'frightened' and 'frightens.'"

Task b. "Circle the **letters** that make the words different." ([e], [d], [s])

Task c. "What **sounds** do these letters make?" (/d/, /z/)

2.5 by/be

Task a. "Say 'by.' Instead of /long I/, say /long E/. What's your new word?" (be) "Write/copy 'by' and 'be.'"

Task b. "Circle the **letters** that make the words different." ([y], [e])

Task c. "What **sounds** do these letters make?" (/long I/, /long E/)

3. Substituting the middle sound or letter in words.

NOTE: *Use lined paper or copy the sheet of lined paper included in the back of this book.*

Stimulus items:

3.1 let/lit

Task a. "Say 'let.' Instead of /short E/, say /short I/. What's your new word?" (lit) "Write/copy 'let' and 'lit.'"

Task b. "Circle the **letters** that make the words different." ([e], [i])

Task c. "What **sounds** do these letters make?" (/short E/, /short I/)

3.2 wake/woke

Task a. "Say 'wake.' Instead of /long A/, say /long O/. What's your new word?" (woke) "Write/copy 'wake' and 'woke.'"

Task b. "Circle the **letters** that make the words different." ([a], [o])

Task c. "What **sounds** do these letters make?" (/long A/, /long O/)

3.3 had/hid

Task a. "Say 'had.' Instead of /short A/, say /short I/. What's your new word?" (hid) "Write/copy 'had' and 'hid.'"

Task b. "Circle the **letters** that make the words different." ([a], [i])

Task c. "What **sounds** do these letters make?" (/short A/, /short I/)

3.4 soon/sun

Task a. "Say 'soon.' Instead of /oo/, say /short U/. What's your new word?" (sun) "Write/copy 'soon' and 'sun.'"

Task b. "Circle the **letters** that make the words different." ([o], [o], [u])

Task c. "What **sounds** do these letters make?" (/oo/, /short U/)

3.5 toad/tied

Task a. "Say 'toad.' Instead of /long O/, say /long I/. What's your new word?" (tied) "Write/copy 'toad' and 'tied.'"

Task b. "Circle the **letters** that make the words different." ([o], [a], [i], [e])

Task c. "What **sounds** do these letters make?" (/long O/, /long I/)

4. Supplying the initial sound or letter in words.

NOTE: *Use lined paper or copy the sheet of lined paper included in the back of this book.*

Stimulus items:

4.1 for/or

Task a. "Say 'for,' say 'or.' What sound did you hear in 'for' that is missing in 'or'?" (/f/) "Now we'll change the **letter**. Write/copy 'for' and 'or.'"

Task b. "Circle the beginning **letter** that makes the words different." **([f])**

Task c. "What **sound** does this letter make?" **(/f/)**

4.2 asleep/sleep

Task a. "Say 'asleep,' say 'sleep.' What sound did you hear in 'asleep' that is missing in 'sleep'?" (/short U/) "Now we'll change the **letter.** Write/copy 'asleep' and 'sleep.'"

Task b. "Circle the beginning **letter** that makes the words different." ([a])

Task c. "What **sound** does this letter make?" (/short U/)

4.3 ran/an

Task a. "Say 'ran,' say 'an.' What sound did you hear in 'ran' that is missing in 'an'?" (/r/) "Now we'll change the **letter.** Write/copy 'ran' and 'an.'"

Task b. "Circle the beginning **letter** that makes the words different." ([r])

Task c. "What **sound** does this letter make?" (/r/)

4.4 ground/round

Task a. "Say 'ground,' say 'round.' What sound did you hear in 'ground' that is missing in 'round'?" (/g/) "Now we'll change the **letter.** Write/copy 'ground' and 'round.'"

Task b. "Circle the beginning **letter** that makes the words different." ([g])

Task c. "What **sound** does this letter make?" (/g/)

4.5 start/tart

Task a. "Say 'start,' say 'tart.' What sound did you hear in 'start' that is missing in 'tart'?" (/s/) "Now we'll change the **letter.** Write/copy 'start' and 'tart.'"

Task b. "Circle the beginning **letter** that makes the words different." ([s])

Task c. "What **sound** does this letter make?" (/s/)

5. Supplying the final sound or letter in words.

NOTE: *Use lined paper or copy the sheet of lined paper included in the back of this book.*

Stimulus items:

5.1 seeds/seed

Task a. "Say 'seeds,' say 'seed.' What sound did you hear in 'seeds' that is missing in 'seed'?" (/z/) "Now we'll change the **letter.** Write/copy 'seeds' and 'seed.'"

Task b. "Circle the ending/last **letter** that makes the words different." ([s])

Task c. "What **sound** does this letter make?" (/z/)

5.2 plants/plant

Task a. "Say 'plants,' say 'plant.' What sound did you hear in 'plants' that is missing in 'plant'?" (/s/) "Now we'll change the **letter.** Write/copy 'plants' and 'plant.'"

Task b. "Circle the ending/last **letter** that makes the words different." ([s])

Task c. "What **sound** does this letter make?" (/s/)

5.3 played/play

Task a. "Say 'played,' say 'play.' What sound did you hear in 'played' that is missing in 'play'?" (/d/) "Now we'll change the **letters**. Write/copy 'played' and 'play.'"

Task b. "Circle the ending/last **letters** that make the words different." ([e], [d])

Task c. "What **sound** do these letters make?" (/d/)

5.4 start/star

Task a. "Say 'start,' say 'star.' What sound did you hear in 'start' that is missing in 'star'?" (/t/) "Now we'll change the **letter**. Write/copy 'start' and 'star.'"

Task b. "Circle the ending/last **letter** that makes the word different." ([t])

Task c. "What **sound** does this letter make?" (/t/)

5.5 looked/look

Task a. "Say 'looked,' say 'look.' What sound did you hear in 'looked' that is missing in 'look'?" (/t/) "Now we'll change the **letters**. Write/copy 'looked' and 'look.'"

Task b. "Circle the ending/last **letters** that make the words different." ([e], [d])

Task c. "What **sound** do these letters make?" (/t/)

6. Switching the first sound and letter in words (ADVANCED).

NOTE: *Use lined paper or copy the sheet of lined paper included in the back of this book.*

Stimulus items:

6.1 did not

Task a. "Say 'did,' say 'not.' What sound do you hear at the beginning of 'did'?" (/d/) "What sound do you hear at the beginning of 'not'?" (/n/) "Switch the first sounds in those words." (nid dot) "Now we'll change the **letters**. Write/copy 'did not' and 'nid dot.'"

Task b. "Circle the beginning **letters** that change the words." ([d], [n])

Task c. "What **sounds** do those letters make?" (/d/, /n/)

6.2 his garden

Task a. "Say 'his,' say 'garden.' What sound do you hear at the beginning of 'his'?" (/h/) "What sound do you hear at the beginning of 'garden'?" (/g/) "Switch the first sounds in those words." (gis harden) "Now we'll change the **letters**. Write/copy 'his garden' and 'gis harden.'"

Task b. "Circle the beginning **letters** that change the words." ([h], [g])

Task c. "What **sounds** do those letters make?" (/h/, /g/)

6.3 this noise

Task a. "Say 'this,' say 'noise.' What sound do you hear at the beginning of 'this'?" (/voiced th/) "What sound do you hear at the beginning of 'noise'?" (/n/) "Switch the first sounds in those words." (nis thoise) "Now we'll change the **letters**. Write/copy 'this noise' and 'nis thoise.'"

Task b. "Circle the beginning **letters** that change the words." ([t], [h], [n])

Task c. "What **sounds** do those letters make?" (/voiced th/, /n/)

6.4 my seeds

Task a. "Say 'my,' say 'seeds.' What sound do you hear at the beginning of 'my'?" (/m/) "What sound do you hear at the beginning of 'seeds'?" (/s/) "Switch the first sounds in those words." (sy meeds) "Now we'll change the **letters**. Write/copy 'my seeds' and 'sy meeds.'"

Task b. "Circle the beginning **letters** that change the words." ([m], [s])

Task c. "What **sounds** do those letters make?" (/m/, /s/)

6.5 next day

Task a. "Say 'next,' say 'day.' What sound do you hear at the beginning of 'next'?" (/n/) "What sound do you hear at the beginning of 'day'?" (/d/) "Switch the first sounds in those words." (dext nay) "Now we'll change the **letters**. Write/copy 'next day' and 'dext nay.'"

Task b. "Circle the beginning **letters** that change the words." ([n], [d])

Task c. "What **sounds** do those letters make?" (/n/, /d/)

Phonological Awareness Activities to Use with *Tortillas and Lullabies*.

Text version used for selection of stimulus items:

Reiser, L., and Valientes, C. (Illustrator). (1998). *Tortillas and Lullabies.* New York: HarperCollins Children's Books/HarperCollins Publishers.

Phonological Awareness Activities at the Word Level

1. Counting words.

What to say to the student: "We're going to count words."

> EXAMPLE "How many words do you hear in this sentence (or phrase): 'my great-grandmother'?" (3)

> **NOTE:** *Use pictured items and/or manipulatives if necessary. Use any of the following stimulus phrases or sentences and/or others you select from the story. The correct answers are in parentheses.*

Stimulus items:

made tortillas (2)

my grandmother (2)

for my grandmother (3)

for my mother (3)

the same, but different (4)

tortillas for my doll (4)

It was the same. (4)

flowers for my mother (4)

a dress for my doll (5)

My mother made tortillas for me. (6)

2. Identifying the missing word from a list.

What to say to the student: "Listen to the words I say. I'll say them again. You tell me which word I leave out."

> **EXAMPLE** "Listen to the words I say: 'doll,' 'bed,' 'time.' I'll say them again. Tell me which one I leave out: 'doll,' 'bed.'" (time)

NOTE: *Use pictured items and/or manipulatives if necessary. Use any of the following stimulus words and/or others you select from the story. The correct answers are in parentheses.*

Stimulus set #1	Stimulus set #2
dress, head	dress (head)
great, doll	doll (great)
gathered, sang, pictures	gathered, pictures (sang)
down, customs, jump	customs, jump (down)
mother, sang, sitting	mother, sang (sitting)
lavado, house, lullaby	lavado, lullaby (house)
everyday, coyote, dress, different	coyote, dress, different (everyday)
there, cantaba, was, tortillas	there, was, tortillas (cantaba)
jump, little, washing, love	jump, little, love (washing)
flowers, received, mamá, grandmother	flowers, received, mamá (grandmother)

3. Identifying the missing word in a phrase or sentence.

What to say to the student: "Listen to the sentence I read. Tell me which word is missing the second time I read the sentence."

> **EXAMPLE** "'I made tortillas.' Listen again and tell me which word I leave out: '_____ made tortillas.'" (I)

NOTE: *Use pictured items and/or manipulatives if necessary. Use any of the following stimulus sentences and/or others you select from the story. The correct answers are in parentheses.*

Stimulus items:

My grandmother. My _____. (grandmother)

But different. _____ different. (But)

Sang a lullaby. Sang a _____. (lullaby)

My mother washed. My _____ washed. (mother)

A dress for me. A _____ for me. (dress)

Flowers for my mother. Flowers for _____ mother. (my)

My doll gathered flowers. My doll _____ flowers. (gathered)

My great-grandmother made tortillas. My _____ -grandmother made tortillas. (great)

Every time it was the same. _____ time it was the same. (Every)

I made tortillas for my doll. I made _____ for my doll. (tortillas)

4. Supplying the missing word as an adult reads.

What to say to the student: "I want you to help me read the story. You fill in the words I leave out."

> **EXAMPLE**   "Tortillas and _____." (lullabies)

> **NOTE:** *Use pictured items and/or manipulatives if necessary. Use any of the following stimulus sentences and/or others you select from the story. The correct answers are in parentheses.*

Stimulus items:

I made _____. (tortillas)

My _____ made tortillas. (mother, grandmother, great-grandmother)

For _____ doll. (my)

My grandmother gathered _____. (flowers)

I sang a lullaby to my _____. (doll)

Every _____ it was the same. (time)

Sitting _____ to sew. (down)

There are _____ I have to do. (things)

My great-grandmother sang a _____ to my grandmother. (lullaby)

My grandmother washed a _____ for my mother. (dress)

5. Rearranging words.

What to say to the student: "I'll say some words out of order. You put them in the right order so they make sense."

> **EXAMPLE**   " 'and lullabies tortillas.' Put those words in the right order." (tortillas and lullabies)

> **NOTE:** *Use pictured items and/or manipulatives if necessary. Use any of the following stimulus words and/or others you select from the story. The correct answers are in parentheses. This word-level activity can be more difficult than some of the syllable- or phoneme-level activities because of the memory load. If your students are only able to deal with two or three words to be rearranged, add more two- and three-word samples from the story and omit the four-word level items.*

Stimulus items:

different but (but different)

mother for my (for my mother)

mother my washed. (My mother washed.)

my tortillas made grandmother. (My grandmother made tortillas.)

sitting to sew down (sitting down to sew)

me for a dress (a dress for me)

dress a my doll for (a dress for my doll)

it same was time every the. (Every time it was the same.)

my lullaby sang grandmother a. (My grandmother sang a lullaby.)

sang my grandmother great (sang my great-grandmother)

Phonological Awareness Activities at the Syllable Level

1. Syllable counting.

What to say to the student: "We're going to count syllables (or parts) of words."

> **EXAMPLE**   "How many syllables do you hear in '_____'?" (stimulus word)
> (e.g., "How many syllables do you hear in 'bed'?") (1)

> **NOTE:** *Use pictured items and/or manipulatives if necessary. Use any of the following stimulus words and/or others you select from the story. Use any group of 10 stimulus items you select per teaching set.*

Stimulus items:

One-syllable words: but, bed, by, book, time, to, doll, dress, do, down, don't, great, my, made, me, same, sang, sew, squash, si, says, for, hush, have, head, house, how, love, was, washed, will, what, with, things, thing, the, there, then, this, that, your, you, and, I, it, a, out, eat, if, is, all

Two-syllable words: para, pretty, pictures, dresses, casa, customs, gathered, given, mother, mamá, mother's, madre, matters, sitting, received, flowers, funny, freely, little, washing, into, about

Three-syllable words: tortillas, cantaba, coyote, grandmother, grandmother's, families, lavado, lullabies, lullaby

2. Initial syllable deleting.

What to say to the student: "We're going to leave out syllables (or parts of words)."

> **EXAMPLE**   "Say '_____.'" (stimulus word) "Say it again without '_____.'"
> (stimulus syllable) (e.g., "Say 'grandmother.' Say it again without 'grand.'")
> (mother)

> **NOTE:** *Use pictured items and/or manipulatives if necessary. Use any of the following stimulus words and/or others you select from the story. The correct answers are in parentheses.*

Stimulus items:

"Say 'mamá' without 'ma.'" (ma)

"Say 'received' without 're.'" (ceived)

"Say 'madre' without 'ma.'" (dre)

"Say 'lullaby' without 'lull.'" (aby)

"Say 'tortilla' without 'tor.'" (tilla)

"Say 'washing' without 'wash.'" (ing)

"Say 'sitting' without 'sit.'" (ing)

"Say 'dresses' without 'dress.'" (uz)

"Say 'cantaba' without 'can.'" (taba)

"Say 'joyously' without 'joy.'" (ously)

3. Final syllable deleting.

What to say to the student: "We're going to leave out syllables (or parts of words)."

> **EXAMPLE**   "Say '_____.'" (stimulus word) "Say it again without '_____.'" (stimulus syllable) (e.g., "Say 'freely' without 'lee.'") (free)

> **NOTE:** *Use pictured items and/or manipulatives if necessary. Use any of the following stimulus words and/or others you select from the story. The correct answers are in parentheses.*

Stimulus items:

"Say 'customs' without 'tums.'" (cus)

"Say 'washing' without 'ing.'" (wash)

"Say 'flowers' without 'ers.'" (flau)

"Say 'everyday' without 'day.'" (every)

"Say 'joyously' without 'lee.'" (joyous)

"Say 'madre' without 'dre.'" (ma)

"Say 'pictures' without 'churs.'" (pick)

"Say 'mamá' without 'ma.'" (ma)

"Say 'lullabies' without 'byes.'" (lulla)

"Say 'sitting' without 'ing.'" (sit)

4. Initial syllable adding.

What to say to the student: "Now let's add syllables (or parts) to words."

> **EXAMPLE**   "Add '_____'" (stimulus syllable) "to the beginning of '_____.'" (stimulus syllable) (e.g., "Add 'grand' to the beginning of 'mother.'") (grandmother)

> **NOTE:** *Use pictured items and/or manipulatives if necessary. Use any of the following stimulus words and/or others you select from the story. The correct answers are in parentheses.*

Stimulus items:

"Add 'ma' to the beginning of 'ma.'" (mamá)

"Add 'grand' to the beginning of 'mother's.'" (grandmother's)

"Add 'free' to the beginning of 'Lee.'" (freely)

"Add 'joy' to the beginning of 'ously.'" (joyously)

"Add 'can' to the beginning of 'taba.'" (cantaba)

"Add 'pick' to the beginning of 'churs.'" (pictures)

"Add 'sit' to the beginning of 'ing.'" (sitting)

"Add 'uh' to the beginning of 'bout.'" (about)

"Add 'ma' to the beginning of 'dray.'" (madre)

"Add 're' to the beginning of 'ceived.'" (received)

5. Final syllable adding.

What to say to the student: "Now let's add syllables (or parts) to words."

> EXAMPLE   "Add '_____'" (stimulus syllable) "to the end of '_____.'" (stimulus syllable) (e.g., "Add 'Lee' to the end of 'free.'") (freely)

NOTE: *Use pictured items and/or manipulatives if necessary. Use any of the following stimulus words and/or others you select from the story. The correct answers are in parentheses.*

Stimulus items:

"Add 'byes' to the end of 'lulla.'" (lullabies)

"Add 'ing' to the end of 'wash.'" (washing)

"Add 'Lee' to the end of 'joyous.'" (joyously)

"Add 'ma' to the end of 'ma.'" (mamá)

"Add 'bout' to the end of 'uh.'" (about)

"Add 'uz' to the end of 'dress.'" (dresses)

"Add 'ers' to the end of 'flau.'" (flowers)

"Add 'bye' to the end of 'lulla.'" (lullaby)

"Add 'day' to the end of 'every.'" (everyday)

"Add 'dray' to the end of 'ma.'" (madre)

6. Syllable substituting.

What to say to the student: "Let's make up some new words."

> EXAMPLE   "Say '_____.'" (stimulus word) "Instead of '_____'" (stimulus syllable), "say '_____.'" (stimulus syllable) (e.g., "Say 'madre.' Instead of 'dray,' say 'ma.' The new word is 'mamá.'")

NOTE: *Use pictured items and/or manipulatives if necessary. Use of the following stimulus words and/or others you select from the story. The correct answers are in parentheses.*

Stimulus items:

"Say 'washing.' Instead of 'wash,' say 'wish.'" (wishing)

"Say 'everyday.' Instead of 'day,' say 'where.'" (everywhere)

"Say 'sitting.' Instead of 'ing,' say 'er.'" (sitter)

"Say 'lullaby.' Instead of 'bye,' say 'byes.'" (lullabies)

"Say 'customs.' Instead of 'cus,' say 'long I.'" (items)

"Say 'freely.' Instead of 'Lee,' say 'dum.'" (freedom)

"Say 'everyday.' Instead of 'day,' say 'one.'" (everyone)

"Say 'grandmother's.' Instead of 'grand,' say 'step.'" (stepmother's)

"Say 'flowers.' Instead of 'flau,' say 'pow.'" (powers)

"Say 'about.' Instead of 'bout,' say 'frayed.'" (afraid)

Phonological Awareness Activities at the Phoneme Level

1. Counting sounds.

What to say to the student: "We're going to count sounds in words."

> **EXAMPLE** "How many sounds do you hear in this word: 'bed'?" (3)

> **NOTE:** *Use pictured items and/or manipulatives if necessary. Use any of the following stimulus words and/or others you select from the story. Be sure to give the letter sound and not the letter name. Use any group of 10 stimulus items you select per teaching set.*

Stimulus items:

Stimulus words with one sound: *a, I*

Stimulus words with two sounds: by, to, do, my, me, sew, si, the, you, it, eat, if, is, all

Stimulus words with three sounds: but, bed, book, time, doll, made, same, sang, says, hush, have, head, love, was, will, what, with, then, this, that, and, one

Stimulus words with four sounds: dress, don't, casa, great, jump, mother, mamá, funny, little, washed, into

Stimulus words with five sounds: pretty, coyote, mother's, madre, matters, squash, freely

Stimulus words with six sounds: pictures, received, family, lavado, lullaby

Stimulus words with seven sounds: cantaba, customs, families, lullabies

Stimulus words with nine sounds: grandmother

2. Sound categorization or identifying a rhyme oddity.

What to say to the student: "Guess which word I say does not rhyme with the other three words."

> **EXAMPLE** "Tell me which word doesn't rhyme with the other three words: '_____,' '_____,' '_____,' '_____.'" (stimulus words) (e.g., "'bed,' 'head,' 'read,' 'time.' Which word doesn't rhyme?") (time)

> **NOTE:** *Use pictured items if necessary. Use any of the following stimulus words and/or others you select from the story. The correct answers are in parentheses.*

Stimulus items:

    jump, stump, pump, doll (doll)

    same, sang, name, game (sang)

    funny, bunny, little, honey (little)

    doll, great, call, mall (great)

    lullaby, sitting, knitting, pitting (lullaby)

    things, rings, cantaba, wings (cantaba)

    mamá, dresses, messes, presses (mamá)

    flowers, powers, mother, showers (mother)

    house, little, mouse, grouse (little)

    made, paid, grade, squash (squash)

3. Matching rhyme.

What to say to the student: "We're going to think of rhyming words."

> **EXAMPLE** "Which word rhymes with '_____'?" (stimulus word) (e.g., "Which word rhymes with 'dress': 'bed,' 'time,' 'same,' 'mess'?") (mess)

NOTE: *Use pictured items if necessary. Use any of the following stimulus words and/or others you select from the story. The correct answers are in parentheses.*

Stimulus items:

    madre: head, made, jump, padre (padre)

    down: gown, squash, washed, family (gown)

    funny: flowers, little, money, washing (money)

    mother: joyously, brother, about, mamá (brother)

    hush: every, sitting, gathered, brush (brush)

    sitting: knitting, everyday, flowers, mother (knitting)

    eat: jump, feet, all, my (feet)

    sew: grandmother, me, go, washing (go)

    dresses: little, messes, lavado, received (messes)

    flowers: coyote, washed, little, powers (powers)

4. Producing rhyme.

What to say to the student: "Now we'll say rhyming words."

> **EXAMPLE** "Tell me a word that rhymes with '_____.'" (stimulus word) (e.g., "Tell me a word that rhymes with 'time.' You can make up a word if you want.") (climb, lime, pime)

NOTE: *Use pictured items if necessary. Use any of the following stimulus words and/or others you select from the story (i.e., you say a word from the list below and the student is to think of a rhyming word). Use any group of 10 stimulus items you select per teaching set.*

Stimulus items:

/p/: pictures, para, pretty

/b/: bed, but, by, book

/t/: time, to, tortillas

/d/: dress, do, doll, dresses, down, don't

/k/: casa, customs, cantaba

/g/: given, great, gathered

/dz/ (as the first sound in jelly): jump

/m/: my, made, mamá, me, madre, matters

/s/: same, sang, sitting, sew, si, says

/f/: for, flowers, funny, freely

/h/: hush, have, head, house, how

/r/: received

/l/: little, love, lullaby, lavado

/w/, /wh/: was, washing, will, what

/voiceless th/: things, thing

/voiced th/: the, there, then, this, that

/y/ (as in yellow): you, your

vowels: and, I, it, one, out, eat, if, is, all

5. Sound matching (initial).

What to say to the student: "Now we'll listen for the first sound in words."

> **EXAMPLE** "Listen to this sound: / /." (stimulus sound). "Guess which word I say begins with that sound: '_____,' '_____,' '_____,' '_____.'" (stimulus words) (e.g., "Listen to this sound: /p/. Guess which word I say begins with that sound: 'doll,' 'para,' 'time,' 'casa.'") (para)

NOTE: *Give the letter sound, not the letter name. Use pictured items if necessary. Use any of the following stimulus words and/or others you select from the story. The correct answers are in parentheses.*

Stimulus items:

/m/: jump, mamá, squash, for (mamá)

/d/: tortillas, washing, jump, down (down)

/p/: pretty, received, lavado, funny (pretty)

/h/: great, hush, things, sang (hush)

/f/: same, love, flowers, house (flowers)

/l/: sang, lavado, head, coyote (lavado)

/k/: dresses, mother, washed, cantaba (cantaba)

/s/: sitting, customs, madre, freely (sitting)

/voiced th/: received, how, this, every (this)

/dz/ (as the first sound in jelly): head, joyously, mamá, casa (joyously)

6. Sound matching (final).

What to say to the student: "Now we'll listen for the last sound in words."

> **EXAMPLE** "Listen to this sound: / /" (stimulus sound). "Guess which word I say ends with that sound: '_____,' '_____,' '_____,' '_____.'" (stimulus words) (e.g., "Listen to this sound: /k/. Guess which word I say ends with that sound: 'book,' 'bed,' 'jump,' 'same.'") (book)

> **NOTE:** *Give the letter sound, not the letter name. Use pictured items and/or manipulatives if necessary. Use any of the following stimulus words and/or others you select from the story. The correct answers are in parentheses.*

Stimulus items:

/f/: if, time, made, don't (if)

/n/: dress, doll, down, there (down)

/z/: para, head, families, time (families)

/ng/: washing, down, made, pretty (washing)

/r/: given, mamá, grandmother, squash (grandmother)

/oo/: says, you, every, my (you)

/s/: house, lullaby, was, hush (house)

/m/: given, cantaba, eat, same (same)

/v/: if, love, things, made (love)

/t/: and, mother, washed, dress (washed)

7. Identifying the initial sound in words.

What to say to the student: "I'll say a word two times. Tell me what sound is missing the second time: '_____,' '_____.'" (stimulus words)

> **EXAMPLE** "What sound do you hear in '_____'" (stimulus word) "that is missing in '_____'?" (stimulus word) (e.g., "What sound do you hear in 'bed' that is missing in 'Ed'?") (/b/)

> **NOTE:** *Give the letter sound, not the letter name. Use pictured items and/or manipulatives if necessary. Use any of the following stimulus words and/or others you select from the story. The correct answers are in parentheses.*

Stimulus items:

"doll, all. What sound do you hear in 'doll' that is missing in 'all'?" (/d/)

"great, rate. What sound do you hear in 'great' that is missing in 'rate'?" (/g/)

"time, I'm. What sound do you hear in 'time' that is missing in 'I'm'?" (/t/)

"love, of. What sound do you hear in 'love' that is missing in 'of'?" (/l/)

"about, bout. What sound do you hear in 'about' that is missing in 'bout'?" (/short U/)

"mother, other. What sound do you hear in 'mother' that is missing in 'other'?" (/m/)

"will, ill. What sound do you hear in 'will' that is missing in 'ill'?" (/w/)

"made, aid. What sound do you hear in 'made' that is missing in 'aid'?" (/m/)

"there, air. What sound do you hear in 'there' that is missing in 'air'?" (/voiced th/)

"same, aim. What sound do you hear in 'same' that is missing in 'aim'?" (/s/)

8. Identifying the final sound in words.

What to say to the student: "I'll say a word two times. Tell me what sound is missing the second time: '_____,' '_____.'" (stimulus words)

> EXAMPLE "What sound do you hear in '_____'" (stimulus word) "that is missing in '_____'?" (stimulus word) (e.g., "What sound do you hear in 'great' that is missing in 'grey'?") (/t/)

> **NOTE:** *Give the letter sound, not the letter name. Use pictured items and/or manipulatives if necessary. Use any of the following stimulus words and/or others you select from the story. The correct answers are in parentheses.*

Stimulus items:

"made, may. What sound do you hear in 'made' that is missing in 'may'?" (/d/)

"every, ever. What sound do you hear in 'every' that is missing in 'ever'?" (/long E/)

"lullabies, lullaby. What sound do you hear in 'lullabies' that is missing in 'lullaby'?" (/z/)

"house, how. What sound do you hear in 'house' that is missing in 'how'?" (/s/)

"washed, wash. What sound do you hear in 'washed' that is missing in 'wash'?" (/t/)

"mamá, mom. What sound do you hear in 'mamá' that is missing in 'mom'?" (/ah/)

"gathered, gather. What sound do you hear in 'gathered' that is missing in 'gather'?" (/d/)

"funny, fun. What sound do you hear in 'funny' that is missing in 'fun'?" (/long E/)

"time, tie. What sound do you hear in 'time' that is missing in 'tie'?" (/m/)

"tortillas, tortilla. What sound do you hear in 'tortillas' that is missing in 'tortilla'?" (/s/)

9. Segmenting the initial sound in words.

What to say to the student: "Listen to the word I say and tell me the first sound you hear."

> EXAMPLE "What's the first sound in '_____'?" (stimulus word) (e.g., "What's the first sound in 'bed'?") (/b/)

> **NOTE:** *Give the letter sound, not the letter name. Use pictured items and/or manipulatives if necessary. Use any of the following stimulus words and/or others you select from the story. Use any group of 10 stimulus items you select per teaching set.*

Stimulus items:

/p/: para, pretty, pictures

/b/: but, bed, by, book

/t/: tortillas, time, to

/d/: doll, different, dress, do, dresses, down, don't

/k/: cantaba, coyote, casa, customs

/g/: great, grandmother, gathered, grandmother's, given

/dz/ (as in jelly): jump, joyously

/m/: my, made, mother, mamá, me, mother's, madre, matters

/s/: same, sang, sitting, sew, squash, si, says

/f/: for, flowers, funny, freely, family, families

/h/: hush, have, head, house, how

/r/: received

/l/: lavado, lullabies, lullaby, little, love

/w/, /wh/: was, washing, washed, will, what, with

/voiceless th/: things, thing

/voiced th/: the, there, then, this, that

/y/ (as in yellow): your, you

vowels: and, every, it, into, eat, if, is, about, everyday, all

10. Segmenting the final sound in words.

What to say to the student: "Listen to the word I say and tell me the last sound you hear."

> **EXAMPLE** "What's the last sound in the word '_____'?" (stimulus word) (e.g., "What's the last sound in the word 'paint'?") (/t/)

> **NOTE:** *Give the letter sound, not the letter name. Use pictured items and/or manipulatives if necessary. Use any of the following stimulus words and/or others you select from the story. Use any group of 10 stimulus items you select per teaching set.*

Stimulus items:

/p/: jump

/t/: but, different, don't, great, washed, what, that, it, out, eat, about

/d/: bed, gathered, made, received, head, and

/k/: book

/m/: time, same

/n/: down, given, then, one

/ng/: sang, sitting, washing, thing

/s/: dress, house, this

/z/: pictures, dresses, customs, grandmother's, mother's, matters, says, flowers, families, lullabies, was, things, is

/f/: if

/v/: have, love

/r/: grandmother, mother, for, there, your

/l/: doll, little, will, all

/sh/: squash, hush

/voiceless th/: with

/long A/: everyday

/long E/: pretty, coyote, joyously, si, funny, freely, family, every

/long I/: by, my, lullaby

/long O/: sew, lavado

/short U/: the

/oo/: to, do, you, into

11. Generating words from the story beginning with a particular sound.

What to say to the student: "Let's think of words from the story that start with certain sounds."

> **EXAMPLE** "Tell me a word from the story that starts with / /." (stimulus sound) (e.g., the sound /p/) (paintbrush)

> **NOTE:** *Give the letter sound, not the letter name. Use pictured items if necessary. Use any of the following stimulus words and/or others you select from the story. You say the sound (e.g., a voiceless /p/ sound), and the student is to say a word from the story that begins with that sound. Use any group of 10 stimulus items you select per teaching set.*

Stimulus items:

/p/: para, pretty, pictures

/b/: but, bed, by, book

/t/: tortillas, time, to

/d/: doll, different, dress, do, dresses, down, don't

/k/: cantaba, coyote, casa, customs

/g/: great, grandmother, gathered, grandmother's, given

/dz/ (as in jelly): jump, joyously

/m/: my, made, mother, mamá, me, mother's, madre, matters

/s/: same, sang, sitting, sew, squash, si, says

/f/: for, flowers, funny, freely, family, families

/h/: hush, have, head, house, how

/r/: received

/l/: lavado, lullabies, lullaby, little, love

/w/, /wh/: was, washing, washed, will, what, with

/voiceless th/: things, thing

/voiced th/: the, there, then, this, that

/y/ (as in yellow): your, you

vowels: and, every, it, into, eat, if, is, about, everyday, all

12. Blending sounds in monosyllabic words divided into onset–rime beginning with a two-consonant cluster + rime.

What to say to the student: "Now we'll put sounds together to make words."

> **EXAMPLE** "Put these sounds together to make a word: / / + / /." (stimulus sounds) "What's the word?" (e.g., "sch + ool: What's the word?") (school)

> **NOTE:** *Give the letter sound, not the letter name. Use pictured items and/or manipulatives if necessary. Use any of the following stimulus words and/or others you select from the story. The correct answers are in parentheses.*

Stimulus items:

dr + ess (dress)

fr + iend (friend)

gr + and (grand)

fr + ee (free)

gr + eat (great)

Sourcebook users are encouraged to add stimulus items into this activity from curriculum materials they may be using with *Tortillas and Lullabies.*

13. Blending sounds in monosyllabic words divided into onset–rime beginning with a single consonant + rime.

What to say to the student: "Let's put sounds together to make words."

> **EXAMPLE** "Put these sounds together to make a word: / / + / /." (stimulus sounds) "What's the word?" (e.g., "/b/ + ed: What's the word?") (bed)

> **NOTE:** *Give the letter sound, not the letter name. Use pictured items and/or manipulatives if necessary. Use any of the following stimulus words and/or others you select from the story. The correct answers are in parentheses.*

Stimulus items:

/b/ + ook (book)

/s/ + ame (same)

/dz/ (as in jelly) + ump (jump)

/s/ + ang (sang)

/h/ + ush (hush)

/voiceless th/ + ings (things)

/m/ + ade (made)

/l/ + ove (love)

/w/ + as (was)

/voiced th/ + en (then)

14. Blending sounds to form a monosyllabic word beginning with a continuant sound.

What to say to the student: "We'll put sounds together to make words."

EXAMPLE "Put these sounds together to make a word: / / + / / + / /." (stimulus sounds) (e.g., /s/ /long E/) (si)

NOTE: *Give the letter sound, not the letter name. Use pictured items and/or manipulatives if necessary. Use any of the following stimulus words and/or others you select from the story. The correct answers are in parentheses.*

Stimulus items:

/l/ /short U/ /v/ (love)

/s/ /long A/ /m/ (same)

/r/ /long O/ /m/ /d/ (roamed)

/h/ /short U/ /sh/ (hush)

/w/ /short I/ /l/ (will)

/y/ (as in yellow) /oo/ (you)

/h/ /short E/ /d/ (head)

/s/ /long O/ (sew)

/voiced th/ /short E/ /n/ (then)

/m/ /long A/ /d/ (made)

15. Blending sounds to form a monosyllabic word beginning with a noncontinuant sound.

What to say to the student: "We'll put sounds together to make words."

EXAMPLE "Put these sounds together to make a word: / / + / / + / /." (stimulus sounds) (e.g., /b/ /short E/ /d/) (bed)

NOTE: *Give the letter sound, not the letter name. Use pictured items and/or manipulatives if necessary. Use any of the following stimulus words and/or others you select from the story. The correct answers are in parentheses.*

Stimulus items:

/b/ /long I/ (by)

/t/ /long I/ /m/ (time)

/k/ /long E/ /p/ (keep)

/t/ /oo/ (to)

/b/ /short U/ /t/ (but)

/d/ /long O/ /n/ /t/ (don't)

/dz/ (as the first sound in jelly) /short U/ /m/ /p/ (jump)

/d/ /ah/ /l/ (doll)

/b/ /ew/ (as in wood) /k/ (book)

/d/ /oo/ (do)

16. Substituting the initial sound in words.

What to say to the student: "We're going to change beginning/first sounds in words."

> **EXAMPLE** "Say '_____.'" (stimulus word) "Instead of / /" (stimulus sound), "say / /." (stimulus sound) (e.g., "Say 'bed.' Instead of /b/, say /r/. What's your new word?") (red)

> **NOTE:** *Give the letter sound, not the letter name. Use pictured items and/or manipulatives if necessary. Use any of the following stimulus words and/or others you select from the story. The correct answers are in parentheses.*

Stimulus items:

"Say 'time.' Instead of /t/, say /l/." (lime)

"Say 'jump.' Instead of /dz/ (as in jelly), say /b/." (bump)

"Say 'madre.' Instead of /m/, say /p/." (padre)

"Say 'sang.' Instead of /s/, say /r/." (rang)

"Say 'will.' Instead of /w/, say /m/." (mill)

"Say 'matters.' Instead of /m/, say /b/." (batters)

"Say 'that.' Instead of /voiced th/, say /p/." (pat)

"Say 'funny.' Instead of /f/, say /m/." (money)

"Say 'great.' Instead of /g/, say /t/." (trait)

"Say 'dresses.' Instead of /d/, say /p/." (presses)

17. Substituting the final sound in words.

What to say to the student: "We're going to change ending/last sounds in words."

> **EXAMPLE** "Say '_____.'" (stimulus word) "Instead of / /" (stimulus sound), "say / /." (stimulus sound) (e.g., "Say 'bed.' Instead of /d/, say /t/. What's your new word?") (bet)

> **NOTE:** *Give the letter sound, not the letter name. Use pictured items and/or manipulatives if necessary. Use any of the following stimulus words and/or others you select from the story. The correct answers are in parentheses.*

Stimulus items:

"Say 'me.' Instead of /long E/, say /long I/." (my)

"Say 'gathered.' Instead of /d/, say /z/." (gathers)

"Say 'same.' Instead of /m/, say /v/." (save)

"Say 'pictures.' Instead of /z/, say /d/." (pictured)

"Say 'was.' Instead of /z/, say /n/." (one)

"Say 'squash.' Instead of /sh/, say /t/." (squat)

"Say 'mamá.' Instead of /ah/, say /long E/." (mommy)

"Say 'to.' Instead of /oo/, say /long E/." (tea)

"Say 'have.' Instead of /v/, say /t/." (hat)

"Say 'flowers.' Instead of /z/, say /d/." (flowered)

18. Segmenting the middle sound in monosyllabic words.

What to say to the student: "Tell me the middle sound in the word I say."

> **EXAMPLE** "What's the middle sound in the word '_____'?" (stimulus word) (e.g., "What's the middle sound in the word 'was'?") (/short U/)

> **NOTE:** *Give the letter sound, not the letter name. Use pictured items and/or manipulatives if necessary. Use any of the following stimulus words and/or others you select from the story. The correct answers are in parentheses.*

Stimulus items:

but (/short U/)

that (/short A/)

bed (/short E/)

what (/short U/)

book (/ew/ as in wood)

time (/long I/)

same (/long A/)

says (/short E/)

will (/short I/)

have (/short A/)

19. Substituting the middle sound in words.

What to say to the student: "We're going to change the middle sound in words."

> **EXAMPLE** "Say '_____.'" (stimulus word) "Instead of / /" (stimulus sound), "say / /." (stimulus sound) (e.g., "Say 'bed.' Instead of /short E/, say /short I/. What's your new word?") (bid)

NOTE: *Give the letter sound, not the letter name. Use pictured items and/or manipulatives if necessary. Use any of the following stimulus words and/or others you select from the story. The correct answers are in parentheses.*

Stimulus items:

"Say 'but.' Instead of /short U/, say /short E/." (bet)

"Say 'time.' Instead of /long I/, say /long E/." (team)

"Say 'doll.' Instead of /ah/, say /short I/." (dill)

"Say 'same.' Instead of /long A/, say /long E/." (seem)

"Say 'book.' Instead of /ew/ (as in wood), say /long I/." (bike)

"Say 'these.' Instead of /long E/, say /long O/." (those)

"Say 'love.' Instead of /short U/, say /long E/." (leave)

"Say 'will.' Instead of /short I/, say /ew/ (as in wood)." (wool)

"Say 'was.' Instead of /short U/, say /short I/." (wiz)

"Say 'freely.' Instead of /long E/, say /short I/." (frilly)

20. Identifying all sounds in monosyllabic words.

What to say to the student: "Now tell me all the sounds you hear in the word I say."

> **EXAMPLE**   "What sounds do you hear in the word '_____'?" (stimulus word) (e.g., "What sounds do you hear in the word 'bed'?") (/b/ /short E/ /d/)

NOTE: *Give the letter sound, not the letter name. Use pictured items and/or manipulatives if necessary. Use any of the following stimulus words and/or others you select from the story. The correct answers are in parentheses.*

Stimulus items:

but (/b/ /short U/ /t/)

doll (/d/ /ah/ /l/)

time (/t/ /long I/ /m/)

great (/g/ /r/ /long A/ /t/)

sew (/s/ /long O/)

same (/s/ /long A/ /m/)

jump (/dz/ (as in jelly) /short U/ /m/ /p/)

washed (/w/ /ah/ /sh/ /t/)

squash (/s/ /k/ /w/ /ah/ /sh/)

don't (/d/ /long O/ /n/ /t/)

21. Deleting sounds within words.

What to say to the student: "We're going to leave out sounds in words."

> **EXAMPLE**   "Say '_____'" (stimulus word) "without / /." (stimulus sound) (e.g., "Say 'pretty' without /r /.") (pitty) Say: "The word that is left—'pitty'—is a real word. Sometimes, the word won't be a real word."

NOTE: *Give the letter sound, not the letter name. Use pictured items and/or manipulatives if necessary. Use any of the following stimulus words and/or others you select from the story. The correct answers are in parentheses.*

Stimulus items:

"Say 'don't' without /n/." (dote)
"Say 'great' without /r/." (gate)
"Say 'washed' without /sh/." (watt)
"Say 'pictures' without /k/." (pitchers)
"Say 'grandmother's' without /m/." (grandother's)
"Say 'dress' without /r/." (dess)
"Say 'lullaby' without /b/." (lulla-eye)
"Say 'squash' without /k/." (swash)
"Say 'squash' without /w/." (skahsh)
"Say 'flowers' without /l/." (fowers)

22. Substituting consonants in words having a two-sound cluster.

What to say to the student: "We're going to substitute sounds in words."

> EXAMPLE "Say '_____.'" (stimulus word) "Instead of / /" (stimulus sound), "say / /." (stimulus sound) (e.g., "Say 'tree.' Instead of /t/, say /f/.") (free) Say: "Sometimes, the new word will be a made-up word."

NOTE: *Give the letter sound, not the letter name. Use pictured items and/or manipulatives if necessary. Use any of the following stimulus words and/or others you select from the story. The correct answers are in parentheses.*

Stimulus items:

"Say 'dress.' Instead of /d/, say /p/." (press)
"Say 'great.' Instead of /g/, say /f/." (freight)
"Say 'great.' Instead of /g/, say /t/." (trait)
"Say 'great.' Instead of /g/, say /k/." (crate)
"Say 'grandmother.' Instead of /r/, say /l/." (glandmother)
"Say 'freely.' Instead of /f/, say /k/." (kreelie)
"Say 'dresses.' Instead of /d/, say /p/." (presses)
"Say 'flowers.' Instead of /f/, say /k/." (clowers)
"Say 'little.' Instead of /t/, say /b/." (libble)
"Say 'gathered.' Instead of /d/, say /z/." (gathers)

23. Phoneme reversing.

What to say to the student: "We're going to say words backward."

> EXAMPLE "Say the word '_____'" (stimulus word) "backward." (e.g., "Say 'bed' backward.") (deb)

NOTE: *This is a difficult phoneme-level task and should only be done with older students. Give the letter sound, not the letter name. Use pictured items and/or manipulatives if necessary. Use any of the following stimulus words and/or others you select from the story. The correct answers are in parentheses.*

Stimulus items:

but (tub)

eat (tea)

these (zeethe)

my (I'm)

time (might)

made (dame)

love (vull)

doll (laud)

same (mace)

squash (shawks)

24. Phoneme switching.

What to say to the student: "We're going to switch the first sounds in two words."

> **EXAMPLE** "Switch the first sounds in '_____' and '_____.'" (stimulus words) (e.g., "Switch the first sounds in 'to' and 'my.'") (moo tie)

NOTE: *This is a difficult phoneme-level task and should only be done with older students. Give the letter sound, not the letter name. Use pictured items and/or manipulatives if necessary. Use any of the following stimulus words and/or others you select from the story. The correct answers are in parentheses.*

Stimulus items:

my doll (dye mall)

for my (more fye)

tortillas for (fortillas tor)

the same (suh thame)

but different (dut bifferent)

to sew (sue toe)

for me (more fee)

dress for (fress door)

sitting down (ditting soun)

to do (do to)

25. Pig Latin.

What to say to the student: "We're going to speak a secret language by using words from the story. In pig Latin, you take off the first sound of a word, put it at the end of the word, and add an 'ay' sound."

EXAMPLE "Say 'bed' in pig Latin." (edbay)

NOTE: *This is a difficult phoneme-level task and should only be done with older students. Use pictured items and/or manipulatives if necessary. Use any of the following stimulus words and/or others you select from the story. The correct answers are in parentheses.*

Stimulus items:

book (ookbay)

casa (asacay)

made (ademay)

dresses (ressesday)

tortillas (ortillastay)

given (ivengay)

love (ovelay)

little (ittlelay)

para (arapay)

grandmother (randmothergay)

From Phonological Awareness into Print

NOTE: *Only five examples per activity are included in this resource due to space. You are encouraged to add many more words into this section that you feel your student(s) is(are) ready to write.*

1. Substituting the initial sound or letter in words.

NOTE: *Use lined paper or copy the sheet of lined paper included in the back of this book.*

Stimulus items:

1.1 to/do

Task a. "Say 'to.' Instead of /t/, say /d/. What's your new word?" (do) "Write/copy 'to' and 'do.'"

Task b. "Circle the **letters** that make the words different." ([t], [d])

Task c. "What **sounds** do these letters make?" (/t/, /d/)

1.2 but/rut

Task a. "Say 'but.' Instead of /b/, say /r/. What's your new word?" (rut) "Write/copy 'but' and 'rut.'"

Task b. "Circle the **letters** that make the words different." ([b], [r])

Task c. "What **sounds** do these letters make?" (/b/, /r/)

1.3 sang/rang

Task a. "Say 'sang.' Instead of /s/, say /r/. What's your new word?" (rang) "Write/copy 'sang' and 'rang.'"

Task b. "Circle the **letters** that make the words different." ([s], [r])

Task c. "What **sounds** do these letters make?" (/s/, /r/)

1.4 house/mouse

    Task a. "Say 'house.' Instead of /h/, say /m/. What's your new word?" (mouse) "Write/ copy 'house' and 'mouse.'"

    Task b. "Circle the **letters** that make the words different." ([h], [m])

    Task c. "What **sounds** do these letters make?" (/h/, /m/)

1.5 matters/batters

    Task a. "Say 'matters.' Instead of /m/, say /b/. What's your new word?" (batters) "Write/copy 'matters' and 'batters.'"

    Task b. "Circle the **letters** that make the words different." ([m], [b])

    Task c. "What **sounds** do these letters make?" (/m/, /b/)

2. Substituting the final sound or letter in words.

    NOTE: *Use lined paper or copy the sheet of lined paper included in the back of this book.*

Stimulus items:

2.1 bed/bet

    Task a. "Say 'bed.' Instead of /d/, say /t/. What's your new word?" (bet) "Write/copy 'bed' and 'bet.'"

    Task b. "Circle the **letters** that make the words different." ([d], [t])

    Task c. "What **sounds** do these letters make?" (/d/, /t/)

2.2 hush/hut

    Task a. "Say 'hush.' Instead of /sh/, say /t/. What's your new word?" (hut) "Write/ copy 'hush' and 'hut.'"

    Task b. "Circle the **letters** that make the words different." ([s], [h], [t])

    Task c. "What **sounds** do these letters make?" (/sh/, /t/)

2.3 have/had

    Task a. "Say 'have.' Instead of /v/, say /d/. What's your new word?" (had) "Write/copy 'have' and 'had.'"

    Task b. "Circle the **letters** that make the words different." ([v], [e], [d])

    Task c. "What **sounds** do these letters make?" (/v/, /d/)

2.4 pictures/pictured

    Task a. "Say 'pictures.' Instead of /z/, say /d/. What's your new word?" (pictured) "Write/copy 'pictures' and 'pictured.'"

    Task b. "Circle the **letters** that make the words different." ([s], [d])

    Task c. "What **sounds** do these letters make?" (/z/, /d/)

2.5 by/be

    Task a. "Say 'by.' Instead of /long I/, say /long E/. What's your new word?" (be) "Write/copy 'by' and 'be.'"

    Task b. "Circle the **letters** that make the words different." ([y], [e])

    Task c. "What **sounds** do these letters make?" (/long I/, /long E/)

3. Substituting the middle sound or letter in words.

NOTE: *Use lined paper or copy the sheet of lined paper included in the back of this book.*

Stimulus items:

3.1 but/bit

Task a. "Say 'but.' Instead of /short U/, say /short I/. What's your new word?" (bit) "Write/copy 'but' and 'bit.'"

Task b. "Circle the **letters** that make the words different." ([u], [i])

Task c. "What **sounds** do these letters make?" (/short U/, /short I/)

3.2 bed/bid

Task a. "Say 'bed.' Instead of /short E/, say /short I/. What's your new word?" (bid) "Write/copy 'bed' and 'bid.'"

Task b. "Circle the **letters** that make the words different." ([e], [i])

Task c. "What **sounds** do these letters make?" (/short E/, /short I/)

3.3 doll/dull

Task a. "Say 'doll.' Instead of /ah/, say /long U/. What's your new word?" (dull) "Write/copy 'doll' and 'dull.'"

Task b. "Circle the **letters** that make the words different." ([o], [u])

Task c. "What **sounds** do these letters make?" (/ah/, /short U/)

3.4 head/hid

Task a. "Say 'head.' Instead of /short E/, say /short I/. What's your new word?" (hid) "Write/copy 'head' and 'hid.'"

Task b. "Circle the **letters** that make the words different." ([e], [a], [i])

Task c. "What **sounds** do these letters make?" (/short E/, /short I/)

3.5 made/mid

Task a. "Say 'made.' Instead of /long A/, say /short I/. What's your new word?" (mid) "Write/copy 'made' and 'mid.'"

Task b. "Circle the **letters** that make the words different." ([a], [e], [i])

Task c. "What **sounds** do these letters make?" (/long A/, /short I/)

4. Supplying the initial sound or letter in words.

NOTE: *Use lined paper or copy the sheet of lined paper included in the back of this book.*

Stimulus items:

4.1 for/or

Task a. "Say 'for,' say 'or.' What sound did you hear in 'for' that is missing in 'or'?" (/f/) "Now we'll change the **letter**. Write/copy 'for' and 'or.'"

Task b. "Circle the beginning **letter** that makes the words different." ([f])

Task c. "What **sound** does this letter make?" (/f/)

4.2 will/ill

Task a. "Say 'will,' say 'ill.' What sound did you hear in 'will' that is missing in 'ill'?" (/w/) "Now we'll change the **letter.** Write/copy 'will' and 'ill.'"

Task b. "Circle the beginning **letter** that makes the words different." ([w])

Task c. "What **sound** does this letter make?" (/w/)

4.3 that/at

Task a. "Say 'that,' say 'at.' What sound did you hear in 'that' that is missing in 'at'?" (/voiced th/) "Now we'll change the **letters.** Write/copy 'that' and 'at.'"

Task b. "Circle the beginning **letters** that make the words different." ([t], [h])

Task c. "What **sound** do these letters make?" (/voiced th/)

4.4 about/bout

Task a. "Say 'about,' say 'bout.' What sound did you hear in 'about' that is missing in 'bout'?" (/short U/) "Now we'll change the **letter.** Write/copy 'about' and 'bout.'"

Task b. "Circle the beginning **letter** that makes the words different." ([a])

Task c. "What **sound** does this letter make?" (/short U/)

4.5 made/ade

Task a. "Say 'made,' say 'ade.' What sound did you hear in 'made' that is missing in 'ade'?" (/m/) "Now we'll change the **letter.** Write/copy 'made' and 'ade.'"

Task b. "Circle the beginning **letter** that makes the words different." ([m])

Task c. "What **sound** does this letter make?" (/m/)

5. Supplying the final sound or letter in words.

NOTE: *Use lined paper or copy the sheet of lined paper included in the back of this book.*

Stimulus items:

5.1 tortillas/tortilla

Task a. "Say 'tortillas,' say 'tortilla.' What sound did you hear in 'tortillas' that is missing in 'tortilla'?" (/s/) "Now we'll change the **letter.** Write/copy 'tortillas' and 'tortilla.'"

Task b. "Circle the ending/last **letter** that makes the words different." ([s])

Task c. "What **sound** does this letter make?" (/s/)

5.2 and/an

Task a. "Say 'and,' say 'an.' What sound did you hear in 'and' that is missing in 'an'?" (/d/) "Now we'll change the **letter.** Write/copy 'and' and 'an.'"

Task b. "Circle the ending/last **letter** that makes the words different." ([d])

Task c. "What **sound** does this letter make?" (/d/)

5.3 gathered/gather

Task a. "Say 'gathered,' say 'gather.' What sound did you hear in 'gathered' that is missing in 'gather'?" (/d/) "Now we'll change the **letters.** Write/copy 'gathered' and 'gather.'"

Task b. "Circle the ending/last **letters** that make the words different." ([e], [d])

Task c. "What **sound** do these letters make?" (/d/)

5.4 mother's/mother

Task a. "Say 'mother's,' say 'mother.' What sound did you hear in 'mother's' that is missing in 'mother'?" (/z/) "Now we'll change the **letter**. Write/copy 'mother's' and 'mother.'"

Task b. "Circle the ending/last **letter** that makes the word different." (['s])

Task c. "What **sound** does this letter make?" (/z/)

5.5 washed/wash

Task a. "Say 'washed,' say 'wash.' What sound did you hear in 'washed' that is missing in 'wash'?" (/t/) "Now we'll change the **letters**. Write/copy 'washed' and 'wash.'"

Task b. "Circle the ending/last **letters** that make the words different." ([e], [d])

Task c. "What **sound** do these letters make?" (/t/)

6. Switching the first sound and letter in words (ADVANCED).

NOTE: *Use lined paper or copy the sheet of lined paper included in the back of this book.*

Stimulus items:

6.1 to do

Task a. "Say 'to,' say 'do.' What sound do you hear at the beginning of 'to'?" (/t/) "What sound do you hear at the beginning of 'do'?" (/d/) "Switch the first sounds in those words." (do to) "Now we'll change the **letters**. Write/copy 'to do' and 'do to.'"

Task b. "Circle the beginning **letters** that change the words." ([t], [d])

Task c. "What **sounds** do those letters make?" (/t/, /d/)

6.2 mother sang

Task a. "Say 'mother,' say 'sang.' What sound do you hear at the beginning of 'mother'?" (/m/) "What sound do you hear at the beginning of 'sang'?" (/s/) "Switch the first sounds in those words." (sother mang) "Now we'll change the **letters**. Write/copy 'mother sang' and 'sother mang.'"

Task b. "Circle the beginning **letters** that change the words." ([m], [s])

Task c. "What **sounds** do those letters make?" (/m/, /s/)

6.3 funny little

Task a. "Say 'funny,' say 'little.' What sound do you hear at the beginning of 'funny'?" (/f/) "What sound do you hear at the beginning of 'little'?" (/l/) "Switch the first sounds in those words." (lunny fittle) "Now we'll change the **letters**. Write/copy 'funny little' and 'lunny fittle.'"

Task b. "Circle the beginning **letters** that change the words." ([f], [l])

Task c. "What **sounds** do those letters make?" (/f/, /l/)

6.4 don't jump

Task a. "Say 'don't,' say 'jump.' What sound do you hear at the beginning of 'don't'?" (/d/) "What sound do you hear at the beginning of 'jump'?" (/dz/ as in jelly) "Switch the first sounds in those words." (jon't dump) "Now we'll change the **letters.** Write/copy 'don't jump' and 'jon't dump.'"

Task b. "Circle the beginning **letters** that change the words." ([d], [j])

Task c. "What **sounds** do those letters make?" (/d/, /dz/ as in jelly)

6.5 same but

Task a. "Say 'same,' say 'but.' What sound do you hear at the beginning of 'same'?" (/s/) "What sound do you hear at the beginning of 'but'?" (/b/) "Switch the first sounds in those words." (bame sut) "Now we'll change the **letters.** Write/copy 'same but' and 'bame sut.'"

Task b. "Circle the beginning **letters** that change the words." ([s], [b])

Task c. "What **sounds** do those letters make?" (/s/, /b/)

CHAPTER 14

Phonological Awareness Activities to Use with *The Three Little Pigs*

Text version used for selection of stimulus items:

Zemach, M. (2002). *The Three Little Pigs.* In *Open Court Readers Level 1 Book 2.* Columbus, Ohio: McGraw-Hill.

Phonological Awareness Activities at the Word Level

1. Counting words.

What to say to the student: "We're going to count words."

> **EXAMPLE** "How many words do you hear in this sentence (or phrase): 'three pigs'?" (2)

> **NOTE:** *Use pictured items and/or manipulatives if necessary. Use any of the following stimulus phrases or sentences and/or others you select from the story. The correct answers are in parentheses.*

Stimulus items:

momma pig (2)

little pig (2)

first little pig (3)

load of sticks (3)

Build me a house. (4)

right down the road (4)

I'll blow your house down. (5)

He huffed and he puffed. (5)

No, I won't let you in. (6)

This made the wolf very angry. (6)

2. Identifying the missing word from a list.

What to say to the student: "Listen to the words I say. I'll say them again. You tell me which word I leave out."

> **EXAMPLE** "Listen to the words I say: 'pig,' 'third,' 'yum.' I'll say them again. Tell me which one I leave out: 'pig,' 'third.'" (yum)

> **NOTE:** *Use pictured items and/or manipulatives if necessary. Use any of the following stimulus words and/or others you select from the story. The correct answers are in parentheses.*

Stimulus set #1	Stimulus set #2
chimney, pig	pig (chimney)
wolf, sticks, meadow	wolf, meadow (sticks)
huff, tomorrow, apple	tomorrow, apple (huff)
barrel, riding, three	barrel, three (riding)
straight, gathering, together	straight, gathering (together)
knocking, momma, angrier	momma, angrier (knocking)
turnips, hurried, puff	turnips, puff (hurried)
basket, himself, roared	basket, himself (roared)
three, cooking, houses	cooking, houses (three)
going, please, banging	going, banging (please)

3. Identifying the missing word in a phrase or sentence.

What to say to the student: "Listen to the sentence I read. Tell me which word is missing the second time I read the sentence."

> **EXAMPLE** "'three little pigs.' Listen again and tell me which word I leave out: 'three _____ pigs.'" (little)

> **NOTE:** *Use pictured items and/or manipulatives if necessary. Use any of the following stimulus sentences and/or others you select from the story. The correct answers are in parentheses.*

Stimulus items:

first little pig. first little _____. (pig)

Give me some straw. Give me some _____. (straw)

Build good, strong houses. Build good, _____ houses. (strong)

Now goodbye my sons, goodbye. Now goodbye my _____, goodbye. (sons)

I'll blow your house down. I'll blow your _____ down. (house)

No, no I won't let you in. No, no I _____ let you in. (won't)

"Right down the road" said the wolf. "Right down the _____" said the wolf. (road)

Long ago there lived three little pigs. Long ago there _____ three little pigs. (lived)

Not by the hair of my chinny-chin-chin. Not by the _____ of my chinny-chin-chin. (hair)

So the man gave him some bricks. So the man gave him _____ bricks. (some)

4. Supplying the missing word as an adult reads.

What to say to the student: "I want you to help me read the story. You fill in the words I leave out."

> **EXAMPLE** "little _____." (pig)

> **NOTE:** *Use pictured items and/or manipulatives if necessary. Use any of the following stimulus sentences and/or others you select from the story. The correct answers are in parentheses.*

Stimulus items:

Go into the _____. (world)

Build good, strong _____. (houses)

built a house of _____. (sticks, straw, bricks)

the big _____ wolf. (bad)

He huffed and he _____. (puffed)

a _____ of turnips. (field)

He blew the house _____. (down)

"I'll come for you at ten _____." (o'clock)

I know where there's an apple _____. (tree)

"I've had enough of your _____." (tricks)

5. Rearranging words.

What to say to the student: "I'll say some words out of order. You put them in the right order so they make sense."

> **EXAMPLE** " 'pigs three.' Put those words in the right order." (three pigs)

> **NOTE:** *Use pictured items and/or manipulatives if necessary. Use any of the following stimulus words and/or others you select from the story. The correct answers are in parentheses. This word-level activity can be more difficult than some of the syllable- or phoneme-level activities because of the memory load. If your students are only able to deal with two or three words to be rearranged, add more two- and three-word samples from the story and omit the four-word level items.*

Stimulus items:

soup wolf for supper (wolf soup for supper)

he fell into the soup of pot. (He fell into the pot of soup.)

little up got pig (little pig got up)

this made the angry really wolf. (This made the wolf really angry.)

I got myself a turnips of basket. (I got myself a basket of turnips.)

himself built a house good, strong (built himself a good, strong house)

he met a man a load with of sticks. (He met a man with a load of sticks.)

he huffed and puffed and down the blew house. (He huffed and puffed and blew the house down.)

not by the hair of chinny-chin-chin my. (Not by the hair of my chinny-chin-chin.)

momma told them to out into the go world. (Momma told them to go out into the world.)

Phonological Awareness Activities at the Syllable Level

1. Syllable counting.

What to say to the student: "We're going to count syllables (or parts) of words."

> **EXAMPLE** "How many syllables do you hear in '_____'?" (stimulus word) (e.g., "How many do you hear syllables in 'pig'?") (1)

> **NOTE:** *Use pictured items and/or manipulatives if necessary. Use any of the following stimulus words and/or others you select from the story. Use any group of 10 stimulus items you select per teaching set.*

Stimulus items:

One-syllable words: pig, pigs, please, puff, pot, build, built, but, by, blow, blew, bricks, back, big, told, time, ten, tree, tricks, day, door, down, came, come, go, good, give, got, chin, just, met, man, me, made, much, now, no, not, know, next, nine, nice, night, strong, sons, straw, sir, some, sticks, safe, saw, straight, soup, see, first, field, fair, fell, house, who, hair, huff, hide, hill, right, road, roof, long, let, load, when, watch, wolf, one, won't, well, where, three, third, threw, their, them, then, this, that, your, yum, you, up

Two-syllable words: basket, barrel, banging, before, turnips, toward, cooking, goodbye, going, chimney, momma, morning, meadow, knocking, supper, faster, himself, hurried, little, world, angry, enough, o'clock, along, across, until, apple

Three-syllable words: tomorrow, together, gathering, angrier, already

2. Initial syllable deleting.

What to say to the student: "We're going to leave out syllables (or parts of words)."

> **EXAMPLE** "Say '_____.'" (stimulus word) "Say it again without '_____.'" (stimulus syllable) (e.g., "Say 'until.' Say it again without 'un.'") (til)

> **NOTE:** *Use pictured items and/or manipulatives if necessary. Use any of the following stimulus words and/or others you select from the story. The correct answers are in parentheses.*

Stimulus items:

"Say 'goodbye' without 'good.'" (bye)

"Say 'himself' without 'him.'" (self)

"Say 'supper' without 'sup.'" (-er)

"Say 'knocking' without 'knock.'" (-ing)

"Say 'already' without 'all.'" (ready)

"Say 'meadow' without 'med.'" (oh)

"Say 'chimney' without 'chim.'" (knee)

"Say 'tomorrow' without 'to.'" (morrow)

"Say 'basket' without 'bass.'" (ket)

"Say 'together' without 'to.'" (gether)

3. Final syllable deleting.

What to say to the student: "We're going to leave out syllables (or parts of words)."

> **EXAMPLE** "Say '_____.'" (stimulus word) "Say it again without '_____.'"
> (stimulus syllable) (e.g., "Say 'before' without 'fore.'") (be)

> **NOTE:** *Use pictured items and/or manipulatives if necessary. Use any of the following stimulus words and/or others you select from the story. The correct answers are in parentheses.*

Stimulus items:

"Say 'toward' without 'ward.'" (to)

"Say 'riding' without 'ing.'" (ride)

"Say 'hurried' without 'eed.'" (her)

"Say 'cooking' without 'ing.'" (cook)

"Say 'gathering' without 'ing.'" (gather)

"Say 'angry' without 'ree.'" (ang)

"Say 'turnips' without 'ips." (turn)

"Say 'supper' without '-er.'" (sup)

"Say 'chimney' without 'knee.'" (chim)

"Say 'goodbye' without 'bye.'" (good)

4. Initial syllable adding.

What to say to the student: "Now let's add syllables (or parts) to words."

> **EXAMPLE** "Add '_____'" (stimulus syllable) "to the beginning of '_____.'"
> (stimulus syllable) (e.g., "Add 'good' to the beginning of 'bye.'") (goodbye)

> **NOTE:** *Use pictured items and/or manipulatives if necessary. Use any of the following stimulus words and/or others you select from the story. The correct answers are in parentheses.*

Stimulus items:

"Add 'chim' to the beginning of 'knee.'" (chimney)

"Add 'ma' to the beginning of '-muh.'" (momma)

"Add 'all' to the beginning of 'ready.'" (already)

"Add 'him' to the beginning of 'self.'" (himself)

"Add 'knock' to the beginning of '-ing.'" (knocking)

"Add 'seck' to the beginning of '-und.'" (second)

"Add 'to' to the beginning of 'morrow.'" (tomorrow)

"Add 'morn' to the beginning of '-ing.'" (morning)

"Add 'to' to the beginning of 'gether.'" (together)

"Add 'bare' to the beginning of '-ul.'" (barrel)

5. Final syllable adding.

What to say to the student: "Now let's add syllables (or parts) to words."

> **EXAMPLE** "Add '_____'" (stimulus syllable) "to the end of '_____.'" (stimulus syllable) (e.g., "Add 'ree' to the end of 'ang.'") (angry)

NOTE: *Use pictured items and/or manipulatives if necessary. Use any of the following stimulus words and/or others you select from the story. The correct answers are in parentheses.*

Stimulus items:

"Add '-er' to the end of 'angry.'" (angrier)

"Add 'fore' to the end of 'be.'" (before)

"Add '-ing' to the end of 'bang.'" (banging)

"Add 'knee' to the end of 'chim.'" (chimney)

"Add 'to' to the end of 'in.'" (into)

"Add 'ward' to the end of 'to.'" (toward)

"Add 'knee' to the end of 'chin.'" (chinny)

"Add '-ing' to the end of 'go.'" (going)

"Add '-er' to the end of 'sup.'" (supper)

"Add '-ing' to the end of 'gather.'" (gathering)

6. Syllable substituting.

What to say to the student: "Let's make up some new words."

> **EXAMPLE** "Say '_____.'" (stimulus word) "Instead of '_____'" (stimulus syllable), "say '_____.'" (stimulus syllable) (e.g., "Say 'jumper.' Instead of 'jump,' say 'camp.' The new word is 'camper.'")

NOTE: *Use pictured items and/or manipulatives if necessary. Use of the following stimulus words and/or others you select from the story. The correct answers are in parentheses.*

Stimulus items:

"Say 'banging.' Instead of 'bang,' say 'cook.'" (cooking)

"Say 'himself.' Instead of 'him,' say 'her.'" (herself)

"Say 'chimney.' Instead of 'chim,' say 'chin.'" (chinny)

"Say 'angrier.' Instead of 'er,' say 'est'.'" (angriest)

"Say 'going.' Instead of 'go,' say 'do.'" (doing)

"Say 'turnip.' Instead of 'ip,' say 'ing.'" (turning)

"Say 'seven.' Instead of 'sev,' say 'hev.'" (heaven)

"Say 'basket.' Instead of '-et,' say '-ing.'" (basking)

"Say 'couldn't.' Instead of 'could,' say 'would.'" (wouldn't)

"Say 'angry.' Instead of '-ree,' say '-er.'" (anger)

Phonological Awareness Activities at the Phoneme Level

1. Counting sounds.

What to say to the student: "We're going to count sounds in words."

> **EXAMPLE** "How many sounds do you hear in this word: 'pig'?" (3)

> **NOTE:** *Use pictured items and/or manipulatives if necessary. Use any of the following stimulus words and/or others you select from the story. Be sure to give the letter sound and not the letter name. Use any group of 10 stimulus items you select per teaching set.*

Stimulus words with two sounds: by, day, go, me, now, no, sir, see, saw, who, you, up, I'll

Stimulus words with three sounds: pig, puff, but, blow, blew, back, big, time, ten, tree, down, came, good, give, got, chin, met, man, made, much, knock, not, nine, nice, night, some, soup, fell, house, huff, puff, hide, hill, right, road, roof, let, load, when, three, third, threw, then, than, that, apple

Stimulus words with four sounds: pigs, please, puffed, build, told, called, cooked, chinny, just, momma, meadow, sons, straw, supper, first, field, rolled, little, leaped, wolf, won't

Stimulus words with five sounds: bricks, turnip, tricks, chimney, jumped, next, sticks, straight, faster

2. Sound categorization or identifying a rhyme oddity.

What to say to the student: "Guess which word I say doesn't rhyme with the other three words."

> **EXAMPLE** "Tell me which word doesn't rhyme with the other three words: '_____,' '_____,' '_____,' '_____.'" (stimulus words) (e.g., "'pig,' 'rig,' 'world,' 'fig.' Which word doesn't rhyme?") (world)

> **NOTE:** *Use pictured items if necessary. Use any of the following stimulus words and/or others you select from the story. The correct answers are in parentheses.*

Stimulus items:

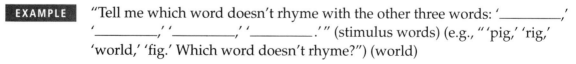

strong, wrong, hurried, song (hurried)

bricks, sticks, ticks, chimney (chimney)

gathering, tree, free, three (gathering)

yum, blow, thumb, tum (blow)

straight, crate, second, freight (second)

chin, fin, tomorrow, grin (tomorrow)

road, toad, sewed, basket (basket)

wolf, straw, caw, raw (wolf)

soup, morning, loop, hoop (morning)

leaped, pigs, cheeped, peeped (pigs)

3. Matching rhyme.

What to say to the student: "We're going to think of rhyming words."

> **EXAMPLE** "Which word rhymes with '_____'?" (stimulus word) (e.g., "Which word rhymes with 'pig': 'seven,' 'three,' 'big,' 'blew'?") (big)

NOTE: *Use pictured items if necessary. Use any of the following stimulus words and/or others you select from the story. The correct answers are in parentheses.*

Stimulus items:

down: chimney, puffed, pigs, town (town)

chin: together, barrel, fin, turnips (fin)

strong: wrong, straight, huffed, gathering (wrong)

three: apples, turnips, meadow, tree (tree)

bricks: momma, jumped, tricks, chimney (tricks)

soup: leaped, hoop, turnip, tomorrow (hoop)

yum: banging, thumb, goodbye, meadow (thumb)

little: brittle, puffed, hurried, knocking (brittle)

banging: wolf, pigs, hanging, supper (hanging)

ate: barrel, tomorrow, chimney, gate (gate)

4. Producing rhyme.

What to say to the student: "Now we'll say rhyming words."

> **EXAMPLE** "Tell me a word that rhymes with '_____.'" (stimulus word) (e.g., "Tell me a word that rhymes with 'pig.' You can make up a word if you want.") (fig)

NOTE: *Use pictured items if necessary. Use any of the following stimulus words and/or others you select from the story (i.e., you say a word from the list below and the student is to think of a rhyming word). Use any group of 10 stimulus items you select per teaching set.*

Stimulus items:

/p/: pigs, pig, please, puff, pot, puffed

/b/: build, built, but, by, blow, blew, bricks, back, basket, big, barrel, banging, before

/t/: told, time, turnips, ten, tomorrow, together, tree, toward, tricks

/d/: day, door, down, didn't

/k/: came, come, couldn't, cooking, called, cooked, climbed

/g/: go, good, goodbye, going, gathering, give, got

/ch/: chin, chinny, chimney

/dz/ (as in gem): just, jumped

/m/: momma, met, man, me, made, morning, meadow, much

/n/: now, knocking, no, not, know, next, nine, nice, night

/s/: strong, sons, straw, sir, some, second, sticks, safe, seven, saw, straight, soup, see, saw, supper

/f/: first, field, fair, fell, faster

/v/: very

/h/: happily, house, houses, who, himself, hair, huff, huffed, hurried, hide, hill

/r/: right, road, rolled, riding, roared, roof

/l/: long, little, lived, let, load, leaped

/w/, /wh/: when, world, watch, wolf, one, won't, well, where, we'll

/voiceless th/: three, third, threw

/voiced th/: their, them, then, this, there's, than, that

/y/ (as in yellow): your, yum, you

/short A/: asked, apple

/short U/: along, up, across, until

/long A/: ate

/long E/: enough

/long I/: I, I'll

/ah/: already

5. Sound matching (initial).

What to say to the student: "Now we'll listen for the first sound in words."

> **EXAMPLE** "Listen to this sound: / /." (stimulus sound). "Guess which word I say begins with that sound: '_____,' '_____,' '_____,' '_____.'" (stimulus words) (e.g., "Listen to this sound: /w/. Guess which word I say begins with that sound: 'pig,' 'basket,' 'already,' 'wolf.'") (wolf)

NOTE: *Give the letter sound, not the letter name. Use pictured items if necessary. Use any of the following stimulus words and/or others you select from the story. The correct answers are in parentheses.*

Stimulus items:

/short A/: turnips, apple, together, momma (apple)

/s/: roared, chimney, sticks, tomorrow (sticks)

/m/: straw, huffed, gathering, meadow (meadow)

/b/: supper, barrel, straight, lived (barrel)

/h/: already, turnips, huffed, goodbye (huffed)

/voiceless th/: banging, three, faster, couldn't (three)

/n/: knocking, chinny, wolf, himself (knocking)

/f/: jumped, hurried, first, bricks (first)

/t/: houses, straight, turnips, cooking (turnips)

/dz/ (as in gem): tomorrow, leaped, jumped, puffed (jumped)

6. Sound matching (final).

What to say to the student: "Now we'll listen for the last sound in words."

> **EXAMPLE** "Listen to this sound: / /." (stimulus sound) "Guess which word I say ends with that sound: '_____,' '_____,' '_____,' '_____.'" (stimulus words) (e.g., "Listen to this sound: /s/. Guess which word I say ends with that sound: 'home,' 'door,' 'bricks,' 'called.'") (bricks)

> **NOTE:** *Give the letter sound, not the letter name. Use pictured items and/or manipulatives if necessary. Use any of the following stimulus words and/or others you select from the story. The correct answers are in parentheses.*

Stimulus items:

/r/: houses, faster, second, morning (faster)

/t/: knocking, pot, tomorrow, barrel (pot)

/r/: meadow, nine, sticks, angrier (angrier)

/long O/: chinny, tomorrow, momma, across (tomorrow)

/z/: apples, rolled, straight, myself (apples)

/d/: angriest, roar, climbed, basket (climbed)

/f/: please, wolf, puffed, o'clock (wolf)

/long E/: meadow, knocked, gathering, happily (happily)

/s/: house, climbed, please, until (house)

/l/: rolled, huffed, yum, barrel (barrel)

7. Identifying the initial sound in words.

What to say to the student: "I'll say a word two times. Tell me what sound is missing the second time: '_____,' '_____.'" (stimulus words)

> **EXAMPLE** "What sound do you hear in '_____'" (stimulus word) "that is missing in '_____'?" (stimulus word) (e.g., "What sound do you hear in 'no' that is missing in 'oh'?") (/n/)

> **NOTE:** *Give the letter sound, not the letter name. Use pictured items and/or manipulatives if necessary. Use any of the following stimulus words and/or others you select from the story. The correct answers are in parentheses.*

Stimulus items:

"soup, oop. What sound do you hear in 'soup' that is missing in 'oop'?" (/s/)

"very, airy. What sound do you hear in 'very' that is missing in 'airy'?" (/v/)

"charms, arms. What sound do you hear in 'charms' that is missing in 'arms'?" (/ch/)

"roar, oar. What sound do you hear in 'roar' that is missing in 'oar'?" (/r/)

"yum, um. What sound do you hear in 'yum' that is missing in '-um'?" (/y/ as in yellow)

"man, an. What sound do you hear in 'man' that is missing in 'an'?" (/m/)

"nice, ice. What sound do you hear in 'nice' that is missing in 'ice'?" (/n/)

"got, ought. What sound do you hear in 'got' that is missing in 'ought'?" (/g/)

"slow, low. What sound do you hear in 'slow' that is missing in 'low'?" (/s/)

"across, cross. What sound do you hear in 'across' that is missing in 'cross'?" (/uh/)

8. Identifying the final sound in words.

What to say to the student: "I'll say a word two times. Tell me what sound is missing the second time: '_____,' '_____.'" (stimulus words)

> **EXAMPLE** "What sound do you hear in '_____'" (stimulus word) "that is missing in '_____'?" (stimulus word) (e.g., "What sound do you hear in 'things' that is missing in 'thing'?") (/z/)

> **NOTE:** *Give the letter sound, not the letter name. Use pictured items and/or manipulatives if necessary. Use any of the following stimulus words and/or others you select from the story. The correct answers are in parentheses.*

Stimulus items:

"lived, live. What sound do you hear in 'lived' that is missing in 'live'?" (/d/)

"time, tie. What sound do you hear in 'time' that is missing in 'tie'?" (/m/)

"built, bill. What sound do you hear in 'built' that is missing in 'bill'?" (/t/)

"asked, ask. What sound do you hear in 'asked' that is missing in 'ask'?" (/t/)

"rolled, roll. What sound do you hear in 'rolled' that is missing in 'roll'?" (/d/)

"pot, pa. What sound do you hear in 'pot' that is missing in 'pa'?" (/t/)

"house, how. What sound do you hear in 'house' that is missing in 'how'?" (/s/)

"I'll, I. What sound do you hear in 'I'll' that is missing in 'I'?" (/l/)

"safe, say. What sound do you hear in 'safe' that is missing in 'say'?" (/f/)

"here's, here. What sound do you hear in 'here's' that is missing in 'here'?" (/z/)

9. Segmenting the initial sound in words.

What to say to the student: "Listen to the word I say and tell me the first sound you hear."

> **EXAMPLE** "What's the first sound in '_____'?" (stimulus word) (e.g., "What's the first sound in 'wolf'?") (/w/)

NOTE: *Give the letter sound, not the letter name. Use pictured items and/or manipulatives if necessary. Use any of the following stimulus words and/or others you select from the story. Use any group of 10 stimulus items you select per teaching set.*

Stimulus items:

/p/: pigs, pig, please, puff, pot, puffed

/b/: build, built, but, by, blow, blew, bricks, back, basket, big, barrel, banging, before

/t/: told, time, turnips, ten, tomorrow, together, tree, toward, tricks

/d/: day, door, down, didn't

/k/: came, come, couldn't, cooking, called, cooked, climbed

/g/: go, good, goodbye, going, gathering, give, got

/ch/: chin, chinny, chimney

/dz/ (as in gem): just, jumped

/m/: momma, met, man, me, made, morning, meadow, much

/n/: now, knocking, no, not, know, next, nine, nice, night

/s/: strong, sons, straw, sir, some, second, sticks, safe, seven, saw, straight, soup, see, supper

/f/: first, field, fair, fell, faster

/v/: very

/h/: happily, house, houses, who, himself, hair, huff, huffed, hurried, hide, hill

/r/: right, road, rolled, riding, roared, roof

/l/: long, little, lived, let, load, leaped

/w/, /wh/: when, world, watch, wolf, one, won't, well, where, we'll

/voiceless th/: three, third, threw

/voiced th/: their, them, then, this, there's, than, that

/y/ (as in yellow): your, yum, you

/short A/: asked, apple

/short U/: along, up, across, until

/long A/: ate

/long E/: enough

/long I/: I, I'll

/ah/: already

10. Segmenting the final sound in words.

What to say to the student: "Listen to the word I say and tell me the last sound you hear."

> **EXAMPLE** "What's the last sound in the word '_____'?" (stimulus word) (e.g., "What's the last sound in the word 'wolf'?") (/f/)

NOTE: *Give the letter sound, not the letter name. Use pictured items and/or manipulatives if necessary. Use any of the following stimulus words and/or others you select from the story. Use any group of 10 stimulus items you select per teaching set.*

Stimulus items:

/p/: up, soup

/t/: out, first, met, built, let, won't, not, ate, huffed, puffed, just, couldn't, asked, right, next, got, basket, eight, jumped, straight, knocked, pot, didn't, get, leaped, cooked, that, night

/d/: lived, told, world, build, good, called, said, second, load, third, made, field, road, hurried, had, climbed, hide, rolled, toward, roared

/k/: o'clock, back

/g/: big

/ch/: watch

/m/: came, them, time, some, him, come, yum

/n/: when, man, one, in, chin, then, down, ten, ran, soon, town, seven, than

/ng/: long, strong, going, along, gathering, knocking, morning, picking, cooking, banging, riding

/s/: house, sticks, bricks, this, turnips, nice, across, chase, tricks

/z/: pigs, houses, always, sons, was, please, his, apples, here's

/f/: wolf, huff, puff, himself, safe, myself, enough, roof

/v/: give, gave

/r/: door, hair, where, together, far, after, fair, over, faster, angrier, before, your, supper

/l/: little, well, I'll, we'll, apple, until, barrel, fell, hill

/voiceless th/: with

/long A/: day, away

/long E/: three, happily, me, hinny, yummy, angry, only, already, very, tree, busy, see, really, chimney

/long I/: goodbye, my, by

/long O/: ago, go, so, no, blow, know, tomorrow, meadow

/uh/: momma

/oo/: into, you, blew, threw, onto

/ow/: now

/ah/: straw, saw

11. Generating words from the story beginning with a particular sound.

What to say to the student: "Let's think of words from the story that start with certain sounds."

> **EXAMPLE** "Tell me a word from the story that starts with / /." (stimulus sound) (e.g., the sound /s/) (strong)

> **NOTE:** *Give the letter sound, not the letter name. Use pictured items if necessary. Use any of the following stimulus words and/or others you select from the story. You say the sound (e.g., a voiceless /p/ sound), and the student is to say a word from the story that begins with that sound. Use any group of 10 stimulus items you select per teaching set.*

Stimulus items:

/p/: pigs, pig, please, puff, pot, puffed

/b/: build, built, but, by, blow, blew, bricks, back, basket, big, barrel, banging, before

/t/: told, time, turnips, ten, tomorrow, together, tree, toward, tricks

/d/: day, door, down, didn't

/k/: came, come, couldn't, cooking, called, cooked, climbed

/g/: go, good, goodbye, going, gathering, give, got

/ch/: chin, chinny, chimney

/dz/ (as in gem): just, jumped

/m/: momma, met, man, me, made, morning, meadow, much

/n/: now, knocking, no, not, know, next, nine, nice, night

/s/: strong, sons, straw, sir, some, second, sticks, safe, seven, saw, straight, soup, see, supper

/f/: first, field, fair, fell, faster

/v/: very

/h/: happily, house, houses, who, himself, hair, huff, huffed, hurried, hide, hill

/r/: right, road, rolled, riding, roared, roof

/l/: long, little, lived, let, load, leaped

/w/, /wh/: when, world, watch, wolf, one, won't, well, where, we'll

/voiceless th/: three, third, threw

/voiced th/: their, them, then, this, there's, than, that

/y/ (as in yellow): your, yum, you

/short A/: asked, apple

/short U/: along, up, across, until

/long A/: ate

/long E/: enough

/long I/: I, I'll

/ah/: already

12. Blending sounds in monosyllabic words divided into onset/rime beginning with a two-consonant cluster + rime.

What to say to the student: "Now we'll put sounds together to make words."

EXAMPLE "Put these sounds together to make a word: / / + / /." (stimulus sounds) "What's the word?" (e.g., "dr + ag: What's the word?") (drag)

NOTE: *Give the letter sound, not the letter name. Use pictured items and/or manipulatives if necessary. Use any of the following stimulus words and/or others you select from the story. The correct answers are in parentheses.*

Stimulus items:

st + rong (strong)

pl + ease (please)

st + icks (sticks)

bl + oh (blow)

br + icks (bricks)

tr + ee (tree)

ch + in (chin)

st + raw (straw)

bl + oo (blew)

kl + I'm (climb)

13. Blending sounds in monosyllabic words divided into onset/rime beginning with a single consonant + rime.

What to say to the student: "Let's put sounds together to make words."

EXAMPLE   "Put these sounds together to make a word: / / + / /." (stimulus sounds) "What's the word?" (e.g., "/s/ + oop: What's the word?") (soup)

NOTE: *Give the letter sound, not the letter name. Use pictured items and/or manipulatives if necessary. Use any of the following stimulus words and/or others you select from the story. The correct answers are in parentheses.*

Stimulus items:

/p/ + ig (pig)

/l/ + oad (load)

/b/ + low (blow)

/f/ + eeld (field)

/m/ + an (man)

/n/ + ext (next)

/w/ + olf (wolf)

/f/ + ell (fell)

/dz/ (as in gem)/ + ump (jump)

/t/ + ime (time)

14. Blending sounds to form a monosyllabic word beginning with a continuant sound.

What to say to the student: "We'll put sounds together to make words."

EXAMPLE   "Put these sounds together to make a word: / / + / / + / /." (stimulus sounds) (e.g., /s/ /uh/ /n/ /z/) (sons)

NOTE: *Give the letter sound, not the letter name. Use pictured items and/or manipulatives if necessary. Use any of the following stimulus words and/or others you select from the story. The correct answers are in parentheses.*

Stimulus items:

/m/ /short A/ /n/ (man)

/s/ /t/ /r/ /ah/ /n/ /g/ (strong)

/l/ /short I/ /v/ /d/ (lived)

/y/ /uh/ /m/ (yum)

/n/ /short E/ /k/ /s/ /t/ (next)

/voiceless th/ /r /d/ (third)

/w/ /short E/ /n/ (when)

/r/ /oo/ /f/ (roof)

/n/ /long I/ /n/ (nine)

/h/ /ou/ /s/ (house)

15. Blending sounds to form a monosyllabic word beginning with a noncontinuant sound.

What to say to the student: "We'll put sounds together to make words."

> EXAMPLE "Put these sounds together to make a word: / / + / / + / /." (stimulus sounds) (e.g., /k/ /long A/ /m/) (came)

NOTE: *Give the letter sound, not the letter name. Use pictured items and/or manipulatives if necessary. Use any of the following stimulus words and/or others you select from the story. The correct answers are in parentheses.*

Stimulus items:

/d/ /long A/ (day)

/t/ /long O/ /l/ /d/ (told)

/dz/ (as in gem) /uh/ /s/ /t/ (just)

/b/ /short I/ /l/ /d/ (build)

/ch/ /short I/ /n/ (chin)

/p/ /ah/ /t/ (pot)

/t/ /r/ /long E/ (tree)

/p/ /l/ /long E/ /z/ (please)

/k/ /ah/ /l/ /d/ (called)

/p/ /uh/ /f/ /t/ (puffed)

16. Substituting the initial sound in words.

What to say to the student: "We're going to change beginning/first sounds in words."

EXAMPLE "Say '_____.'" (stimulus word) "Instead of / /" (stimulus sound), "say / /." (stimulus sound) (e.g., "Say 'gave.' Instead of /g/, say /s/. What's your new word?") (save)

NOTE: *Give the letter sound, not the letter name. Use pictured items and/or manipulatives if necessary. Use any of the following stimulus words and/or others you select from the story. The correct answers are in parentheses.*

Stimulus items:

"Say 'fair.' Instead of /f/, say /h/." (hair)

"Say 'three.' Instead of /voiceless th/, say /t/." (tree)

"Say 'pig.' Instead of /p/, say /d/." (dig)

"Say 'chase.' Instead of /ch/, say /r/." (race)

"Say 'house.' Instead of /h/, say /m/." (mouse)

"Say 'third.' Instead of /voiceless th/, say /b/." (bird)

"Say 'puffed.' Instead of /p/, say /h/." (huffed)

"Say 'jumped.' Instead of /dz/ (as in gem), say /b/." (bumped)

"Say 'town.' Instead of /t/, say /d/." (down)

"Say 'bricks.' Instead of /b/, say /t/." (tricks)

17. Substituting the final sound in words.

What to say to the student: "We're going to change ending/last sounds in words."

EXAMPLE "Say '_____.'" (stimulus word) "Instead of / /" (stimulus sound), "say / /." (stimulus sound) (e.g., "Say 'made.' Instead of /d/, say /k/. What's your new word?") (make)

NOTE: *Give the letter sound, not the letter name. Use pictured items and/or manipulatives if necessary. Use any of the following stimulus words and/or others you select from the story. The correct answers are in parentheses.*

Stimulus items:

"Say 'please.' Instead of /z/, say /d/." (plead)

"Say 'man.' Instead of /n/, say /p/." (map)

"Say 'load.' Instead of /d/, say /n/." (loan)

"Say 'build.' Instead of /d/, say /t/." (built)

"Say 'time.' Instead of /m/, say /t/." (tight)

"Say 'chin.' Instead of /n/, say /p/." (chip)

"Say 'down.' Instead of /n/, say /t/." (doubt)

"Say 'called.' Instead of /d/, say /z/." (calls)

"Say 'jumped.' Instead of /t/, say /s/." (jumps)

"Say 'field.' Instead of /d/, say /z/." (feels)

18. Segmenting the middle sound in monosyllabic words.

What to say to the student: "Tell me the middle sound in the word I say."

EXAMPLE   "What's the middle sound in the word '_____'?" (stimulus word) (e.g., "What's the middle sound in the word 'some'?") (/uh/)

NOTE: *Give the letter sound, not the letter name. Use pictured items and/or manipulatives if necessary. Use any of the following stimulus words and/or others you select from the story. The correct answers are in parentheses.*

Stimulus items:

back (/short A/)

house (/ow/)

road (/long O/)

knock (/ah/)

made (/long A/)

load (/long O/)

tree (/r/)

hill (/short I/)

huff (/uh/)

time (/long I/)

19. Substituting the middle sound in words.

What to say to the student: "We're going to change the middle sound in words."

EXAMPLE   "Say '_____.'" (stimulus word) "Instead of / /" (stimulus sound), "say / /." (stimulus sound) (e.g., "Say 'ten.' Instead of /short E/, say /short A/. What's your new word?") (tan)

NOTE: *Give the letter sound, not the letter name. Use pictured items and/or manipulatives if necessary. Use any of the following stimulus words and/or others you select from the story. The correct answers are in parentheses.*

Stimulus items:

"Say 'pig.' Instead of /short I/, say /uh/." (pug)

"Say 'pot.' Instead of /ah/, say /short I/." (pit)

"Say 'roof.' Instead of /oo/, say /uh/." (rough)

"Say 'time.' Instead of /long I/, say /long E/." (team)

"Say 'yum.' Instead of /uh/, say /short A/." (yam)

"Say 'nine.' Instead of /long I/, say /long O/." (known)

"Say 'met.' Instead of /short E/, say /short A/." (mat)

"Say 'right.' Instead of /long I/, say /long A/." (rate)

"Say 'leap.' Instead of /long E/, say /short I/." (lip)

"Say 'brick.' Instead of /short I/, say /long A/." (break)

20. Identifying all sounds in monosyllabic words.

What to say to the student: "Now tell me all the sounds you hear in the word I say."

> **EXAMPLE** "What sounds do you hear in the word '_____'?" (stimulus word) (e.g., "What sounds do you hear in the word 'pot'?") (/p/ /ah/ /t/)

> **NOTE:** *Give the letter sound, not the letter name. Use pictured items and/or manipulatives if necessary. Use any of the following stimulus words and/or others you select from the story. The correct answers are in parentheses.*

Stimulus items:

pig (/p/ /short I/ /g/)

man (/m/ /short A/ /n/)

huff (/h/ /uh/ /f/)

straw (/s/ /t/ /r/ /ah/)

chin (/ch/ /short I/ /n/)

sticks (/s/ /t/ /short I/ /k/ /s/)

yum (/y/ /uh/ /m/)

bricks (/b/ /r/ /short I/ /k/ /s/)

strong (/s/ /t/ /r/ /ah/ /ng/)

road (/r/ /long O/ /d/)

21. Deleting sounds within words.

What to say to the student: "We're going to leave out sounds in words."

> **EXAMPLE** "Say '_____'" (stimulus word) "without / /." (stimulus sound) (e.g., "Say 'grew' without /r/.") (goo) Say: "The word that is left—'goo'—is a real word. Sometimes, the word won't be a real word."

> **NOTE:** *Give the letter sound, not the letter name. Use pictured items and/or manipulatives if necessary. Use any of the following stimulus words and/or others you select from the story. The correct answers are in parentheses.*

Stimulus items:

"Say 'please' without /l/." (peas)

"Say 'stick' without /t/." (sick)

"Say 'blow' without /l/." (bow with a /long O/)

"Say 'tree' without /r/." (tee)

"Say 'basket' without /k/." (basset)

"Say 'blew' without /l/." (boo)

"Say 'tricks' without /r/." (ticks)

"Say 'chimney' without /m/." (chinny)

"Say 'next' without /k/." (nest)

"Say 'asked' without /s/." (act)

22. Substituting consonants in words having a two-sound cluster.

What to say to the student: "We're going to substitute sounds in words."

> **EXAMPLE** "Say '_____.'" (stimulus word) "Instead of / /" (stimulus sound), "say / /." (stimulus sound) (e.g., "Say 'stop.' Instead of /t/, say /l/.") (slop) Say: "Sometimes, the new word won't be a real word."

NOTE: *Give the letter sound, not the letter name. Use pictured items and/or manipulatives if necessary. Use any of the following stimulus words and/or others you select from the story. The correct answers are in parentheses.*

Stimulus items:

"Say 'blow.' Instead of /l/, say /r/." (bro)

"Say 'blew.' Instead of /l/, say /r/." (brew)

"Say 'bricks.' Instead of /b/, say /t/." (tricks)

"Say 'ask.' Instead of /k/, say /p/." (asp)

"Say 'climb.' Instead of /l/, say /r/." (crime)

"Say 'tricks.' Instead of /t/, say /b/." (bricks)

"Say 'field.' Instead of /d/, say /z/." (feels)

"Say 'tricks.' Instead of /k/, say /p/." (trips)

"Say 'sticks.' Instead of /k/, say /f/." (stiffs)

"Say 'build.' Instead of /d/, say /t/." (built)

23. Phoneme reversing.

What to say to the student: "We're going to say words backward."

> **EXAMPLE** "Say the word '_____'" (stimulus word) "backward." (e.g., "Say 'but' backward.") (tub)

NOTE: *This is a difficult phoneme-level task and should only be done with older students. Give the letter sound, not the letter name. Use pictured items and/or manipulatives if necessary. Use any of the following stimulus words and/or others you select from the story. The correct answers are in parentheses.*

Stimulus items:

pot (top)

nice (sign)

road (door)

let (tell)

much (chum)

made (dame)

came (make)

face (safe)

day (aid)

nine (nine)

24. Phoneme switching.

What to say to the student: "We're going to switch the first sounds in two words."

> **EXAMPLE** "Switch the first sounds in '_____' and '_____.'" (stimulus words) (e.g., "Switch the first sounds in 'big' and 'pig.'") (pig big)

> **NOTE:** *This is a difficult phoneme-level task and should only be done with older students. Give the letter sound, not the letter name. Use pictured items and/or manipulatives if necessary. Use any of the following stimulus words and/or others you select from the story. The correct answers are in parentheses.*

Stimulus items:

man who (han moo)

pig built (big pilt)

chin hair (hin chair)

momma pig (pomma mig)

huff puff (puff huff)

house down (douse hown)

turnip basket (burnip tasket)

next morning (mext norning)

down hill (hown dill)

cooked soup (sooked coup)

25. Pig Latin.

What to say to the student: "We're going to speak a secret language by using words from the story. In pig Latin, you take off the first sound of a word, put it at the end of the word, and add an 'ay' sound."

> **EXAMPLE** "Say 'day' in pig Latin." (ayday)

> **NOTE:** *This is a difficult phoneme-level task and should only be done with older students. Use pictured items and/or manipulatives if necessary. Use any of the following stimulus words and/or others you select from the story. The correct answers are in parentheses.*

Stimulus items:

pig (igpay)

wolf (uulfway)

house (ousehay)

momma (ommamay)

chin (inchay)

little (ittlelay)

knocking (ockingnay)

morning (orningmay)

turnips (urnipstay)

barrel (arrelbay)

From Phonological Awareness into Print

NOTE: *Only five examples per activity are included in this resource due to space. You are encouraged to add many more words into this section that you feel your student(s) is(are) ready to write.*

1. Substituting the initial sound or letter in words.

NOTE: *Use lined paper or copy the sheet of lined paper included in the back of this book.*

Stimulus items:

1.1 pig/big

Task a. "Say 'pig.' Instead of /p/, say /b/. What's your new word?" (big) "Write/copy 'pig' and 'big.'"

Task b. "Circle the **letters** that make the words different." ([p], [b])

Task c. "What **sounds** do these letters make?" (/p/, /b/)

1.2 yum/tum

Task a. "Say 'yum.' Instead of /y/ (as in yellow), say /t/. What's your new word?" (tum) "Write/copy 'yum' and 'tum.'"

Task b. "Circle the **letters** that make the words different." ([y], [t])

Task c. "What **sounds** do these letters make?" (/y/ as in yellow, /t/)

1.3 nice/rice

Task a. "Say 'nice.' Instead of /n/, say /r/. What's your new word?" (rice) "Write/copy 'nice' and 'rice.'"

Task b. "Circle the **letters** that make the words different." ([n], [r])

Task c. "What **sounds** do these letters make?" (/n/, /r/)

1.4 hair/fair

Task a. "Say 'hair.' Instead of /h/, say /f/. What's your new word?" (fair) "Write/copy 'hair' and 'fair.'"

Task b. "Circle the **letters** that make the words different." ([h], [f])

Task c. "What **sounds** do these letters make?" (/h/, /f/)

1.5 fell/bell

Task a. "Say 'fell.' Instead of /f/, say /b/. What's your new word?" (bell) "Write/copy 'fell' and 'bell.'"

Task b. "Circle the **letters** that make the words different." ([f], [b])

Task c. "What **sounds** do these letters make?" (/f/, /b/)

2. Substituting the final sound or letter in words.

NOTE: *Use lined paper or copy the sheet of lined paper included in the back of this book.*

Stimulus items:

2.1 man/mat

Task a. "Say 'man.' Instead of /n/, say /t/. What's your new word?" (mat) "Write/copy 'man' and 'mat.'"

Task b. "Circle the **letters** that make the words different." ([n], [t])

Task c. "What **sounds** do these letters make?" (/n/, /t/)

2.2 load/loan

Task a. "Say 'load.' Instead of /d/, say /n/. What's your new word?" (loan) "Write/copy 'load' and 'loan.'"

Task b. "Circle the **letters** that make the words different." ([d], [n])

Task c. "What **sounds** do these letters make?" (/d/, /n/)

2.3 built/build

Task a. "Say 'built.' Instead of /t/, say /d/. What's your new word?" (build) "Write/copy 'built' and 'build.'"

Task b. "Circle the **letters** that make the words different." ([t], [d])

Task c. "What **sounds** do these letters make?" (/t/, /d/)

2.4 chin/chip

Task a. "Say 'chin.' Instead of /n/, say /p/. What's your new word?" (chip) "Write/copy 'chin' and 'chip.'"

Task b. "Circle the **letters** that make the words different." ([n], [p])

Task c. "What **sounds** do these letters make?" (/n/, /p/)

2.5 road/roam

Task a. "Say 'road.' Instead of /d/, say /m/. What's your new word?" (roam) "Write/copy 'road' and 'roam.'"

Task b. "Circle the **letters** that make the words different." ([d], [m])

Task c. "What **sounds** do these letters make?" (/d/, /m/)

3. Substituting the middle sound or letter in words.

NOTE: *Use lined paper or copy the sheet of lined paper included in the back of this book.*

Stimulus items:

3.1 man/men

Task a. "Say 'man.' Instead of /short A/, say /short E/. What's your new word?" (men) "Write/copy 'man' and 'men.'"

Task b. "Circle the **letters** that make the words different." ([a], [e])

Task c. "What **sounds** do these letters make?" (/short A/, /short E/)

3.2 sticks/stacks

Task a. "Say 'sticks.' Instead of /short I/, say /short A/. What's your new word?" (stacks) "Write/copy 'sticks' and 'stacks.'"

Task b. "Circle the **letters** that make the words different." ([i], [a])

Task c. "What **sounds** do these letters make?" (/short I/, /short A/)

3.3 time/tame

Task a. "Say 'time.' Instead of /long I/, say /long A/. What's your new word?" (tame). Write/copy 'time' and 'tame.'"

Task b. "Circle the **letters** that make the words different." ([i], [a])

Task c. "What **sounds** do these letters make?" (/long I/, /long A/)

3.4 hill/hall

Task a. "Say 'hill.' Instead of /short I/, say /ah/. What's your new word?" (hall) "Write/copy 'hill' and 'hall.'"

Task b. "Circle the **letters** that make the words different." ([i], [a])

Task c. "What **sounds** do these letters make?" (/short I/, /ah/)

3.5 pig/pug

Task a. "Say 'pig.' Instead of /short I/, say /uh/. What's your new word?" (pug) "Write/copy 'pig' and 'pug.'"

Task b. "Circle the **letters** that make the words different." ([i], [u])

Task c. "What **sounds** do these letters make?" (/short I/, /uh/)

4. Supplying the initial sound or letter in words.

NOTE: *Use lined paper or copy the sheet of lined paper included in the back of this book.*

Stimulus items:

4.1 man/an

Task a. "Say 'man,' say 'an.' What sound did you hear in 'man' that is missing in 'an'?" (/m/) "Now we'll change the **letter**. Write/copy 'man' and 'an.'"

Task b. "Circle the beginning **letter** that makes the words different." ([m])

Task c. "What **sound** does this letter make?" (/m/)

4.2 now/ow

> **Task a.** "Say 'now,' say 'ow.' What sound did you hear in 'now' that is missing in 'ow'?" (/n/) "Now we'll change the **letter.** Write/copy 'now' and 'ow.'"
>
> **Task b.** "Circle the beginning **letter** that makes the words different." ([n])
>
> **Task c.** "What **sound** does this letter make?" (/n/)

4.3 nice/ice

> **Task a.** "Say 'nice,' say 'ice.' What sound did you hear in 'nice' that is missing in 'ice'?" (/n/) "Now we'll change the **letter.** Write/copy 'nice' and 'ice.'"
>
> **Task b.** "Circle the beginning **letter** that makes the words different." ([n])
>
> **Task c.** "What **sound** does this letter make?" (/n/)

4.4 hair/air

> **Task a.** "Say 'hair,' say 'air.' What sound did you hear in 'hair' that is missing in 'air'?" (/h/) "Now we'll change the **letter.** Write/copy 'hair' and 'air.'"
>
> **Task b.** "Circle the beginning **letter** that makes the words different." ([h])
>
> **Task c.** "What **sound** does this letter make?" (/h/)

4.5 blow/low

> **Task a.** "Say 'blow,' say 'low.' What sound did you hear in 'blow' that is missing in 'low'?" (/b/) "Now we'll change the **letter.** Write/copy 'blow' and 'low.'"
>
> **Task b.** "Circle the beginning **letter** that makes the words different." ([b])
>
> **Task c.** "What **sound** does this letter make?" (/b/)

5. Supplying the final sound or letter in words.

> **NOTE:** *Use lined paper or copy the sheet of lined paper included in the back of this book.*

Stimulus items:

5.1 bricks/brick

> **Task a.** "Say 'bricks,' say 'brick.' What sound did you hear in 'bricks' that is missing in 'brick'?" (/s/) "Now we'll change the **letter.** Write/copy 'bricks' and 'brick.'"
>
> **Task b.** "Circle the ending/last **letter** that makes the words different." ([s])
>
> **Task c.** "What **sound** does this letter make?" (/s/)

5.2 pigs/pig

> **Task a.** "Say 'pigs,' say 'pig.' What sound did you hear in 'pigs' that is missing in 'pig'?" (/z/) "Now we'll change the **letter.** Write/copy 'pigs' and 'pig.'"
>
> **Task b.** "Circle the ending/last **letter** that makes the words different." ([s])
>
> **Task c.** "What **sound** does this letter make?" (/z/)

5.3 lived/live

> **Task a.** "Say 'lived,' say 'live.' What sound did you hear in 'lived' that is missing in 'live'?" (/d/) "Now we'll change the **letter.** Write/copy 'lived' and 'live.'"

Task b. "Circle the ending/last **letter** that make the words different." ([d])

Task c. "What **sound** does this letter make?" (/d/)

5.4 turnips/turnip

Task a. "Say 'turnips,' say 'turnip.' What sound did you hear in 'turnips' that is missing in 'turnip'?" (/s/) "Now we'll change the **letter**. Write/copy 'turnips' and 'turnip.'"

Task b. "Circle the ending/last **letter** that makes the word different." ([s])

Task c. "What **sound** does this letter make?" (/s/)

5.5 sons/son

Task a. "Say 'sons,' say 'son.' What sound did you hear in 'sons' that is missing in 'son'?" (/z/) "Now we'll change the **letter**. Write/copy 'sons' and 'son.'"

Task b. "Circle the ending/last **letter** that makes the words different." ([s])

Task c. "What **sound** does this letter make?" (/z/)

6. Switching the first sound and letter in words (ADVANCED).

NOTE: *Use lined paper or copy the sheet of lined paper included in the back of this book.*

Stimulus items:

6.1 little pig

Task a. "Say 'little,' say 'pig.' What sound do you hear at the beginning of 'little'?" (/l/) "What sound do you hear at the beginning of 'pig'?" (/p/) "Switch the first sounds in those words." (pittle lig) "Now we'll change the **letters**. Write/copy 'little pig' and 'pittle lig.'"

Task b. "Circle the beginning **letters** that change the words." ([l], [p])

Task c. "What **sounds** do those letters make?" (/l/, /p/)

6.2 house down

Task a. "Say 'house' say 'down.' What sound do you hear at the beginning of 'house'?" (/h/) "What sound do you hear at the beginning of 'down'?" (/d/) "Switch the first sounds in those words." (douse hown) "Now we'll change the **letters**. Write/copy 'house down" and 'douse hown.'"

Task b. "Circle the beginning **letters** that change the words." ([h], [d])

Task c. "What **sounds** do those letters make?" (/h/, /d/)

6.3 momma pig

Task a. "Say 'momma,' say 'pig.' What sound do you hear at the beginning of 'momma'?" (/m/) "What sound do you hear at the beginning of 'pig'?" (/p/) "Switch the first sounds in those words." (pomma mig) "Now we'll change the **letters**. Write/copy 'momma pig' and 'pomma mig.'"

Task b. "Circle the beginning **letters** that change the words." ([m], [p])

Task c. "What **sounds** do those letters make?" (/m/, /p/)

6.4 down hill

Task a. "Say 'down,' say 'hill.' What sound do you hear at the beginning of 'down'?" (/d/) "What sound do you hear at the beginning of 'hill'?" (/h/) "Switch the first sounds in those words." (hown dill) "Now we'll change the **letters.** Write/copy 'down hill' and 'hown dill.'"

Task b. "Circle the beginning **letters** that change the words." ([d], [h])

Task c. "What **sounds** do those letters make?" (/d/, /h/)

6.5 huffed puffed

Task a. "Say 'huffed,' say 'puffed.' What sound do you hear at the beginning of 'huffed'?" (/h/) "What sound do you hear at the beginning of 'puffed'?" (/p/) "Switch the first sounds in those words." (puffed huffed). "Now we'll change the **letters.** Write/copy 'huffed puffed' and 'puffed huffed.'"

Task b. "Circle the beginning **letters** that change the words." ([h], [p])

Task c. "What **sounds** do those letters make?" (/h/, /p/)

Forms for Tracking Student Performance

RECORD SHEET #1

Record Sheet #1 is suggested as one way of tracking a student's performance on the various phonological awareness activities. A check mark (✓), date, and/or percentage (reflecting accuracy) can be recorded in the box intersecting a particular story with an activity.

STUDENT: _____

STORIES	Benny's Pennies	Bunny Cakes	Chicken Soup With Rice	Chrysanthemum	From Head to Toe	Home for a Bunny	Liang and the Magic Paintbrush	Mice Squeak, We Speak	Miss Bindergarten Gets Ready for Kindergarten	The Garden	Tortillas and Lullabies	The Three Little Pigs
ACTIVITIES												
WORD LEVEL												
1. Counting words												
2. ID missing words												
3. ID missing words phrase/sentence												
4. Supplying word												
5. Rearranging words												
SYLLABLE LEVEL												
1. Counting syllables												
2. Initial syllable deleting												
3. Final syllable deleting												
4. Initial syllable adding												

5. Final syllable adding									
6. Syllable substituting									
PHONEME LEVEL									
1. Counting sounds									
2. Sound categorization									
3. Matching rhyme									
4. Producing rhyme									
5. Initial sound matching									
6. Final sound matching									
7. ID initial sound									
8. ID final sound									
9. Segmenting initial sound									
10. Segmenting final sound									
11. Generating words									
12. Blending sounds: onset/rime with a two-consonant beginning									

(Continued)

13. Blending sounds: onset/rime with a single consonant beginning											
14. Blending sounds beginning with a continuant sound											
15. Blending sounds beginning with a noncontinuant sound											
16. Substituting initial sound											
17. Substituting final sound											
18. Segmenting middle sound											
19. Substituting middle sound											
20. ID all sounds											
21. Deleting sounds within words											
22. Substituting consonant in a two-sound cluster											
23. Phoneme reversing											
24. Phoneme switching											
25. Pig Latin											

FROM PHONOLOGICAL AWARENESS TO PRINT										
1. Substituting initial sound/letter in words										
2. Substituting final sound/letter in words										
3. Substituting middle sound/letter in words										
4. Supplying initial sound/letter in words										
5. Supplying final sound/letter in words										
6. Switching first sound/letter in words										

RECORD SHEET #2

Record Sheet #2 is suggested as one way of tracking a student's performance on the various phonological awareness activities. A check mark (✓), date, percentage (reflecting accuracy), and/or specific notes can be recorded on the lines next to activities.

Student: _____ Story: _____

Phonological Awareness Activities at the Word Level

1. Counting words: _____
2. Identifying the missing word from a list: _____
3. Identifying the missing word in a phrase or sentence: _____
4. Supplying the missing word as an adult reads: _____
5. Rearranging words: _____

Phonological Awareness Activities at the Syllable Level

1. Syllable counting: _____
2. Initial syllable deleting: _____
3. Final syllable deleting: _____
4. Initial syllable adding: _____
5. Final syllable adding: _____
6. Syllable substituting: _____

Phonological Awareness Activities at the Phoneme Level

1. Counting sounds: _____
2. Sound categorization or identifying rhyme oddity: _____
3. Matching rhyme: _____
4. Producing rhyme: _____
5. Sound matching (initial): _____
6. Sound matching (final): _____
7. Identifying the initial sound in words: _____
8. Identifying the final sound in words: _____
9. Segmenting the initial sound in words: _____
10. Segmenting the final sound in words: _____
11. Generating words from the story beginning with a particular sound: _____
12. Blending sounds in monosyllabic words divided into onset/rime beginning with a two-consonant cluster + rime: _____
13. Blending sounds in monosyllabic words divided into onset/rime beginning with a single consonant + rime: _____

14. Blending sounds to form a monosyllabic word beginning with a continuant sound: _____

15. Blending sounds to form a monosyllabic word beginning with a noncontinuant sound: _____

16. Substituting the initial sound in words: _____

17. Substituting the final sound in words: _____

18. Segmenting the middle sound in monosyllabic words: _____

19. Substituting the middle sound in words: _____

20. Identifying all sounds in monosyllabic words: _____

21. Deleting the sounds within words: _____

22. Substituting the consonant in words having a two-sound cluster: _____

23. Phoneme reversing: _____

24. Phoneme switching: _____

25. Pig Latin: _____

From Phonological Awareness into Print Awareness

1. Substituting the initial sound/letter in words: _____

2. Substituting the final sound/letter in words: _____

3. Substituting the middle sound/letter in words: _____

4. Supplying the initial sound/letter in words: _____

5. Supplying the final sound/letter in words: _____

6. Switching the first sound/letter in words: _____

References

American Speech-Language-Hearing Association. (2001). *Roles and responsibilities of speech-language pathologists with respect to reading and writing in children and adolescents.* Washington, DC: Author.

Cabell, S. Q., Justice, L. M., Kaderavek, J. N., Turnbull, K. P., & Breit-Smith, A. (2009). *Emergent literacy: Lessons for success.* San Diego: Plural Publishing.

California State Department of Education. (1998). *California language arts content standards.* Sacramento: California State Department of Education.

Goldsworthy, C. (1998, 2012). *Sourcebook of phonological awareness activities: Children's classic literature.* San Diego: Singular Publishing Group.

Goldsworthy, C. (2001, 2012). *Sourcebook of phonological awareness training: Children's core literature.* San Diego: Singular Publishing Group.

Goldsworthy, C. (2003). *Developmental reading disabilities: A language based treatment approach.* San Diego: Singular Publishing Group.

Goldsworthy, C. (2010, 2012). *Linking the strands of language and literacy: A resource manual.* San Diego: Plural Publishing.

Goldsworthy, C., & Pieretti, R. (2004, 2013). *Sourcebook of phonological awareness activities v. III: Children's core literature grades 3 through 5.* New York: Thomson-Delmar.

Hodson, B. W., & Edwards, M. L. (1997). *Perspectives in applied phonology.* Gaithersburg, MD: Aspen Publishers.

Justice, L. M. (2007, August). *Evidence-based intervention: Approaches for emergent literacy.* Presentation at Leading Best Practices in Language and Literacy Conference, Monterey, CA.

Moats, L. C., Furry, A. R., & Brownell, N. (1998) *Learning to read: Components of beginning reading instruction K-8.* Sacramento: California State Board of Education.

National Center on Education and the Economy. (1999). *Primary literacy standards.* Washington, DC: National Center on Education and the Economy.

National Early Literacy Panel. (2004, November). *The National Early Literacy Panel: A research synthesis on early literacy development.* Presentation to the National Association of Early Childhood Specialists, Anaheim, CA.

National Reading Panel (NRP). (2000). *Teaching children to read: An evidence-based assessment of the scientific research literature on reading and its implications for reading instruction: Report of the subgroups* (NIH Publication No. 00-4754). Washington, DC: National Institutes of Health and National Institute of Child Health and Human Development.

Perfetti, C.A. (1991). Representations and awareness in the acquisition of reading competence. In L. Rieben & C. A. Perfetti (Eds.), *Learning to read: Basic research and its implications* (pp. 33–46). Hillsdale, NJ: Lawrence Erlbaum.

Snow, C. E., Burns, M. S., & Griffin, P. (1998). *Preventing reading difficulties in young children.* Washington, DC: National Academy Press.

Stackhouse, J. (1997). Phonological awareness: Connecting speech and literacy problems. In B. W. Hodson & M. L. Edwards (Eds.), *Perspectives in applied phonology* (pp. 157–196). Gaithersburg, MD: Aspen Publishers.

Torgesen, J. K., & Mathes, P. G. (2000). *A basic guide to understanding, assessing, and teaching phonological awareness.* Austin, TX: Pro-Ed.

WORKSHEETS FOR PHONOLOGICAL AWARENESS INTO PRINT ACTIVITIES